Designing and Delivering Dementia Services

Designing and Delivering Dementia Services

Edited by

Hugo de Waal, MD, FRCPsych, FHEA

Lead Consultant, Norfolk Dementia Care Academy, Norwich, UK
Associate Postgraduate Dean, East of England Deanery, Cambridge, UK

Constantine Lyketsos, MD, MHS

Elizabeth Plank Althouse Professor
Director of the Johns Hopkins Memory and Alzheimer's Treatment Center
Johns Hopkins Medicine, Maryland, USA

David Ames, BA, MD, FRCPsych, FRANZCP

Director, National Ageing Research Institute
University of Melbourne Professor of Ageing and Health
Victoria, Australia

John O'Brien, BA, BM BCh, MA, FRCPsych, MD

Department of Psychiatry
University of Cambridge
Cambridge, UK

WILEY Blackwell

This edition first published 2013, © 2013 by John Wiley & Sons, Ltd

Registered office: John Wiley & Sons, Ltd, The Atrium, Southern Gate, Chichester, West Sussex, PO19 8SQ, UK

Editorial offices: 9600 Garsington Road, Oxford, OX4 2DQ, UK
The Atrium, Southern Gate, Chichester, West Sussex, PO19 8SQ, UK
111 River Street, Hoboken, NJ 07030-5774, USA

For details of our global editorial offices, for customer services and for information about how to apply for permission to reuse the copyright material in this book please see our website at www.wiley.com/wiley-blackwell.

The right of the author to be identified as the author of this work has been asserted in accordance with the UK Copyright, Designs and Patents Act 1988.

Library of Congress Cataloging-in-Publication Data
Designing and delivering dementia services / edited by Hugo de Waal ... [et al.].
       p. ; cm.
   Includes bibliographical references and index.
   ISBN 978-1-119-95349-4 (cloth)
   I. De Waal, Hugo (Hugo Eduard), 1956-
   [DNLM: 1. Dementia–therapy.   2. Mental Health Services–organization & administration.   3. Patient-Centered Care–economics. WM 30.1]
   362.1968'3–dc23
               2013005830

A catalogue record for this book is available from the British Library.

Wiley also publishes its books in a variety of electronic formats. Some content that appears in print may not be available in electronic books.

Cover image: iStock © Robert Adrian Hillman
Cover design by Sarah Dickinson

Set in 10/12 pt Times Roman by Toppan Best-set Premedia Limited
Printed and bound in Malaysia by Vivar Printing Sdn Bhd

1   2013

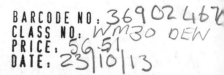

Contents

Foreword

On Smiling

Guerrilla activity – that's what it was some 50 years ago, when a few psychiatrists in a few countries started informally to grapple with constructing local services for old people. Today, dementia, until quite recently hardly noted as a public health issue, is almost everywhere seen as the huge challenge that it is.

In this 'bench-book', workers will find not only new ideas from all over the world, but often, almost as importantly, corroboration that they are on the right track; other readers, I hope, dipping casually, may find themselves stimulated towards work in this fascinating field.

We see here much heartening progress, not least in improving physical environments for dementia care. Almost gone in my country are the slums in which most such care took place. Now, gifted architects, designers and electronics specialists have been drawn in alongside health staff, to great effect. Collaboration between services is beginning to become real. In many countries, 'minimum standards' have been promulgated, though enforcement is still far from stringent. And we have taught that good care must be preceded by meticulous diagnosis and be accompanied by open-minded continuing reassessment.

But alas, the shortcomings in care which originally stimulated many pioneers to enter this field [1] have not gone away. Despite the accumulation of skills and experience and despite monitoring, scandals still hit the media almost weekly – and many don't reach the media. What is to be done to prevent such tragedies? Erving Goffman [2] long ago taught those of us who work in what he called 'the tinkering trades' ('tinkering' with the minds and bodies of human beings) that collective care of groups of vulnerable people has an inherent tendency to routineism and to depersonalisation, even leaving aside underfunding and understaffing.

Good, humane and respectful care seems to me largely to rest on the following pillars: first, a basic adequacy (not necessarily an abundance) of resources, in settings that are appropriate to needs. Next, effective education of professional and non-professional staff (and it is the latter that often present the biggest challenge to educators). Then, and crucially, the importance of senior staff as 'role models'. They must not only set standards, but must demonstrate them by their own behaviour, even in small details. They should give to all staff a sense of ownership of the enterprise, and pride in it. Readiness to listen and to attend to views and problems presented from 'below' – these are powerful determinants of good care, even in otherwise unprivileged settings.

Finally and seriously, I urge that we train ourselves and our staff to *smile* in response to calls from patients and relatives, even when we are hard-pressed. If the big supermarkets can train their staff to smile when customers accost them, even when they are busy on other tasks, why can't we? Smiling is the great under-tapped resource!

Tom Arie, CBE
Professor Emeritus of Health Care of the Elderly
University of Nottingham
Ageing and Disability Research Unit
The Medical School
Queen's Medical Centre
Nottingham, UK

References

1. University of Glasgow (2008) Guthrie trust witness seminar on old age psychiatry. Available at: http://www.gla.ac.uk/media/media_196526_en.pdf (last accessed on 27 March 2013).
2. Goffman E (1961) *Asylums*. New York: Doubleday.

Preface

Dementia is rightly no longer considered a normal and inevitable part of the ageing process, nor an affliction for which there are no meaningful interventions. It is now appropriately recognised, at least by all enlightened practioners, as a major brain illness for which considerable benefits can be accorded by a prompt and full assessment and diagnosis, followed by the provision of appropriate services, which would include subtype specific treatment and support. Debates on what should or should not be considered part of normal ageing are now superseded by research attempting to define the boundaries of conditions such as 'mild cognitive impairment', not because it is thought 'normal' or indeed 'mild', but because it indicates someone is at higher risk of developing outright dementia.

Dementia is an especially devastating illness, because at its heart it represents an organic failure of the most complex organ and so directly affects characteristics of someone's being in a way not seen in any other 'organ failure'. Dementia erodes one's understanding of the world, including self and personhood (recently Julian Hughes wrote about this with great clarity in *Thinking through Dementia*,[1] an exploration which charts those matters in detail). It is no wonder that the symptoms of dementia are bewildering to the person with the illness, as well as to everyone around them. For this reason in particular, services cannot just be diagnostically driven; to be of high quality they need to be 'person-centred'.

In compiling this text, the editors sought to be advocates of high-quality dementia services, a role we share with many practitioners. However, the book cannot prescribe what a 'good service' exactly should look like, for the reasons above. On top of the fact that services need to be responsive to patients and carers, they need to fit in with the wider construction of local healthcare systems. Furthermore, those who champion dementia services will have no choice but to engage in the process of securing resources in competition with other worthwhile causes.

That leads to the conundrum of designing services with on one hand the individual foremost in mind, while forming part of a complex health discourse on the other. How to advise on such service design in general terms? The first unavoidable truism is that dementia care services must be flexible. Any service which has to say 'no, we can't meet that need' is already not person-centred. The second and opposite truism is that there is no point in the approach 'we can do whatever it is you need us to do' if it can't be lived up to. A balance must be struck between a service being manageable and affordable (which likely predicts a degree of inflexibility) and being able to respond to someone's personhood, given someone's predicament. In other words, without the latter, the service won't work for someone; without the former, the service won't work for anyone.

In putting this book together we felt it was important to 'set the scene' in order to refresh our minds on the components of high-quality dementia care, particularly if supported by evidence, and taking into account the history of how we have arrived where we are. The two chapters in Section I provide a comprehensive account of this backdrop.

---

[1] Julian C Hughes. (2011) *Thinking through Dementia*. New York: Oxford University Press.

The contributors in Section II explore in detail service design, bearing in mind the likely needs people may have in different stages of dementia and at different levels of severity (and ignoring willfully the effect of diagnostic subtypes on those needs, as we focus on problems, challenges and needs, rather than on symptoms). The exception is the chapter on services for younger people with dementia, designated by age group, rather than severity of illness. This recognises the particular impact of age, when it relates to the responsibilities, hopes and expectations someone may have, who is likely still working and supporting a family.

As we pointed out above, while it is impossible to isolate a diagnosis of dementia from the person, neither is it possible to consider service design without taking into account the wider political, economical and healthcare context. Section III provides insight into those issues from a number of viewpoints. We are grateful to the senior officials of various Alzheimer's Associations and Societies for sharing their experiences. In this section attention is given to the crucial role national or governmental strategies can play, an issue echoed in many contributions from around the world in Section IV. Anyone wondering how to foster such strategies will be able to get several very pragmatic tips in Chapter 9. However, as noted, services do not exist in a vacuum and often have to compete in an economic reality, which is less than fortuitous in many countries. It is therefore of increasing relevance to identify how a service lives up to its 'investment'. Chapter 10 provides vital knowledge and expertise in these – more 'hard-nosed' – issues.

We thought it would be foolish not to learn from others: in Section IV we collated contributions from around the world. While many themes appear universal, every country in our list describes initiatives and lessons learned, which may be of use to others.

Finally in Section V we address additional pragmatic considerations relevant to service design. In Chapter 15 we provide advice to any practitioner who wants to take initiative and improve the environment of people with dementia. We present a relatively simple example of how to construct a 'business case' as we think it helpful to anyone who wants to 'make the case'. In the hope that a wide range of practitioners will read this book, we furthermore present a more complicated case study on what a business case might look like if it proposes services with a number of objectives, to be delivered by a variety of agencies. We comment on potential errors to illustrate how to read and interpret a business case in general.

Given the growing demand for services, every contribution in this book expresses concern that resources are at best projected to stagnate at current levels. This means that everyone needs to do more with less. We feel strongly that the dementia 'workforce' (including informal and family carers) cannot meet that demand unless it develops into a workforce which is as effective and efficient as possible. This implies workforce planning and development: Chapter 16 analyses in detail essential aspects and components of such planning. We put emphasis on experiential learning, as we believe that a workforce which trains and educates while providing care is more likely to be of high quality. It allows for the possibility that the workforce generates more capacity in the healthcare system in a cascading fashion.

Lastly, Chapter 17 heralds the future: pointing out the impact physical environments have on people's well-being, it describes the opportunities technological advances, such as telehealth, may present. Interestingly, it stresses that technology can only be used effectively if it takes full account of the person it is meant to assist: an insight that takes us full circle.

Hugo de Waal
Constantine Lyketsos
David Ames
John O'Brien
Norwich (UK), Baltimore (USA), Melbourne (Australia), Cambridge (UK)
December 2012

Contributors

Ricardo F. Allegri Memory and Aging Center, Instituto de Investigaciones Neurológicas Raúl Carrea (FLENI), Buenos Aires, Argentina

David Ames, BA, MD, FRCPsych, FRANZCP Professor of Ageing and Health, and Director, National Ageing Research Institute, National Ageing Research Institute, Royal Melbourne Hospital, Parkville, Victoria, Australia

June Andrews Director of the Dementia Services Development Centre, School of Applied Social Science, University of Stirling, Stirling, Scotland, UK

Pablo M. Bagnati Memory and Aging Center, Instituto de Investigaciones Neurológicas Raúl Carrea (FLENI), Buenos Aires, Argentina

Christian Bakker Health Care Psychologist. Radboud University Nijmegen, the Netherlands

Sube Banerjee Professor of Dementia, Centre for Dementia Studies, Brighton and Sussex Medical School, University of Sussex, Brighton, UK

Brigitta Baran, MD, PhD Department of Psychiatry and Psychotherapy, Faculty of Medicine, Semmelweis University, Budapest, Hungary

Betty S. Black, PhD Associate Professor, Department of Psychiatry and Behavioral Sciences, the Johns Hopkins University School of Medicine and the Johns Hopkins Berman Institute of Bioethics, Johns Hopkins Hospital, Baltimore, Maryland, USA

John Beaumont Former professor, School of Management, University of Bath, Bath, UK; Applied Management Systems, University of Stirling, Stirling, Scotland, UK

Mary Blazek, MD Clinical Assistant Professor, Department of Psychiatry, Geriatric Psychiatry Section, University of Michigan Medical School, Ann Arbor, Michigan, USA

Cassio M. C. Bottino Old Age Research Group (PROTER), Institute and Department of Psychiatry, University of São Paulo, São Paulo, Brazil

Christopher M. Callahan, MD Indiana University Center for Aging Research and the Regenstrief Institute, Inc., Indianapolis, Indiana, USA

Andrew Chidgey Head of Policy and Public Affairs, Alzheimer's Society, London, UK

Tiffany Chow, MD, MSc Assistant Professor of Psychiatry, Department of Medicine, Geriatric Psychiatry Division, University of Toronto, Toronto, Canada

Claudia Cooper, PhD Mental Health Sciences Unit, University College London, London, UK

David Conn, MBBCh, BAO, FRCPC Associate Professor, Department of Psychiatry, University of Toronto, Toronto, Canada

Stephen Curran, MRCPsych, PhD Consultant in Old Age Psychiatry, South West Yorkshire

Partnership NHS Foundation Trust, Wakefield, UK; Professor of Old Age Psychiatry, Centre for Health and Social Care Research, School of Human and Health Sciences, University of Huddersfield, Huddersfield, UK

Colleen Doyle Principal Research Fellow, National Ageing Research Institute, Royal Melbourne Hospital, Melbourne, Victoria, Australia

Engin Eker, MD Professor, Faculty of Medicine, Department of Geriatric Medicine and National Alzheimer Foundation, Bezmialem Vakif University, Istanbul, Turkey

Eleanor Flynn, MB BS, BTheol, M Ed, Dip Ger Med, FRACGP, FRACMA Senior Lecturer in Medical Education, University of Melbourne, Parkville, Victoria, Australia

Manuel Franco, MD, PhD Associate professor, University of Salamanca, Salamanca, Spain. Head of Psychiatric Department, Zamora Hospital, Zamora, Spain; Director of IBIP Lab, Iberian Research Institute, Intras Foundation, Zamora, Spain

Patricio Fuentes Cognitive Neurology and Dementia Unit, Neurology Service, Hospital of Salvador and Geriatrics Section, Clinical Hospital University of Chile, Santiago, Chile

Gábor Gazdag, MD, PhD Head of the Consultation–Liaison Psychiatric Service, Department of Psychiatry and Psychotherapy, Faculty of Medicine, Semmelweis University, Budapest, Hungary; Head of the Consultation–Liaison Psychiatric Service, Consultation–Liaison Psychiatric Service, Szent István and Szent László Hospitals, Budapest, Hungary

Laura N. Gitlin, PhD Center for Innovative Care in Aging, Department of Community-Public Health, School of Nursing, Baltimore, Maryland, USA; Department of Psychiatry and Behavioral Sciences, Johns Hopkins University, Baltimore, Maryland, USA

Jean Georges Executive Director, Alzheimer Europe, Luxembourg

Meredith Gresham, B.App.Sci.O.T. (Sydney University) Dip Arts Mus. (Qld. Cons.) A. Mus.A. HammondCare's Research Manager, HammondCare Foundation, Sydney, NSW, Australia

Zoltán Hidasi, MD, PhD Department of Psychiatry and Psychotherapy, Faculty of Medicine, Semmelweis University, Budapest, Hungary

Iva Holmerova, MD, PhD Associate Professor, Centre of Gerontology and CELLO-ILC-CZ, Faculty of Humanities, Charles University in Prague, Prague, Czech Republic

Jakub Hort, MD, PhD Associate Professsor, Memory Disorders Clinic, Department of Neurology, 2nd Faculty of Medicine, Charles University in Prague and University Hospital Motol V Úvalu 84, Prague, Czech Republic; Associate Professsor, International Clinical Research Center, St. Anne's University Hospital Brno, Brno, Czech Republic

Aud Johannessen Aldring og Helse, Nasjonalt Kompetansesenter, Oslo, Norway

Roy W. Jones The RICE Centre, Royal United Hospital, Bath, UK

Helen C. Kales, MD Department of Psychiatry, School of Medicine, University of Michigan, Ann Arbor, Michigan, USA

Janet Kavanagh, MS Director of Project Development and Administration, Program for Positive Aging, Department of Psychiatry, University of Michigan Medical School, Ann Arbor, Michigan, USA

Dorothy Kennerley Head of Education and Training, Norfolk & Suffolk Dementia Alliance, Norfolk, Norfolk, UK

Raymond T.C.M. Koopmans Department of Primary and Community Care, Centre for Family Medicine, Geriatric Care and Public Health, Radboud University Nijmegen, Medical Centre, Nijmegen, The Netherlands

Janus L. Kremer Instituto de Neuropsiquiatría Kremer, Córdoba, Argentina

Alexander F. Kurz Department of Psychiatry and Psychotherapy, Klinikum rechts der Isar, Technische Universität München, Munich, Germany

Nicola T. Lautenschlager Academic Unit for Psychiatry of Old Age, Department of Psychiatry, The University of Melbourne, St. George's Campus, St. Vincent's Hospital, Kew, Victoria, Australia; School of Psychiatry and Clinical Neurosciences and WA Centre for Health & Ageing, The University of Western Australia, Perth, Western Australia, Australia

Florence Lébert Centre national de référence des malades Alzheimer jeunes, Université Lille Nord de France, France

Jerzy Leszek, MD Associate Professor of Psychiatry, Department of Psychiatry, Wroclaw Medical University, Wroclaw, Poland; President, Lower Silesian Association of Alzheimer Patients' Families, Wroclaw, Poland

Gill Livingston, MD Mental Health Sciences Unit, University College London, London, UK

Dina Lo Giudice, MB BS, PhD, FRACP Geriatrician, Royal Melbourne Hospital, Parkville, Victoria, Australia

Constantine G. Lyketsos, MD, MHS Department of Psychiatry and Behavioral Sciences and Memory and Alzheimer's Treatment Center, Bayview Campus, Johns Hopkins University, Baltimore, Maryland, USA

Raimundo Mateos, MD, PhD Professor of Psychiatry, Department of Psychiatry (University of Santiago de Compostela, USC) and Psychogeriatric Unit (CHUS University Hospital), School of Medicine, Santiago de Compostela, Spain

Claire Mitchell, MBA Visiting Lecturer, Durham University Business School, Durham, UK

Miharu Nakanishi, PhD, RN Senior Researcher, Research Division, Institute for Health Economics and Policy, Minato-ku, Tokyo, Japan

Florence Pasquier, MD, PhD Professeur des Universités – Praticien-Hospitalier en Neurologie au Centre. Hospitalier et Universitaire de Lille, Lille, France

Lynne Pezzullo Lead Partner, Health Economics and Social Policy, Deloitte Access Economics, Deloitte Touche Tohmatsu, Kingston, ACT, Australia

Peter V. Rabins, MD, MPH Professor, Department of Psychiatry and Behavioral Sciences, the Johns Hopkins University School of Medicine and the Johns Hopkins Berman Institute of Bioethics, Johns Hopkins Hospital, Baltimore, Maryland, USA

Julie Ratcliffe Professor in Health Economics, School of Medicine, Flinders University, Repatriation General Hospital, Daw Park, South Australia, Australia

Glenn Rees CEO, Alzheimer's Australia, Australia

Denise Rettenmaier, MD Ambulatory Care Clinic, Yountville, CA, USA

Louise Robinson Professor of Primary Care and Ageing, Institute of Health and Society, Newcastle University, Newcastle upon Tyne, UK

Tor Rosness   Norwegian Centre for Dementia Research, Department of Geriatric Medicine, Ullevaal University Hospital, Oslo, Norway

Quincy M. Samus   Department of Psychiatry and Behavioral Sciences, Johns Hopkins Bayview, The Johns Hopkins School of Medicine, Baltimore, Maryland, USA

Manuel Sánchez-Pérez, MD   Coordinator of the Psychogeriatric Unit, Unitat de Psiquiatria Geriátrica, Hospital Sagrat Cor., Barcelona, Spain

K.S. Shaji   Professor of Psychiatry, Govt. Medical College, Thrissur, India

Laura M. Struble, PhD, GNP-BC   Clinical Assistant Professor, University of Michigan School of Nursing and the Department of Psychiatry, University of Michigan Medical School, Ann Arbor, Michigan, USA

Guk-Hee Suh, MD, PhD   Professor of Psychiatry, Hallym University Hangang Sacred Heart Hospital, Seoul, Korea

Katerina Sheardova, MD   Assistant Professor, International Clinical Research Center, Department of Neurology, St. Anne's University Hospital Brno, Brno, Czech Republic

Marta Sochocka, MD   Laboratory of Virology, Laboratory of Biomedical Chemistry, Institute of Immunology and Experimental Therapy Polish Academy of Sciences, Wroclaw, Poland

T.P. Sumesh   Assistant Professor of Psychiatry, Govt. Medical College, Thrissur, India

Fernando E. Taragano   Department of Neurosciences, Centro de Estudios Médicos e Investigaciones Clínicas (CEMIC), Buenos Aires, Argentina

Denise Thompson   Department of Primary and Community Care, Centre for Family Medicine, Geriatric Care and Public Health, Radboud University Nijmegen, Medical Centre, Nijmegen, The Netherlands

Ahmet Turan Isik, MD   Professor, National Alzheimer Foundation, Istanbul, Turkey

Marjolein de Vugt   Neuropsychologist, School for Mental Health and Neuroscience, Alzheimer Centrum Limburg, Maastricht University, Maastricht, The Netherlands

Hugo de Waal, MD, FRCPsych, FHEA   Lead Consultant, Norfolk Dementia Care Academy, The Julian Hospital, Norwich, Norfolk, UK.

Lars-Olof Wahlund, MD, PhD   Professor of Geriatic Medicine and Per-Olof Sandman, Professor of Care, Department of Neurobiology, Care Sciences and Society, Section of Clinical Geriatrics and Section of Nursing, Karolinska Institutet, Stockholm, Sweden

Huali Wang, MD   Associate Director of the Dementia Care & Research Centre and Associate Professor of Psychiatry. Institute of Mental Health, Peking University, Beijing, China

John Wattis, FRCPsych   Professor of Psychiatry for Older People, Centre for Health and Social Care Research, School of Human and Health Sciences, University of Huddersfield, Huddersfield, UK

Siegfried Weyerer, PhD   Professor of epidemiology, Zentralinstitut für Seelische Gesundheit, Mannheim, Baden-Württemberg, Deutschland

Adrienne Withall   School of Public Health and Community Medicine, Kensington Campus, University of New South Wales, Australia

Marc Wortmann   Executive Director, Alzheimer's Disease International, London, UK

Atsuhiro Yamada, PhD, MBA   Senior Consultant, Research & Consulting Division, the

Japan Research Institute Ltd, Shinagawa-ku, Tokyo, Japan

Yung-Jen Yang Tsao-Tun Psychiatric Centre, Nan-Tou, Taiwan

Xin Yu, MD Vice Chairman of Chinese Association for Alzheimer's Disease and Professor of Psychiatry. Institute of Mental Health, Peking University, Beijing, China

Section 1

The need for dementia services of excellence: Setting the scene

Chapter 1

The need for dementia care services

Gill Livingston and Claudia Cooper

Mental Health Sciences Unit, University College London, UK

The problem of dementia: A historical perspective

Dementia is largely an age associated disease. It was relatively rare prior to the rapid increase in the average life spans of people in the developed world in the 20th century. Nonetheless, Plato and other writers from ancient Greece and Egypt described a major memory disorder associated with ageing. Philippe Pinel (1745–1826) and Esquirol (1772–1840) were among the first to define dementia: Esquirol described it as 'a cerebral disease characterised by an impairment of sensibility, intelligence and will'. In 1906, Alois Alzheimer first described what came to be known as Alzheimer's disease (AD), a degenerative and severely debilitating neurological disorder. He regarded the condition as a relatively rare form of dementia, generally afflicting patients younger than 65. This belief that senile dementia was an inevitable consequence of ageing and distinct from pre-senile dementia, an unusual disease with specific cerebral pathology occurring by definition in people aged under 65, remained unchallenged until the 1970s. In 1976, Katzmann suggested that many cases of senile dementia were pathologically identical to AD [1]. He called Alzheimer's a 'major killer' and the fourth leading cause of death in the USA. His seminal editorial revolutionised the care of older people with dementia, who could be diagnosed as having a disease, rather than suffering from an inevitable part of normal ageing. This paved the way for the first trials of dementia treatments. In the decade prior to his publication, fewer than 150 articles were published on the topic of AD. There were virtually no trials of pharmacological or non-pharmacological treatments for dementia. Since 1976, research interest in dementia has blossomed, with PubMed recording nearly 9000 publications about Alzheimer's and nearly 20,000 about dementia in 2011 alone.

The need for dementia services

The number of people with dementia is currently estimated as 35 million worldwide, and this number is projected to double every 20 years due to increased lifespan, with numbers reaching 66 million by 2030, 81 million by 2040 and over 115 million by 2050 [2,3]. The largest numbers of people with dementia are currently in China and the developing Western Pacific, Western Europe and the USA [4]. It is estimated to cost $600 billion annually, which is equivalent to 1% of the gross domestic product [5]. Worldwide dementia contributes 4.1% of all disability-adjusted life years and 11.3% of years lived with disability [5].

Designing and Delivering Dementia Services, First Edition. Edited by Hugo de Waal, Constantine Lyketsos, David Ames, and John O'Brien.

Dementia affects the person with the illness, their family and society through loss of memory and independence, challenging behaviour, and often decreased well-being of both the person with dementia and their carer(s). All of these aspects require social and healthcare services and therefore have cost implications. The largest cost is for 24-hour care.

Managing dementia

In the last 15 years, symptomatic treatments for dementia have become available. Alongside these, growing evidence bases of non-pharmacological interventions for dementia and treatment of neuropsychiatric symptoms have developed. While disease-modifying treatments for dementia are not yet available, many promising trials, targeted mainly at beta-amyloid but also, for example, at tau phosphorylation or aggregation and glycogen synthase kinase-3 (GSK-3), are underway and will be reported soon. Meanwhile, developments in the symptomatic treatment of the illness have been drivers to transform dementia care. The benefits of early diagnosis and thus access to treatment are now clear, and this has led to developments in setting up of dementia specific services in the developed world.

Good dementia care has thus changed over the last decades to encompass the provision of active evidence-based treatments, including psychosocial and educational management, as well as drug-based treatment and access to research participation. This chapter will discuss the components of current high-quality, evidence-based dementia care from prevention to diagnosis to end of life care, and how this compares with current service provision.

Screening and prevention of dementia

Management of risk factors

There are many potentially modifiable risks or protective factors for dementia. There is clear evidence from observational studies of the protective effects of cognitive reserve (helped by intellectual or social activities and occupation), Mediterranean diet, exercise or physical activity, and potentially modifiable medical risks, such as midlife obesity, midlife hypertension and hypercholesterolaemia, smoking, diabetes, depression, and stroke [4,6]. Randomised controlled trials have been inconsistent in showing that controlling hypertension reduces the risk of developing dementia, and trials of statins have been negative [4]. Thus, while those measures are potentially important and controlling them has theoretical potential to prevent up to half the incident cases of AD, there is little evidence as to their real-life effect [4,6]. This may be because vascular factors in midlife increase the risk of Alzheimer's and vascular dementia, while the interventions studies have enrolled older people as participants [7]. Although treating hypertension and hypercholesterolaemia are not yet shown to reduce dementia at a population level, reducing risk of cerebrovascular events in those at high risk is clearly a rational step to preserve cognition, as well as being part of good primary care.

Pre-dementia syndromes

There is a growing body of evidence that dementia may be preceded by a period of subjective cognitive impairment without objective impairment [8]. This raises the possibility of screening for pre-dementia syndromes in order to intervene at an early stage. Self-reported memory problems are currently the best single indicator we have of objective cognitive problems [9], but their sensitivity for detecting future dementia appears fairly low. A third of people who screened negative for dementia reported forgetfulness in the past month in a large English survey, and this symptom was not related to age, suggesting that reporting forgetfulness was not a prelude to dementia in most of the younger adults who reported it [10]. Although currently there is little evidence for effective treatment strategies before the clinical dementia syndrome becomes apparent, this would be the logical time to use disease-modifying drugs if they become available, because the pathological changes are thought to precede the clinical picture of neurodegenerative dementias by many years.

Mild cognitive impairment (MCI) is a better indicator of incipient dementia with more than 50% of people with MCI progressing to dementia within 5 years, although some people with MCI remain stable or improve [11]. Patients presenting to memory clinics with MCI have an 18% per annum conversion rate, which is higher than the rates reported in epidemiological studies, and people with poor verbal memory, executive functioning deficits and accompanying neuropsychiatric symptoms are at particularly high risk [11]. Neuropsychiatric symptoms in MCI are common and persistent [12]. Thus one strategy for early diagnosis and intervention is to follow up patients presenting to clinics with MCI: this would also enable clinicians to modify risk factors and treat any neuropsychiatric symptoms.

Raising awareness

Assisting patients and carers to recognise dementia and seek help will equip people to play a more active role in their health care [13], but current evidence suggests that community-based campaigns to raise awareness about seeking help for memory problems are insufficient to promote early assessment and diagnosis of dementia [14]. In the UK, the Alzheimer's Society's 2008 'Worried about your memory?' campaign provided useful information about when to seek help, for example, if your memory (or that of someone you know) is getting worse or impacting on everyday life. Targeting similar information at all adults may improve detection of objective cognitive impairment and common mental disorders. Pre-screening those who are worried about dementia in primary care ensures that specialist memory services are well targeted.

Tackling stigma

Stigma is an important barrier for many in seeking a diagnosis for themselves or their relative [13]. In Japan, a successful campaign to raise public understanding and awareness of dementia included re-labelling dementia from 'Chiho' (an untreatable blockage of intellectual activities, a senile insanity) to 'Ninchisho' (this dementia is thought to be treatable and possibly preventable with computer games, exercise and cardiovascular health – although there may still be stigma attached to it) [15]. This changed the emphasis from long-term care of those who were not able to have social relationships to community care and inclusion. Stigma may increase social isolation in dementia where people avoid those with the illness. It may also operate within services and institutions, with for example people with dementia excluded from services they may benefit from.

Service configuration

In the remainder of the chapter, we will discuss interventions that are evidence-based and the mismatch between these and the services delivered.

Services for people with dementia and their carers have until recently evolved, influenced by historical, national and local agendas, rather than being actively planned with consideration of the evidence. Different professionals and services between and within countries have offered services ranging from diagnosis with immediate discharge to integrated health and social care with ongoing monitoring and help with changing problems. A number of countries, including Norway, the UK, the Netherlands, France, Switzerland and Japan have now developed national strategies for dementia [15]. In addition, there are guidelines for treatment of dementia in the USA, Canada, Germany, Italy, the Netherlands, Spain and Singapore [16–18]. These strategies and guidelines have a common theme, emphasising the importance of awareness, early diagnosis, information provision and advice for people with dementia and their carers with a model of cooperation between primary and secondary care, along the lines of referral to a memory clinic and community care [15,16,19]. Memory clinics, first developed in the USA, began to spread in the early 1980s. These actively designed services seek to introduce help and services earlier than occurred with traditional service models, where early referral of uncomplicated cases of dementia to secondary care, or indeed early diagnosis, were not encouraged, and diagnosis was more likely to occur at a point of crisis. People with dementia who use home care services were 22% less likely to move to a care home in a US 3-year cohort study [20]. Services now try to ensure people with dementia are cared for at home for as long as possible, both because that is what most people choose for themselves and because of cost.

Receiving a diagnosis

The case for early diagnosis

Most people with dementia and their families wish to know the diagnosis, feel relieved by diagnostic certainty and can access drug, psychological and psychosocial treatment that improve the prognosis, and start to plan and make choices about future care [13,21]. In addition, early diagnosis and intervention in dementia facilitates access to specialist services, support and treatment, is cost-effective [22], and reduces crises and care-home admissions [23].

Diagnostic rates

The majority of people with dementia do not have a formal diagnosis. Only 20–50% of people in developed countries with dementia are diagnosed and many less in the developing world. For example, in India, an estimated 90% of people remain undiagnosed [22]. Extrapolated, these figures imply that nearly 80% of the 36 million people worldwide with dementia are not diagnosed, therefore cannot access information to make choices, and have the treatment, care and support available to people with dementia [22]. The proportion of people diagnosed with AD receiving treatment in 2004 in European countries was estimated to vary from 97% in Greece to 3% in Hungary with a mean rate of 30%. Diagnosis and treatment rates vary hugely within as well as between countries [24].

The difficulties of obtaining a diagnosis

Family carers and people with dementia often experience difficulty in obtaining a diagnosis of dementia for their relative, which can take several years. This can result in increased anxiety and carer burden [13,25–27]. The impact of a dementia diagnosis, how it is made and when it is communicated are important. When people with dementia and their families are supported, there is rarely a catastrophic emotional reaction. Instead, one mostly detects patients and carers experiencing a sense of relief at having an explanation on one hand, but sometimes mixed with shock, anger and grief. Often, these emotions are balanced and then replaced with relief, hope and the feelings of being in control of decisions [21,22,28,29].

Barriers to accessing doctors for the diagnosis

Families report that relatives with memory problems often refuse to consult their physician about their memory and deny problems when seen [13]. Other barriers to seeking help include fear of the diagnosis, concerns about stigma and negative responses from other family members [22]. In our recent study involving family carers of people with dementia in England, once the carer had decided that they should seek help, the first point of contact was usually the primary care physician, often despite the care recipient's opposition. Carers overcame this problem in a variety of ways: going to see the doctor together helped, as did the doctor inviting the patient to an appointment. In some cases, families' strategies included manipulation, albeit benign [13]. Once at the doctor's, carers often described difficulties in obtaining the correct diagnosis, with problems either discounted or attributed incorrectly, or the doctor appearing reluctant to refer to specialist services. The patient's lack of insight often contributed to this and sometimes they remained undiagnosed until their behaviour was very risky. Carers commonly found that confidentiality impeded them from receiving information, but if it was clear the care recipient gave permission, then this improved.

Receiving a diagnosis in primary care

Despite attempts, including financial incentives, to improve early diagnosis and documentation of dementia in primary care, detection remains low even after presentation. This may partly relate to the difficulty of diagnosing early dementia and doctors under- or overestimating the prevalence of dementia. This may lead to missed diagnoses or concerns about the effect that identifying the illness may have on their workload [26,30,31]. GPs know about dementia, but may lack experience and confidence in diagnosing it and informing patients [26,31]. There is some evidence that educational interventions in which primary care doctors set their own objectives may increase detection rates [25,32–34]. Some professionals and relatives are concerned that telling people they have a devastating illness for which there is no cure is stigmatising, unhelpful and may be counterproductive, although most people who opt to protect their family members say they would like to know if they had the illness [35,36].

Inequalities in access to care

Socioeconomic barriers

The Inverse Care Law describes a perverse relationship between need and care so that those who most need medical care because of socio-economic deprivation are least likely to receive it [37]. It follows from this that, paradoxically, higher socio-economic groups who are healthier have greater access to services, including new and expensive drug treatments. There is preliminary evidence from the UK and Sweden that this may apply in dementia, with those from higher socio-economic classes being more likely to be prescribed drug treatment for dementia [38–40].

Minority ethnic status

Minority ethnic people with dementia in the USA, the UK and Australia are referred later in their illness then their white counterparts, when they are more cognitively impaired and commonly in crisis [41,42]. This is especially concerning, as some minority ethnic groups have higher rates of dementia than the indigenous population [43–45]. They are also less likely to be involved in trials of dementia drugs than their white counterparts [41]. Socio-economically disadvantaged older people may face a double jeopardy in accessing mental health, including dementia care [46]. Older minority ethnic people with mental illness have been described as experiencing 'triple jeopardy' [47].

Interventions after diagnosis

Information

Information provision alone for people with dementia and their carers does not improve outcomes [39]. When linked with other interventions, such as skills training, telephone support, or providing direct assistance with navigating the medical and social care systems, it can improve neuropsychiatric symptoms and possibly quality of life, although not carer burden [19,48]. Thus, services should provide information alongside other interventions.

Interventions for cognition

Current drug treatments for AD are symptomatic and consist of cholinesterase inhibitors (ChEIs: donepezil, galantamine and rivastigmine) and the N-methyl-D-aspartate (NMDA) inhibitor memantine. ChEIs have a moderate effect on cognition (1·5–2 points on the Mini-Mental State Examination over 6–12 months), with additional short-term (3–6 months) improvement in cognition and global outcome, and some stabilisation of function over this period [4]. Although it was initially thought that ChEIs improved neuropsychiatric symptoms in AD, this has not been confirmed in trials. Memantine improved cognitive performance and function over a 6-month period compared with placebo in those with moderate to severe AD, and there seem to be additive benefits of combining a cholinesterase inhibitor and memantine [4].

Cognitive stimulation therapy is a non-pharmacological treatment that can improve cognition [49]. It is now given as routine care in parts of the UK where, as it can be accessed by people with all types of dementia and those in whom anti-dementia drugs are contraindicated, its availability has extended the proportion of people with a diagnosis of dementia offered an active treatment.

Reducing abuse

One in four older people and one in three with dementia are at risk of abuse, but only a small proportion of this is currently detected [50–52]. Family carers with more anxiety or depressive symptoms are more likely to abuse, and this effect is mediated by the use of dysfunctional coping strategies; over time, without intervention, carer anxiety, depressive symptoms and abusive behaviour increase [53,54], so helping the family carer cope is important for the person with dementia and the carer.

Interventions for family carers

About 40% of family carers for people with dementia have psychological disorders, while others have significant symptoms [55,56]. These reduce carers' quality of life and increase the likelihood of the person with dementia moving to a care home as the carer becomes unable to care. There is excellent research evidence from the USA that six or more sessions of individual behavioural management therapy for family carers centred on the care recipient's behaviour alleviates the carer's depressive symptoms immediately and for up to 32 months, but this has so far not been translated into everyday clinical practice [57]. Teaching caregivers positive coping strategies either individually or in a group also appeared effective in improving caregiver psychological health immediately and for some months afterwards [57]. Overall systematic review finds evidence that individual interventions are more effective than group interventions. We are currently awaiting results of a randomised controlled trial of individual coping interventions in the UK that have been delivered by graduates with a psychology degree rather than clinical psychologists to make them more practical and affordable. In the USA, translation of these effective programmes into community practice has commenced [58]. Education about dementia, group behavioural therapy, respite and supportive therapy do not by themselves improve family carer mental health [57,59].

Interventions for neuropsychiatric symptoms

Clinically significant neuropsychiatric symptoms occur in about one-third of patients with mild dementia, two-thirds with more severe impairment [60–62] and a higher proportion of those in residential care. Agitation is one of the most common symptoms, especially in care homes. It affects nearly half of people with AD [62–64] and generally persists if untreated [64].

Initial interventions

Good clinical practice begins by considering the underlying cause(s) of neuropsychiatric symptoms (e.g. pain, delirium or constipation) and treating these if possible [65,66]. After this psychological and social treatments should be considered. These include avoiding triggers if possible, reducing environmental complexity and distractors like noise, allowing the person with dementia time to do things, educating carers about communication with someone with dementia, explaining to the person with dementia what is happening during tasks that cause agitation, and occupation to prevent agitation resulting from boredom.

Drug treatment

Neuropsychiatric symptoms can be difficult to manage. The potential importance of non-pharmacological approaches has increased due to concerns regarding the undesirable effects of drug treatments for agitation, such as antipsychotics. Initially, evidence indicated that risperidone and olanzapine should not be used for treatment of non-psychotic symptoms in dementia because of increased risk of cerebrovascular adverse events and death. All antipsychotics seem to confer risk, and the increased mortality may be greater with typical than atypical antipsychotics [67,68]. Recent meta-analyses found modest benefits in the treatment of aggression (best evidence for risperidone, then aripiprazole; quetiapine is ineffective) but increased cerebrovascular events and death [69–71]. Therefore, it is recommended that the use of antipsychotic medication for treating agitation or psychosis in people with dementia is limited to those whose behaviour is causing significant distress [72]. The use of both antipsychotics [73] and benzodiazepines [74] in dementia has been associated with increased cognitive decline. In practice, professionals and carers often struggle to implement effective non-pharmacological treatment, and psychotropic drugs are commonly prescribed to manage agitation. Cholinesterase inhibitors seem to be ineffective [75]. In 2009, a UK government-commissioned review found that only 20% of the 180,000 patients with dementia in the UK who were prescribed antipsychotics benefited from them, and antipsychotic over prescribing was linked to 1800 excess deaths a year [76].

Non-pharmacological interventions

Some non-pharmacological treatments reduce neuropsychiatric symptoms [48]. Teaching family carers to modify their interactions with patients has proved effective, with benefits lasting for months [48]. Additionally, eight sessions at home, teaching individual patient/carer dyads to monitor behavioural problems, understand behaviour, improve carer communication, increase pleasant events and enhance carer support was effective at 6 months in improving caregiver mood and care recipient neuropsychiatric symptoms [77]. Behavioural management techniques were particularly effective for depressive symptoms with lasting effects [48]. Training staff in 24-hour care settings about dementia, respecting the person as an individual, and communication and behavioural skills training are effective in reducing mood disturbance, agitation and aggression immediately and over months [78]. This type of intervention, particularly when coupled with increasing pleasant events, may also improve care homes residents' quality of life and theoretically decrease abusive behaviour, as we discuss later, when considering care homes [79]. Music therapy, multi-sensory therapy and possibly sensory stimulation were useful during the treatment session but had no longer-term effects [48].

Social care including care homes

People with dementia need help with their daily living activities, enabling them to live safely and with dignity. This is usually provided at home, mainly by family or friends but also by paid carers, particularly as the illness progresses. Thus, personal care, help with shopping, cooking and finances, as well as assistive technology that detects open doors, lack of movement, gas, water, smoke and falls alarms, prolong the time someone can live at home. Day centres and clubs provide social and cognitive stimulation.

In the UK, a 2011 Equality and Human Rights Commission report into home care by paid carers found evidence of 'systematic failure', physical abuse, neglect, disregard for privacy and dignity and 'dehumanising' care. A high proportion of people receiving home care have dementia, as do most older people in care homes, but most paid carers have little or no training in the psychological care of people with dementia.

Staff often lack understanding of dementia and the associated behavioural difficulties, and relatives may be dissatisfied with staff [80]. Residents want choice, for example, about what, when or where to eat and the possibility of privacy [80,81]. Dementia-specific training and education of staff in all long-term care settings, including induction, should address the management of problem behaviours. This has the potential to improve staff fulfilment and relatives' satisfaction.

There are currently no evidence-based interventions to prevent abuse in care homes, but training in person-centred care and alleviating neuropsychiatric symptoms seems an obvious place to start [78].

Care homes and end of life

Most people with dementia are resident in care homes when they die [82]. People with other terminal conditions, such as cancer or severe cardiovascular disease, are also more likely to live in nursing homes if they have dementia. Dementia is associated with poor nutrition, infections, skin breakdowns, dehydration and recurrent pneumonia [83]. Many staff favour life-prolonging treatments for care home residents as they do not perceive dementia as a terminal illness [84]. Staff often do not talk to relatives about death in advance or explain directly when it is imminent [85,86]. Paid carers in homes may often differ culturally and ethnically from those for whom they care, in US and UK care homes at least, and be focused on preserving life with less use of advance directives to limit treatment [87,88]. This all may lead to inappropriate, aggressive and distressing treatments that fail to prolong life but extend discomfort [89]. Internationally, there is a lack of access to skilled, good quality, basic care or palliative care for people with dementia at the end of their life [89–91]. A recent systematic review found limited evidence that making advanced care plans affected the treatment people with dementia received and concluded it may be too late to discuss them by the time people with dementia are resident in nursing homes settings [92]. Until recently, there were no studies that showed evidence of improved end of life care for patients with dementia, family satisfaction or decreased inappropriate interventions, including hospitalisations, just before expected death [93]. Despite over a decade of research, care and treatment guidelines for people with dementia at the end of life are mainly consensus based and more work is needed [93]. In the USA, one group found educating nursing staff about end of life care in dementia improved family satisfaction [94]. Within the UK, our group have found preliminary results suggesting that tackling attitudes and fears of care home staff may decrease inappropriate hospitalisation and increase family satisfaction [85,95].

Hospital care for people with dementia

Many people in hospital have dementia [96], and both older and younger people with dementia tend to have longer admissions than those without dementia [96,97] and are more likely to die in hospital [98]. In particular, care home residents with advanced dementia are often transferred to hospital at the end of their lives, when this may not be in their best interest or in line with their wishes [99,100]. Hospitalisation may be especially difficult for patients with advanced dementia, as they frequently experience uncomfortable interventions that lack demonstrable benefit and do not improve survival times [99,101].

Conclusions

The advantages of early and active treatment of dementia are now clear and include, but are not limited to, planning and choices for maximising independence and living at home, as well as symptomatic treatments for dementia and non-pharmacological interventions for dementia and associated neuropsychiatric symptoms. This requires dedicated services focused on early diagnosis and treatment that enable people with dementia to stay living well at home as long as possible and also enable their family carers to cope. Trials of disease-modifying anti-dementia drugs are underway. If successful, this will probably lead to further, radical changes in service configuration, possibly with screening programmes focused on the identification of pre-dementia syndromes and home treatments. Most people with dementia in the developed world do not receive a diagnosis and more live in the developing world with little access to dementia diagnosis or these recent advances in treatment: addressing this issue is a major global challenge.

References

1. Katzman R (1976) Prevalence and malignancy of Alzheimer's disease – A major killer. *Archives of Neurology* 33(4):217–218.
2. Ferri CP, Prince M, Brayne C, Brodaty H, Fratiglioni L, Ganguli M, et al. (2005 January) Global prevalence of dementia: a Delphi consensus study. *The Lancet* 366(9503):2112–2117.
3. Prince M (2009) World Alzheimer Report 2009.
4. Ballard C, Gauthier S, Corbett A, Brayne C, Aarsland D, Jones E (2011 March 19) Alzheimer's disease. *The Lancet* 377(9770):1019–1031.
5. Wimo A (2010) World Alzheimer Report 2010: The Global Economic Impact of Dementia.

6. Barnes DE, Yaffe K (2011 September) The projected effect of risk factor reduction on Alzheimer's disease prevalence. *The Lancet Neurology* 10(9):819–828.

7. Fratiglioni L, Qiu C (2011 September) Prevention of cognitive decline in ageing: dementia as the target, delayed onset as the goal. *The Lancet Neurology* 10(9):778–779.

8. Jessen F, Wiese B, Bachmann C, Eifflaender-Gorfer S, Haller F, Kolsch H, et al. (2010 April) Prediction of dementia by subjective memory impairment effects of severity and temporal association with cognitive impairment. *Archives of General Psychiatry* 67(4):414–422.

9. Palmer K, Backman L, Winblad B, Fratiglioni L (2003 February 1) Detection of Alzheimer's disease and dementia in the preclinical phase: population based cohort study. *British Medical Journal* 326(7383):245–247.

10. Cooper C, Bebbington P, Lindesay J, Meltzer H, McManus S, Jenkins R, et al. (2011 November) The meaning of reporting forgetfulness: a cross-sectional study of adults in the English 2007 Adult Psychiatric Morbidity Survey. *Age and Ageing* 40(6):711–717.

11. Gauthier S, Reisberg B, Zaudig M, Petersen RC, Ritchie K, Broich K, et al. (2006 April 15) Mild cognitive impairment. *The Lancet* 367(9518):1262–1270.

12. Ryu SH, Ha JH, Park DH, Yu J, Liyingston G (2011 Mar) Persistence of neuropsychiatric symptoms over six months in mild cognitive impairment in community-dwelling Korean elderly. *International Psychogeriatrics* 23(2):214–220.

13. Livingston G, Leavey G, Manela M, Livingston D, Rait G, Sampson E, et al. (2010 August 18) Making decisions for people with dementia who lack capacity: qualitative study of family carers in UK. *British Medical Journal* 341:c4184.

14. Chan T, van Vlymen J, Dhoul N, de Lugisnan S (2011) Using routinely collected data to evaluate a leaflet campaign to increase the presentation of people with memory problems to general practice: a locality based controlled study. *Informatics in Primary Care* 18(3):189–196.

15. Takeda A, Tanaka N, Chiba T (2010) Review article: prospects of future measures for persons with dementia in Japan. *Psychogeriatrics* 10(2):95–101.

16. Waldemar G, Phung KTT, Burns A, Georges J, Hansen FR, Iliffe S, et al. (2007) Access to diagnostic evaluation and treatment for dementia in Europe. *International Journal of Geriatric Psychiatry* 22(1):47–54.

17. Vasse E, Vernooij-Dassen M, Cantegreil I, Franco M, Dorenlot P, Woods B, et al. (2012) Guidelines for psychosocial interventions in dementia care: a European survey and comparison. *International Journal of Geriatric Psychiatry* 27(1):40–48.

18. Mayeux R (2010 June 4) Early Alzheimer's disease. *The New England Journal of Medicine* 362(23):2194–2201.

19. Corbett A, Stevens J, Aarsland D, Day S, Moniz-Cook E, Woods R, et al. (2012) Systematic review of services providing information and/or advice to people with dementia and/or their caregivers. *International Journal of Geriatric Psychiatry* 27(6):628–636.

20. Gaugler JE, Kane RL, Kane RA, Newcomer R (2005 April) Early community-based service utilization and its effects on institutionalization in dementia caregiving. *The Gerontologist* 45(2):177–185.

21. Robinson L, Gemski A, Abley C, Bond J, Keady J, Campbell S, et al. (2011 Sep) The transition to dementia – individual and family experiences of receiving a diagnosis: a review. *International Psychogeriatrics* 23(7):1026–1043.

22. Prince M, Bryce R, Ferri CP (2012) World Alzheimer Report 2011: The Benefits of Early Diagnosis and Intervention.

23. Banerjee S, Wittenberg R (2009 July) Clinical and cost effectiveness of services for early diagnosis and intervention in dementia. *International Journal of Geriatric Psychiatry* 24(7):748–754.

24. Alzheimers Society, Alzheimers Scotland Mapping the dementia care gap. 11 AD. Available at: http://www.alzheimers.org.uk/dementiamap (last accessed on 21 February 2013).

25. Olafsdottir M, Skoog I, Marcusson J (2000 July) Detection of dementia in primary care: the Linkoping study. *Dementia and Geriatric Cognitive Disorders* 11(4):223–229.

26. Olafsdottir M, Foldevi M, Marcusson J (2001 September) Dementia in primary care: why the low detection rate? *Scandinavian Journal of Primary Health Care* 19(3):194–198.

27. Department of Health (2010) The National Dementia Strategy.

28. Pinner G, Bouman WP (2003 September) Attitudes of patients with mild dementia and their carers towards disclosure of the diagnosis. *International Psychogeriatrics* 15(3):279–288.
29. Carpenter BD, Xiong C, Porensky EK, Lee MM, Brown PJ, Coats M, et al. (2008 March) Reaction to a dementia diagnosis in individuals with Alzheimer's disease and mild cognitive impairment. *Journal of the American Geriatrics Society* 56(3):405–412.
30. Lopponen MK, Isoaho R, Kivela SL (2002 July) Underdocumentation of dementia continues in primary health care – does it matter? A cross-sectional population based study of people aged 65+. *Neurobiology of Aging* 23(1):S139.
31. Turner S, Iliffe S, Downs M, Wilcock J, Bryans M, Levin E, et al. (2004 September) General practitioners' knowledge, confidence and attitudes in the diagnosis and management of dementia. *Age and Ageing* 33(5):461–467.
32. Rait G, Walters K, Bottomley C, Petersen I, Iliffe S, Nazareth I (2010 August 5) Survival of people with clinical diagnosis of dementia in primary care: cohort study. *British Medical Journal* 341.
33. Lopponen M, Raiha I, Isoaho R, Vahlberg T, Kivela SL (2003 November) Diagnosing cognitive impairment and dementia in primary health care – a more active approach is needed. *Age and Ageing* 32(6):606–612.
34. Koch T, Iliffe S (2011 August) Dementia diagnosis and management: a narrative review of changing practice. *The British Journal of General Practice* 61(589):e513–e525.
35. Fahy M, Wald C, Walker Z, Livingston G (2003 July) Secrets and lies: the dilemma of disclosing the diagnosis to an adult with dementia. *Age and Ageing* 32(4):439–441.
36. Pinner G (2000 June) Truth-telling and the diagnosis of dementia. *The British Journal of Psychiatry* 176:514–515.
37. Hart JT (1971) Inverse care law. *The Lancet* 1(7696):405–412.
38. Cooper C, Blanchard M, Selwood A, Livingston G (2010) Antidementia drugs: prescription by level of cognitive impairment or by socio-economic group? *Aging & Mental Health* 14(1):85–89.
39. Johnell K, Weitoft GR, Fastbom J (2008) Education and use of dementia drugs: a register-based study of over 600,000 older people. *Dementia and Geriatric Cognitive Disorders* 25(1):54–59.
40. Matthews FE, McKeith I, Bond J, Brayne C (2007 July) Reaching the population with dementia drugs: what are the challenges? *International Journal of Geriatric Psychiatry* 22(7):627–631.
41. Cooper C, Tandy AR, Balamurali TBS, Livingston G (2010 March) A systematic review and meta-analysis of ethnic differences in use of dementia treatment, care, and research. *The American Journal of Geriatric Psychiatry* 18(3):193–203.
42. Mukadam N, Cooper C, Basit B, Livingston G (2011 September) Why do ethnic elders present later to UK dementia services? A qualitative study. *International Psychogeriatrics* 23(7):1070–1077.
43. Adelman S, Blanchard M, Rait G, Leavey G, Livingston G (2011 August) Prevalence of dementia in African-Caribbean compared with UK-born White older people: two-stage cross-sectional study. *The British Journal of Psychiatry* 199(2):119–125.
44. Livingston G, Leavey G, Kitchen G, Manela M, Sembhi S, Katona C (2001 October) Mental health of migrant elders – the Islington study. *The British Journal of Psychiatry* 179:361–366.
45. Adelman S, Blanchard M, Livingston G (2009 July) A systematic review of the prevalence and covariates of dementia or relative cognitive impairment in the older African-Caribbean population in Britain. *International Journal of Geriatric Psychiatry* 24(7):657–665.
46. Cooper C, Bebbington P, McManus S, Meltzer H, Stewart R, Farrell M, et al. (2010 December) The treatment of common mental disorders across age groups: results from the 2007 Adult Psychiatric Morbidity Survey. *Journal of Affective Disorders* 127(1–3):96–101.
47. Rait G, Burns A, Chew C (1996 November 30) Age, ethnicity, and mental illness: a triple whammy – we need validated assessment instruments for specific communities. *British Medical Journal* 313(7069): 1347–1348.
48. Livingston G, Johnston K, Katona C, Paton J, Lyketsos CG (2005 November) Systematic review of psychological approaches to the management of neuropsychiatric symptoms of dementia. *The American Journal of Psychiatry* 162(11):1996–2021.
49. Spector A, Thorgrimsen L, Woods B, Royan L, Davies S, Butterworth M, et al. (2003 September) Efficacy of an evidence-based cognitive stimulation therapy programme for people with dementia – randomised controlled trial. *The British Journal of Psychiatry* 183:248–254.

50. Cooper C, Selwood A, Livingston G (2008 March) The prevalence of elder abuse and neglect: a systematic review. *Age and Ageing* 37(2):151–160.
51. Cooper C, Selwood A, Blanchard M, Walker Z, Blizard R, Livingston G (2009 January 22) Abuse of people with dementia by family carers: representative cross sectional survey. *British Medical Journal* 338.
52. Cooper C, Selwood A, Livingston G (2009 October) Knowledge, detection, and reporting of abuse by health and social care professionals: a systematic review. *The American Journal of Geriatric Psychiatry* 17(10):826–838.
53. Cooper C, Selwood A, Blanchard M, Walker Z, Blizard R, Livingston G (2010 February) The determinants of family carers' abusive behaviour to people with dementia: results of the CARD study. *Journal of Affective Disorders* 121(1–2):136–142.
54. Cooper C, Blanchard M, Selwood A, Walker Z, Livingston G (2010 June) Family carers' distress and abusive behaviour: longitudinal study. *The British Journal of Psychiatry* 196(6):480–485.
55. Mahoney R, Regan C, Katona C, Livingston G (2005 September) Anxiety and depression in family caregivers of people with Alzheimer disease – the LASER-AD study. *The American Journal of Geriatric Psychiatry* 13(9):795–801.
56. Cooper C, Balamurali TBS, Livingston G (2007 April) A systematic review of the prevalence and covariates of anxiety in caregivers of people with dementia. *International Psychogeriatrics* 19(2):175–195.
57. Selwood A, Johnston K, Katona C, Lyketsos C, Livingston G (2007 August) Systematic review of the effect of psychological interventions on family caregivers of people with dementia. *Journal of Affective Disorders* 101(1–3):75–89.
58. Teri L, McKenzie G, Logsdon RG, McCurry SM, Bollin S, Mead J, et al. (2012 January 12) Translation of two evidence-based programs for training families to improve care of persons with dementia. *The Gerontologist*. doi:10.1093/geront/gnr132.
59. Cooper C, Balamurali TBS, Selwood A, Livingston G (2007 March) A systematic review of intervention studies about anxiety in caregivers of people with dementia. *International Journal of Geriatric Psychiatry* 22(3):181–188.
60. Lyketsos CG, Sheppard JME, Steinberg M, Tschanz JAT, Norton MC, Steffens DC, et al. (2001 November) Neuropsychiatric disturbance in Alzheimer's disease clusters into three groups: the Cache County study. *International Journal of Geriatric Psychiatry* 16(11):1043–1053.
61. Lyketsos CG (2007 June) Neuropsychiatric symptoms (behavioral and psychological symptoms of dementia) and the development of dementia treatments. *International Psychogeriatrics* 19(3):409–420.
62. Ballard CG, Margallo-Lana M, Fossey J, Reichelt K, Myint P, Potkins D, et al. (2001 August) A 1-year follow-up study of behavioral and psychological symptoms in dementia among people in care environments. *The Journal of Clinical Psychiatry* 62(8):631–636.
63. Sommer OH, Kirkevold O, Cvancarova M, Engedal K (2010) Factor analysis of the brief agitation rating scale in a large sample of Norwegian nursing home patients. *Dementia and Geriatric Cognitive Disorders* 29(1):55–60.
64. Ryu SH, Katona C, Rive B, Livingston G (2005 November 1) Persistence of and changes in neuropsychiatric symptoms in Alzheimer disease over 6 months: the LASER-AD study. *The American Journal of Geriatric Psychiatry* 13(11):976–983.
65. Livingston G, Cooper C (2010) Non-pharmacological therapies to manage behavioural and psychological symptoms of dementia: what works and what doesn't In: Ames D, Burns A, O'Brien J (eds), *Dementia*, 4th edn. London: Hodder Arnold, pp. 214–221.
66. Yaffe K (2007 Oct 4) Treatment of neuropsychiatric symptoms in patients with dementia. *The New England Journal of Medicine* 357(14):1441–1443.
67. Committee for the Safety of Medicines (2004) Atypical antipsychotics and stroke. Medicines and Healthcare Regulatory Agencies 2004. Available at: http://www.mhra.gov.uk/Safetyinformation/Safetywarningsalertsandrecalls/Safetywarningsandmessagesformedicines/CON1004298 (last accessed on 21 February 2013).
68. Wang PS, Schneeweiss S, Avorn J, Fischer MA, Mogun H, Solomon DH, et al. (2005 December 1) Risk of death in elderly users of conventional vs. atypical antipsychotic medications. *The New England Journal of Medicine* 353(22):2335–2341.

69. Ballard C, Howard R (2006 Jun) Neuroleptic drugs in dementia: benefits and harm. *Nature Reviews. Neuroscience* 7(6):492–500.
70. Schneider LS, Dagerman K, Insel PS (2006 March) Efficacy and adverse effects of atypical antipsychotics for dementia: meta-analysis of randomized, placebo-controlled trials. *The American Journal of Geriatric Psychiatry* 14(3):191–210.
71. Schneider LS, Dagerman KS, Insel P (2005 October 19) Risk of death with atypical antipsychotic drug treatment for dementia: meta-analysis of randomized placebo-controlled trials. *JAMA* 294(15):1934–1943.
72. National Collaborating Centre for Mental Health (2006) Dementia: a NICE–SCIE Guideline on supporting people with dementia and their carers in health and social care. Social Care Institute for Excellence National Institute for Health and Clinical Excellence 2006. Available at: http://www.nice.org.uk/CG42 (last accessed on 21 June 2010).
73. Ballard C, Margallo-Lana M, Juszczak E, Douglas S, Swann A, Thomas A, et al. (2005 April 16) Quetiapine and rivastigmine and cognitive decline in Alzheimer's disease: randomised double blind placebo controlled trial. *BMJ* 330(7496):874.
74. Bierman EJ, Comijs HC, Gundy CM, Sonnenberg C, Jonker C, Beekman AT (2007 December) The effect of chronic benzodiazepine use on cognitive functioning in older persons: good, bad or indifferent? *International Journal of Geriatric Psychiatry* 22(12):1194–1200.
75. Howard RJ, Juszczak E, Ballard CG, Bentham P, Brown RG, Bullock R, et al. (2007 October 4) Donepezil for the treatment of agitation in Alzheimer's disease. *The New England Journal of Medicine* 357(14):1382–1392.
76. Banerjee S (2010) The Use of Antipsychotic Medication for People with Dementia: Time for Action. A report. Department of Health 2010. Available at: http://www.dh.gov.uk/prod_consum_dh/groups/dh_digitalassets/documents/digitalasset/dh_108302.pdf (last accessed on 21 February 2013).
77. Teri L, McCurry SM, Logsdon R, Gibbons LE (2005 December) Training community consultants to help family members improve dementia care: a randomized controlled trial. *The Gerontologist* 45(6):802–811.
78. Teri L, Huda P, Gibbons L, Young H, van Leynseele J (2005 October) STAR: a dementia-specific training program for staff in assisted living residences. *The Gerontologist* 45(5):686–693.
79. Cooper C, Mukadam N, Katona C, Lyketsos CG, Ames D, Rabins P, et al. (2012 January 16) Systematic review of the effectiveness of non-pharmacological interventions to improve quality of life of people with dementia. *International Psychogeriatrics* 24(6):856–870.
80. Train G, Nurock S, Kitchen G, Manela M, Livingston G (2005 June) A qualitative study of the views of residents with dementia, their relatives and staff about work practice in long-term care settings. *International Psychogeriatrics* 17(2):237–251.
81. Train GH, Nurock SA, Manela M, Kitchen G, Livingston GA (2005 March) A qualitative study of the experiences of long-term care for residents with dementia, their relatives and staff. *Aging & Mental Health* 9(2):119–128.
82. Houttekier D, Cohen J, Bilsen J, Addington-Hall J, Onwuteaka-Philipsen BD, Deliens L (2010 April) Place of death of older persons with dementia. A study in five European Countries. *Journal of the American Geriatrics Society* 58(4):751–756.
83. Volandes AE, Lehmann LS, Cook EF, Shaykevich S, Abbo ED, Gillick MR (2008 May 12) Using video images of dementia in advance care planning (vol 167, pg 828, 2007). *Archives of Internal Medicine* 168(9):995.
84. Mitchell SL, Kiely DK, Hamel M, Morris JN, Park PS, Fries BE (2004 April) Estimating prognosis for nursing home residents with advanced dementia. *Journal of the American Geriatrics Society* 52(4): S175–S176.
85. Livingston G, Pitfield C, Morris J, Manela M, Lewis-Holmes E, Jacobs H (2011 August 22) Care at the end of life for people with dementia living in a care home: a qualitative study of staff experience and attitudes. *International Journal of Geriatric Psychiatry* 27(6):643–650.
86. Caplan GA, Meller A, Squires B, Chan S, Willett W (2006 November) Advance care planning and hospital in the nursing home. *Age and Ageing* 35(6):581–585.
87. Kiely DK, Mitchell SL, Marlow A, Murphy KM, Morris JN (2001 October) Racial and state differences in the designation of advance directives in nursing home residents. *Journal of the American Geriatrics Society* 49(10):1346–1352.

88. Thune-Boyle IC, Stygall J, Keshtgar MR, Davidson TI, Newman SP (2011 July) Religious coping strategies in patients diagnosed with breast cancer in the UK. *Psychooncology* 20(7):771–782.
89. Mitchell SL, Black BS, Ersek M, Hanson LC, Miller SC, Sachs GA, et al. (2012 January 3) Advanced dementia: state of the art and priorities for the next decade. *Annals of Internal Medicine* 156(1):45–U95.
90. Sampson EL, Ritchie CW, Lai R, Raven PW, Blanchard MR (2005 March) A systematic review of the scientific evidence for the efficacy of a palliative care approach in advanced dementia. *International Psychogeriatrics* 17(1):31–40.
91. Sampson EL, Burns A, Richards M (2011 Nov) Improving end-of-life care for people with dementia. *The British Journal of Psychiatry* 199:357–359.
92. Robinson L, Dickinson C, Rousseau N, Beyer F, Clark A, Hughes J, et al. (2011 December 8) A systematic review of the effectiveness of advance care planning interventions for people with cognitive impairment and dementia. *Age and Ageing* 41(2):263–269.
93. van der Steen JT (2010) Dying with dementia: what we know after more than a decade of research. *Journal of Alzheimer's Disease* 22(1):37–55.
94. Arcand M, Monette J, Monette M, Sourial N, Fournier L, Gore B, et al. (2009 January) Educating nursing home staff about the progression of dementia and the comfort care option: impact on family satisfaction with end-of-life care. *Journal of the American Medical Directors Association* 10(1):50–55.
95. Pitfield C, Shahriyarmolki K, Livingston G (2011 February) A systematic review of stress in staff caring for people with dementia living in 24-hour care settings. *International Psychogeriatrics* 23(1):4–9.
96. Mukadam N, Sampson EL (2011 Apr) A systematic review of the prevalence, associations and outcomes of dementia in older general hospital inpatients. *International Psychogeriatrics* 23(3):344–355.
97. Draper B, Karmel R, Gibson D, Peut A, Anderson P (2011) The Hospital Dementia Services Project: age differences in hospital stays for older people with and without dementia. *International Psychogeriatrics* 23(10):1649–1658.
98. Lamberg JL, Person CJ, Mitchell SJ (2004 April) Dying with advanced dementia in long-term care. *Journal of the American Geriatrics Society* 52(4):S99–S100.
99. Lamberg JL, Person CJ, Kiely DK, Mitchell SL (2005 August) Decisions to hospitalize nursing home residents dying with advanced dementia. *Journal of the American Geriatrics Society* 53(8):1396–1401.
100. Waldrop D, Kirkendall AM (2010) Rural-urban differences in end-of-life care: implications for practice. *Social Work in Health Care* 49(3):263–289.
101. Sampson EL, Candy B, Jones L (2009) Enteral tube feeding for older people with advanced dementia. *Cochrane Database of Systematic Reviews* (2):CD007209.

Chapter 2

The historical development and state of the art approach to design and delivery of dementia care services

Christopher M. Callahan[a], Helen C. Kales[b], Laura N. Gitlin[c,d], and Constantine G. Lyketsos[d,e]

[a]Indiana University Center for Aging Research and the Regenstrief Institute, Inc., USA
[b]Department of Psychiatry, School of Medicine, University of Michigan, USA
[c]Center for Innovative Care in Aging, Department of Community-Public Health, School of Nursing, USA
[d]Department of Psychiatry and Behavioral Sciences, Johns Hopkins University, USA
[e]Memory and Alzheimer's Treatment Center, Bayview Campus, Johns Hopkins University, USA

Introduction

Current understanding of dementia has evolved over some two centuries from pre-20th century conceptualisation of senility and dementia [1,2] and Dr Alzheimer's original clinical observations [3] to modern descriptions of potentially causal pathologies [4–6] and assessment methods [7–9]. In a parallel fashion, changes in societal perceptions of dementia have shaped current models of dementia care [10–12].

The history of the study of ageing, including dementia, is characterised by continuous debate regarding which conditions are 'normal' and which are due to disease or deprivation [13] and this debate continues today to at least some degree [14,15]. Medical treatments are still somewhat controversial, and there are no evidence-based strategies to prevent Alzheimer's disease [16].

Thus, the emphasis in dementia care is on trying to formulate evidence-based strategies to design and provide care for people with dementia and to support their carers.

The design of most dementia care services has its roots in generic care services for older adults and healthcare providers and healthcare systems did not distinguish between the two. Until the mid-20th century, most conditions of the ageing brain were considered irreversible, or at least consistent with other inevitable declines in health and vitality. Older adults with declining cognition or mental illness were often institutionalised in asylums or almshouses that provided custodial care, and for many an accurate diagnosis was considered irrelevant because the approach to care was the same regardless [17]. This diagnostic and therapeutic nihilism was decried at least as late as the 1980s [18].

Designing and Delivering Dementia Services, First Edition. Edited by Hugo de Waal, Constantine Lyketsos, David Ames, and John O'Brien.
© 2013 John Wiley & Sons, Ltd. Published 2013 by John Wiley & Sons, Ltd.

Establishing a diagnosis is important for a number of reasons:

- It assigns a culturally accepted reason and label for the patient's or family's concerns.
- It provides an entry and pathway for formal care and it dictates the types of professionals who can provide that care.
- It enables researchers to develop consistent and comparable research.
- It provides clinicians with therapeutic criteria.

The efficacy of any therapies then defines which diagnoses are treatable, in turn providing further rationale for diagnosis. The availability and efficacy of treatments often leads to a recategorisation of conditions believed to be due to normal ageing as opposed to disease or deprivation.

In the 1950s, editorials in the medical literature began to warn of an impending crisis stemming from the confluence of three major social changes:

- the projected growth in the older adult population
- the growing cost of care for older adults with mental illness in asylums, almshouses and hospitals
- the lack of information about which patients with which diagnoses needed what type of care and in what setting [19,20].

As the sheer numbers and plight of these individuals were revealed, families, healthcare professionals, advocates and public policy experts began to ask questions, and it became of paramount importance to begin sorting out which problems of the ageing brain were due to the ageing process itself and which were due to disease or neglect.

Clinical epidemiology

The brief history in the next section begins with large-scale clinical epidemiological studies seeking better to understand the health of older adults. These led to more detailed inquiries into the epidemiology of mental illness among older adults, in turn ushering in large-scale population based studies into risk factors and neuropathology of dementia. Findings from these studies led to research seeking to organise medical, social and financial resources to improve the care of older adults with dementia.

Early surveys of the health of older adults

Our focus on the origins of the current care and treatment paradigm begins with surveys of sickness in the UK following the Second World War. In 1947, Rowntree carried out one of the first community-based surveys of the health of older adults, and he reported four key findings:

1. The small amount of data served to outline how little was known about the ageing population.
2. Most older adults were living independently at home and most of their needs were provided through informal care systems.
3. There was a great deal of unmet social and medical need.
4. A lack of social, economic, recreational, and educational opportunities was contributing to disability and disease in older adults [21].

Studies of this type helped us understand that an important component of the disability associated with ageing is due to social and economic hardship, rather than just ageing or illness. Further investigation of a random sample of Rowntree's original population showed that 11.2% of subjects living in the community had evidence of cognitive impairment, 3.8% were severely cognitively impaired and 3.2% were 'eccentric'. Furthermore, 10% were found to have episodes of depression and 20% reported loneliness [22].

Many of the brain-based problems of ageing were considered irreversible and were often lumped under the heading of 'senility'. From an individual's perspective, the term 'senility' meant the dread of losing one's functional capacity with age and the likelihood of becoming a burden on family resources. From a societal perspective, it also captured a biased picture of the elderly as being 'useless' and a significant drain on social and medical resources [12]. Thus, the prevailing perception of the medical and lay community was that senility, and other brain-based illnesses associated with ageing, inevitably leads to functional decline and eventual institutionalisation and death.

In reviewing the history of dementia care, it is difficult to escape the fact that the cost of institutional care was a major driver of investment into community services and it continues to influence the content, design and quality of care [23]. The magnitude of the burden of care for these older adults has typically been viewed as so extreme that it undermines the quality of care for other conditions and age groups: terms, such as 'bed blockers' (hospitalised older adults, whose discharges are presenting with difficulties), are well known to medical practitioners. However, these early studies began to challenge the notion that all cognitive impairment associated with ageing was irreversible or progressive.

In 1951, Felix Post reported the outcomes of 214 older patients admitted to a psychiatric hospital in the UK. After three years over 50% had died, 20% remained in hospital and nearly 25% had returned to the community [24]. In 1952, Roth and Morrissey published a retrospective review of 150 older adults admitted to a psychiatric hospital in the UK. While they were surprised to find that 50% of admissions were for depression, they suggested that there were clear lines of demarcation between the presenting symptoms and outcomes of patients with affective disorders as opposed to 'senile psychoses' [25]. Early studies such as these catalysed a new field of inquiry into the proper assessment and classification of both cognitive and affective disorders, as well as studies of prevalence and risk factors in community settings. Most importantly, these studies began to fracture the image of irreversible impairment, inevitable institutionalisation and early death for persons with mental illness in old age. They also revealed that a large group of older adults with cognitive impairment live in the community.

Clinical epidemiology of dementia

The early history of senility and dementia begins to coalesce into the current concept of 'Alzheimer's disease' in the 1960s, with further refinements in the methods of clinical epidemiology. In 1964, Martin Roth and colleagues conducted the first prospective studies of mental disorder in old age [26–28]. They assembled random samples of community-dwelling and institutionalised older adults in the same city and reported that 10% of community-dwelling subjects had organic brain syndromes, including 4.9% with 'severe mental deterioration', while 31% of those with psychiatric illness had 'functional psychiatric disorders'. Reflecting on this work many years later, Kay commented:

'Prevalence rates in the community were high; institutional cases were the tip of an iceberg and the burden of care fell on relatives, pointing to the need for community services'. [29]

The same team later described a correlation between post-mortem senile plaques and pre-mortem cognitive function [30,31]. Previously the scientific community debated the similarities and differences between: (1) normal brain ageing and disease; (2) senile psychoses, affective disorders and organic brain disorders and (3) presenile and senile dementia. With these new findings, the focus shifted to the correlation between cognitive function and histological pathology, but findings were inconclusive [32]. Roth et al. attributed some of this to inaccurate or non-standardised clinical diagnoses and later reported that using standardised assessments led to a 'highly significant association' [33].

Armed with the hypothesis that some age-related cognitive decline might be due to disease (with the potential of being treatable), together with some early agreement on diagnostic criteria and improving techniques in neuropathology, investigators conducted multiple population-based studies of cognitive impairment among older adults. Zaccai et al. [34] completed a systematic review of some of these studies. They concluded that major contributions of these studies have been to validate pre-mortem diagnostic criteria, as well as generate various hypotheses for further investigation, such as potential targets for medication and the contributions of various risk factors, for example, genetic predisposition, vascular disease, inflammation, traumatic brain injury and lifestyle factors [35,36].

One example is the Cache County Study in Utah in the USA: more than 5000 adults over 65 were enrolled, undergoing regular clinical assessments, including investigation of blood parameters and genetic samples. An important finding with particular relevance to designing dementia care services was the high prevalence of behavioural and psychological symptoms among community-dwelling subjects with dementia [37,38].

Care needs of persons with dementia

Agreement on research diagnostic criteria of Alzheimer's disease and studying its prevalence in the community is of critical importance, but a very different undertaking from developing care models and a healthcare system capable of responding to unmet care needs. In the 1950s, most patients with early stages of dementia lived in the community and were cared for by family members, a fact that remains true today. For many families, the burden of care was so great that it affected their financial prospects, and this strain was for instance one of the key drivers of the original Medicare and Medicaid legislation in the USA [39], where in the 1960s (in concert with the de-institutionalisation movement) asylums and state mental hospitals began discharging patients with dementia, at the same time that nursing homes were attempting to limit admissions [23,40,41]. Opportunities for early diagnosis and treatment, as well as prevention, were greatest through local community resources, including primary care, so that by 1960, many were calling for a fundamental redesign of the healthcare system to improve community-based care. Kay et al. wrote that:

'The key concepts on which a modern geriatric service must be based are as follows: (a) integration of services on a practical level to make the most efficient possible use of all the facilities available; and (b) early ascertainment of high-risk groups, thus allowing resources to be focused where they are most needed and enabling preventive and therapeutic efforts to be started at an early stage. It is becoming widely recognised that fulfillment of these aims hinges very largely on improving and coordinating the domiciliary services provided by the general practitioner and the local authority'. [42]

They also called for the development of special geriatric units that could support general practitioners caring for older adults [42]: many attributed a whole range of conditions to the inevitable consequences of ageing, resulting in under-recognition and under-reporting of diseases in the elderly [43]. Williamson et al. showed through geriatric clinics that as many as 50% of older adults could be shown to suffer from remediable or treatable conditions [44], a finding frequently repeated since.

The clarion call for a major societal response to Alzheimer's disease was perhaps best captured in 1976 by Robert Katzman, stating:

'Alzheimer's disease and senile dementia are a single process and should, therefore, be considered a single disease'. He added: 'Alzheimer disease may rank as the fourth or fifth most common cause of death in the United States'. [19]

This contributed to the establishment of the Alzheimer's Association in the USA and the National Institute on Ageing [11,45]. Similar alerts to the growing 'epidemic' were published in the UK, calling for more research on the appropriate design of services, as well as efforts to educate providers and families [20]. Specialist care units started to be designed, with an emphasis on accurate diagnosis, proactive treatment and the role of the physical environment in optimising function. Specialist outpatient clinics were developed later and some focused on building capacity for research as well as delivering care and providing information. By the 1980s, expert recommendations started to emerge to guide psychiatrists, neurologists, geriatricians and other practitioners in the diagnosis and management of dementia [10,46–48]. These guidelines were informed primarily by expert opinion, rather than based on clear evidence.

We turn now to the evidence base for state-of-the-art dementia care services, as has accrued since.

Dementia care research

Research into the evidence base for dementia care services falls into three broad categories:

1. psychosocial research, typically focusing on educating caregivers and facilitating access to community services
2. biomedical or pharmacological research focusing on healthcare providers
3. non-pharmacological research into modifiable factors contributing to a patient's excess disability, behavioural symptoms or poor quality of life.

And three more specific ones:

1. detection in primary care
2. case management
3. home-based interventions.

Psychosocial research

Family caregivers (mostly women) have always been and are likely to continue to be the main providers of care, even for those with severe cognitive and functional impairment, but the importance of their role has often not been fully recognised [49]. Little has changed in terms of the importance of the role of families [50], and Maurer et al. observed that 21st century

'disease management would hinge, as it did 100 years ago, on the efforts of a compassionate team of professionals working with [her] and [her] family to achieve the best possible outcome for this incurable, progressive, neurodegenerative disease'. [51]

The history of psychosocial interventions can be broadly characterised as evolving over a number of overlapping and co-occurring phases. Initially, psychosocial intervention research emerged from an understanding of both the importance and the stresses of the generation that is called up to provide care for ageing parents, concurrent with care for young children (the 'sandwich generation', as it is known in the USA). One example is the work of Elaine Brody at the Philadelphia Geriatric

Center in the USA in the 1960s and 1970s [23,40,41,45]. At the time, nursing homes excluded older adults with significant illnesses. By following the 'excluded' older adults and the problems of their caregivers, Brody and colleagues sought to support them and avoid institutionalisation through education and activation of community resources. Various caregiver intervention studies subsequently focused on the benefits of psycho-educational and supportive programmes including respite care and care management. Results from these early efforts were mixed, with individualised approaches demonstrating better outcomes than group interventions [52].

Another example from this initial phase is Lawton and colleagues' project, which found that those offered formal respite care maintained their relative longer in the community, although it was ineffective for caregiver burden and caregiver mental health [53]. The Medicare Alzheimer's Disease Demonstration Project is an example of an attempt to improve caregiver outcomes through case management and subsidised community services, thereby decreasing nursing home usage [54,55]. However, the investigators were unable to demonstrate substantial reductions in caregiver burden, caregiver depression or nursing home placement, and concluded that interventions needed to be reformulated to include coordination with primary care and/or chronic disease management.

Limitations of these early studies include an almost exclusive focus on caregiver burden and depression, poor description of interventions, lack of attention to treatment concordance, and use of global outcome measures that were too distal from the purpose and content of the interventions being tested. Building on these early endeavours, more sophisticated randomised trials were subsequently developed in the mid- to late 1990s, such as the seminal study by Mittleman and colleagues. This team conducted a clinical trial to determine the long-term effectiveness of comprehensive support for spouse-caregivers and their families. The intervention was designed to postpone or prevent nursing home placement. After 8 months, caregivers in the intervention arm were significantly less depressed than controls, nursing home placement was delayed by 1.5 years and this delay was not at the expense of the caregivers' mental health [56–58]. No other studies have replicated this delay in institutionalisation, but the study did have a number of methodological limitations.

Intervention research has continued to advance with more robust randomised trials. One example is the Resources for Enhancing Alzheimer's Caregiver Health (REACH I), with six interventions:

1. psycho-educational group counselling
2. individual counselling
3. skills training in behavioural management
4. problem-solving
5. technology-based education
6. supportive programmes.

The interventions were tested using more rigorous conditions and controls than previous studies and including more racially, ethnically (Caucasian, African-American and Latino), culturally and geographically diverse families. Design improved with detailed treatment fidelity protocols, manualisation and careful documentation of intervention protocols including dose, intensity and caregiver participation levels. The interventions showed a wide range of positive outcomes, including caregiver skills, mastery, efficacy and mental health [59–61]. While REACH I improved testing of caregiver interventions, the focus remained on caregiver mental health and of families at the moderate disease stage.

REACH I was followed by REACH II, investigating the most active ingredients of the REACH I interventions at five sites and focusing on five domains: reducing depression, decreasing burden, improving self-care, enhancing social support and managing problem behaviours. The interventions were tailored to the caregivers and demonstrated improvement for most caregivers in the intervention group. However, it failed to show statistically significant differences in institutionalisation at 6 months [62].

Current research expands the field of interest from early stage of the illness to end of life, with novel approaches and technologies, including some with a dyadic focus in their design [63]. A meta-analysis of 23 high-quality studies showed significant reductions in behavioural symptoms of persons with dementia as well as decreased caregiver stress. This offers important support for such interventions to be integrated into comprehensive dementia care [49], demonstrating that

- it is possible to make small but important gains in caregiver well-being
- dementia caregiving is more distressful than caring for older adults with physical impairments
- intervening with caregivers has a positive impact on quality of life of persons with dementia.

In addition, we now know the active components of successful interventions:

- tailoring interventions to unique and specific concerns of the caregiver
- involving elements such as skill building and education
- actively involving the caregiver in instruction (versus didactic education only)
- guiding interventions by risk or needs assessments and prioritisation of problems in the home
- intervening in the home.

Future research will need to address effects on cost and health utilisation, tailoring interventions and how to incorporate proven interventions in comprehensive dementia care services. An up-to-date overview of such research focusing on relevant health economic aspects by Colleen Doyle and colleagues is to be found in Chapter 10 in this book.

Biomedical or pharmacological research

Between 1975 and 2000, most biomedical research focused on the development of new pharmacological therapies for dementia. Several medications, however modest, have been approved by regulatory agencies around the world. This activity has spurred advances in medical treatment and fuelled improvements in memory assessment services, such as in the UK (see Chapter 14 for a detailed account). As a result, the last decade has seen the development of clinical guidelines for dementia. Many of these, including diagnostic criteria, treatment guidelines and guidance on how to conduct drug treatment trials, emanated from a number of academic research centres. Over time, a great deal of consistency was achieved across the various guidelines from authoritative groups and they have changed little over the past quarter century. However, nearly as soon as these guidelines were developed, scientists began to document the continued low levels of diagnosis and treatment in primary care [64,65], an issue we will focus on in the following section on non-pharmacological research.

Non-pharmacological research

Non-pharmacological interventions encompass a broad range of approaches, from generalised (e.g. caregiver education, carer support, patient exercise and activity programmes) to targeted (e.g. aiming to address specific behaviours or functional concerns, such as safely bathing). They may directly involve the patient (e.g. activity programme) or work through another agent, typically the caregiver (e.g. use of communication techniques) or the physical environment (e.g. reduction of clutter, use of signage). Research into the efficacy of such approaches produced the strongest evidence base for the use of structured activities, exercise, environmental modifications and adult day services [61,66–70]. However, there is inconsistent evidence that non-pharmacological approaches reduce behavioural symptoms, including reminiscence therapy, validation therapy, simulated presence therapy (use of audiotapes by family members), aromatherapy, light therapy and acupuncture [71].

Detection in primary care

Most patients with dementia receive their medical care in the primary care sector, yet most primary care physicians have fewer than 25 of such patients on their lists [72]. Researchers consistently document suboptimal quality of care and poor outcomes and several studies have shown that primary care physicians often either fail to make a diagnosis of dementia or misdiagnose altogether [73]. Reasons for under-detection include:

- a fear of upsetting patients if the perception is there is little to offer to alter the course of the illness
- failure to recognise early symptoms
- attribution of symptoms to co-morbid medical conditions
- discomfort with the care of demented patients or their families
- patients as well as caregivers may under-report problems for fear of precipitating a diagnosis of dementia and/or transfer to a nursing home
- caregivers may fear that the physician will lose interest in caring for the patient.

Thus, early medical interventions focused on improving recognition and treatment. In the UK, Iliffe and colleagues studied the use of brief screening instruments for dementia, depression and problem drinking among adults aged over 75 and showed that screening resulted in a significant increase in the detection of possible dementia, but did not change patterns of treatment or referral. They concluded that 'in the absence of agreed guidelines and resources, information derived from screening instruments may not alter clinical practice' [74]. Subsequent studies increased the intensity of the interventions in primary care by providing better education or improved access to practice guidelines. Various studies tested a variety of educational strategies in primary care, but findings are inconsistent [75–77]. A key weakness in many of these studies has been the lack of measurement of patient-specific outcomes.

Case management

Investigators first studied case management for older adults with dementia in specialist settings. In 2002, Challis and colleagues evaluated intensive case management in a community-based mental health clinic. After 2 years, 51% of the case management participants remained at home, compared with 33% of the comparison group. There were also improvements in caregiver stress, but overall service use increased in the experimental group. This early trial raised issues that remain unanswered today, including: on which patients to focus exceptional resources, how to determine if upfront investments result in downstream savings, where such services should be located and how to integrate this care with the patients' other healthcare needs [78].

Callahan et al. reported a study comparing collaborative care with augmented usual care. Intervention patients received case management by an interdisciplinary team, led by a nurse practitioner working with the patient's family caregiver. The study showed that:

- primary care patients with Alzheimer's disease are highly symptomatic
- intervention patients were more likely to receive cholinesterase inhibitors and antidepressants
- intervention patients were more likely to rate their primary care as very good
- intervention patients had significantly fewer behavioural and psychological symptoms of dementia at 12 months

- intervention caregivers reported significant decreased distress at 12 months and sustained decrease in depression at 18 months [79].

Vickrey et al. investigated arguably the most comprehensive case management approach to dementia care tested to date, with the intervention emphasising linkages with community resources and multi-agency coordination through a dementia care manager. They found large improvements in adherence to quality of care indicators by primary care practitioners [80] and an improved quality of life as reported by patients. Caregiver quality of life did not improve, but the study did not assess behavioural symptoms or cognitive function, physical function, or time to nursing home placement [81].

Home-based interventions

Home-based interventions have tended to focus on preventing functional decline and/or preventing and managing behavioural symptoms of dementia. Teri et al. demonstrated significant improvement in functioning and depression scores among subjects receiving an exercise plus behavioural management intervention, concluding that

> 'caregivers were able to learn how to encourage and supervise exercise participation, and patients participating in this programme achieved increased levels of physical activity, decreased rates of depression, and improved physical health and function'. [67]

Graff et al. investigated the effectiveness of community-based occupational therapy on daily functioning of patients with dementia and the sense of competence of their caregivers. Compensatory strategies were used to adapt activities of daily living to the disabilities of patients and environmental strategies to adapt their physical environment. They reported significant improvement in self-reports of patients' daily functioning and caregiver burden [82] and improvements in patients' mood, quality of life and health status [83]. Gitlin and colleagues similarly found improvements in caregiver well-being, patient functioning and behaviours, using home-based occupational therapy strategies [61,66]. They also investigated a tailored activity programme to reduce dementia-related neuropsychiatric behaviours and improve caregiver well-being and found that intervention caregivers reported reduced problem behaviours and greater activity engagement [84].

In summary, dementia care services have been tested in specialist clinics, primary care clinics and home-based settings, among others. However, there is increasing recognition that care for these patients is distributed across multiple sites, involving various services [85]. In a sense current dementia care services may resemble islands with limited bridges between them. A dementing illness may last a decade or more and usually progresses from early, relatively asymptomatic to severe stages, the latter requiring full care, support and – for many patients – palliative care. There is still limited evidence that new models of care, such as collaborative care or case management, can save money or be even cost-neutral. In addition to financial costs, clinical practices must consider space constraints, patient flow, providers' other roles, the patient-physician relationship, information technology, cultural barriers and the overall organisational acceptance or resistance to change [86–89]. Finally, there are many unmet needs in this patient population, and the dementing illness may only be one disease among many that the older adult faces.

State-of-the-art design of dementia care services

Many groups have published clinical practice guidelines, but these tend to focus on diagnosis, pharmacological and non-pharmacological management and caregiver support. An alternative approach is the recent publication of a Dementia Performance Measurement Set [90], consisting of

10 measures and providing guidelines to improve the quality of care and obtain better patient outcomes, such as staging of dementia, conducting routine cognitive assessments, assessments of neuropsychiatric and depressive symptoms, managing neuropsychiatric symptoms, assessment of and advice about safety concerns, palliative care, advanced care planning, and caregiver education and support.

Recommendations for the design of dementia care services across the continuum of care are not typically included in clinical practice guidelines. The summary below is not an attempt to harmonise recommendations across the different published guidelines or provide recommendations for patient-specific care, but is a description of the state-of-the-art components of best practice, based on the evidence presented in this chapter:

- Active case-finding for cognitive impairment coupled with a second-stage assessment to diagnose dementia and the specific subtype. This requires the use of standardised instruments to evaluate cognitive function.
- Evaluation for treatable conditions contributing to cognitive impairment, including prescription and non-prescription medication.
- Evaluation of remediable causes of excess functional disability, including assessment of home environmental problems and the role of assistive technology.
- Active case-finding and treatment of co-morbid depression and behavioural and psychological symptoms of dementia with an emphasis on non-pharmacological approaches.
- Discussion of the diagnosis, prognosis, and treatment options with the patient and family.
- Referral to patient and caregiver educational programmes and/or community support agencies, such as the local Alzheimer's Association.
- Monitoring and support of the caregiver's emotional and physical health and ongoing education across the progression of the condition.
- Encourage and facilitate patients' continued physical, social and mental activity, including cognitive training.
- Referral to occupational therapy, exercise programmes and other physical activity to minimise the impact of functional decline.
- Specialist referral to neurology, psychiatry, geriatric medicine or memory services for patients with unclear diagnosis, rapid progression of cognitive or functional decline, or poorly controlled behavioural disturbances.
- Consideration for treatment with cholinesterase inhibitors and/or memantine.
- Discussion of advanced care planning, including goals of care, risks and benefits of treatments for other co-morbid conditions and end of life care.
- Facilitated communication among the care providers within the healthcare system and the community.
- Surveillance and tracking of patient outcomes with feedback to the healthcare team.

Although each of these components of best practice is recommended by one or more of the current guidelines, and most have evidence of efficacy from clinical trials, few clinical practices in any setting or country are currently able to deliver this comprehensive approach, and more research is needed on how to implement and evaluate such comprehensive services [88,91,92].

References

1. Boller F, Forbes MM (1998) History of dementia and dementia in history: an overview. *J Neurol Sci* 158:125–133.

2. Berchtold NC, Cotman CW (1998) Evolution in the conceptualization of dementia and Alzheimer's disease: Greco-Roman period to the 1960s. *Neurobiol Aging* 19:173–189.
3. Goedert M, Ghetti B (2007) Alois Alzheimer: his life and times. *Brain Pathol* 17:57–62.
4. Whitehouse PJ, Maurer K, Ballenger JF (2000) *Concepts of Alzheimer Disease: Biological, Clinical, and Cultural Perspectives*. Baltimore, MD: Johns Hopkins University Press.
5. Davies P, Maloney AJ (1976) Selective loss of central cholinergic neurons in Alzheimer's disease. *Lancet* 2:1403.
6. Smith CM, Swash M, Exton-Smith AN, Phillips MJ, Overstall PW, Piper ME, Bailey MR (1978) Choline therapy in Alzheimer's disease. *Lancet* 2:318.
7. Katz S, Ford AB, Moskowitz RW, Jackson BA, Jaffe MW (1963) Studies of illness in the aged. The index of ADL: a standardized measure of biological and psychosocial function. *JAMA* 185:914–919.
8. McKhann G, Drachman D, Folstein M, Katzman R, Price D, et al. (1984) Clinical diagnosis of Alzheimer's disease: report of the NINCDS-ADRDA Work Group under the auspices of Department of Health and Human Services Task Force on Alzheimer's Disease. *Neurology* 34:939–944.
9. Folstein MF, Folstein SE, McHugh PR (1975) 'Mini-Mental State'. A practical method for grading the cognitive state of patients for the clinician. *J Psychiatr Res* 12:189–198.
10. Butler RN (1982) Charting the conquest of senility. *Bull N Y Acad Med* 58:362–381.
11. Fox P (1989) From senility to Alzheimer's disease: the rise of the Alzheimer's disease movement. *Milbank Q* 67:58–102.
12. Ballenger JF (2006) *Self, Senility, and Alzheimer's Disease in Modern America*. Baltimore, MD: Johns Hopkins University Press.
13. Cowdry E (1939) *Problems of Ageing: Biological and Medical Aspects*. Baltimore, MD: Williams & Wilkins Company.
14. Brayne C, Galloway P (1988) Normal ageing, impaired cognitive function, and senile dementia of the Alzheimer's type: a continuum? *Lancet* 1:1265–1267.
15. Brayne C, Fox C, Boustani M (2007) Dementia screening in primary care: is it time? *JAMA* 298:2409–2411.
16. Daviglus ML, Bell CC, Berrettini W, Bowen PE, Connolly ES Jr, et al. (2010) National Institutes of Health State-of-the-Science Conference Statement: preventing Alzheimer disease and cognitive decline. *Ann Intern Med* 153:176–181.
17. Callahan CM, Berrrios GE (2004) *Reinventing Depression: A History of the Treatment of Depression in Primary Care, 1940–2004*. Oxford: Oxford University Press.
18. Cassel CK, Jameton AL (1981) Dementia in the elderly: an analysis of medical responsibility. *Ann Intern Med* 94:802–807.
19. Katzman R (1976) Editorial: the prevalence and malignancy of Alzheimer disease. A major killer. *Arch Neurol* 33:217–218.
20. Dementia – the quiet epidemic (1978) *Br Med J* 6104:1–2.
21. Rowntree BS; Nuffield Foundation, Survey Committee on the Problems of Ageing and the Care of Old People (1947) *Old People: Report of a Survey Committee on the Problems of Ageing and the Care of Old People*. London: Oxford University Press.
22. Sheldon JH (1948) Some aspects of old age. *Lancet* 1:621–624.
23. Brody EM, Lawton MP, Liebowitz B (1984) Senile dementia: public policy and adequate institutional care. *Am J Public Health* 74:1381–1383.
24. Post F (1951) The outcome of mental breakdown in old age. *Br Med J* 1:436–440.
25. Roth M, Morrissey JD (1952) Problems in the diagnosis and classification of mental disorder in old age; with a study of case material. *J Ment Sci* 98:66–80.
26. Kay DWK, Beamish P, Roth M (1964) Old age mental disorders in Newcastle-upon-Tyne. Part I. *Br J Psychiatry* 110:146–158.
27. Kay DWK, Beamish P, Roth M (1964) Old age mental disorders in Newcastle-upon-Tyne. Part II: a study of possible social and medical causes. *Br J Psychiatry* 110:668–682.
28. Garside RF, Kay DWK, Roth M (1965) Old age mental disorders in Newcastle-upon-Tyne. Part III: a factorial study of medical, psychiatric and social characteristics. *Br J Psychiatry* 111:939–946.
29. Kay DWK, Roth M (1993) Mental disorders in an elderly urban population. *Curr Contents* 26.

30. Roth M, Tomlinson BE, Blessed G (1967) The relationship between quantitative measures of dementia and of degenerative changes in the cerebral grey matter of elderly subjects. *Proc R Soc Med* 60: 254–260.
31. Blessed G, Tomlinson BE, Roth M (1968) The association between quantitative measures of dementia and of senile change in the cerebral grey matter of elderly subjects. *Br J Psychiatry* 114:797–811.
32. Rothschild D, Trainor MA (1937) Pathologic changes in senile psychoses and their psychobiologic significance. *Am J Psychiatry* 93:757–788.
33. Roth M, Tomlinson BE, Blessed G (1966) Correlation between scores for dementia and counts of 'senile plaques' in cerebral grey matter of elderly subjects. *Nature* 209:109–110.
34. Zaccai J, Ince P, Brayne C (2006) Population-based neuropathological studies of dementia: design, methods and areas of investigation – a systematic review. *BMC Neurol* 6:2.
35. Hendrie HC (1998) Epidemiology of dementia and Alzheimer's disease. *Am J Geriatr Psychiatry* 6:S3–S18.
36. Blennow K, de Leon MJ, Zetterberg H (2006) Alzheimer's disease. *Lancet* 368:387–403.
37. Tschanz JT, Treiber K, Norton MC, Welsh-Bohmer KA, Toone L, et al. (2005) A population study of Alzheimer's disease: findings from the Cache County Study on Memory, Health, and Aging. *Care Manag J* 6:107–114.
38. Lyketsos CG, Steinberg M, Tschanz JT, Norton MC, Steffens DC, et al. (2000) Mental and behavioral disturbances in dementia: findings from the Cache County Study on Memory in Aging. *Am J Psychiatry* 157:708–714.
39. Clark DO, Maddox GL (1992) Social context and personal expenditures for health care: federal policy and the experience of older adults in the 1970s. *J Aging Soc Policy* 4:179–198.
40. Lawton MP, Brody EM (1969) Assessment of older people: self-maintaining and instrumental activities of daily living. *Gerontologist* 9:179–186.
41. Brody EM, Kleban MH, Lawton MP, Levy R, Waldow A (1972) Predictors of mortality in the mentally-impaired institutionalized aged. *J Chronic Dis* 25:611–620.
42. Kay DW, Roth M, Hall MR (1966) Special problems of the aged and the organization of hospital services. *Br Med J* 2:967–972.
43. Williamson J, Stokoe IH, Gray S, Fisher M, Smith A, et al. (1964) Old people at home. Their unreported needs. *Lancet* 1:1117–1120.
44. Lowther CP, MacLeod RD, Williamson J (1970) Evaluation of early diagnostic services for the elderly. *Br Med J* 3:275–277.
45. Katzman R, Bick K (2000) *Alzheimer Disease: The Changing View*. San Diego, CA: Academic Press.
46. Hendrie HC (1978) Organic Brain Disorders; Classification, the 'Symptomatic' Psychoses, Misdiagnosis.
47. Small GW, Liston EH, Jarvik LF (1981) Diagnosis and treatment of dementia in the aged. *West J Med* 135:469–481.
48. Yesavage J (1979) Dementia: differential diagnosis and treatment. *Geriatrics* 34:51–59.
49. Gitlin LN, Schulz R (2012) Family caregiving of older adults. In: Prohask T, Anderson L, Binstock R (eds), *Public Health for an Aging Society*. Baltimore, MD: Johns Hopkins University Press., pp. 181–204.
50. Pruchno R, Gitlin LN (2012) Family caregiving in late life: shifting paradigms. In: Blieszner R, Bedford VH (eds), *Handbook of Families and Aging*. Westport, CT: Praeger Publishers, pp. 515–543.
51. Maurer K, McKeith I, Cummings J, Ames D, Burns A (2006) Has the management of Alzheimer's disease changed over the past 100 years? *Lancet* 368:1619–1621.
52. Knight BG, Lutzky SM, Macofsky-Urban F (1993) A meta-analytic review of interventions for caregiver distress: recommendations for future research. *Gerontologist* 33:240–248.
53. Lawton MP, Brody EM, Saperstein AR (1989) A controlled study of respite service for caregivers of Alzheimer's patients. *Gerontologist* 29:8–16.
54. Miller R, Newcomer R, Fox P (1999) Effects of the Medicare Alzheimer's Disease Demonstration on nursing home entry. *Health Serv Res* 34:691–714.
55. Newcomer R, Yordi C, DuNah R, Fox P, Wilkinson A (1999) Effects of the Medicare Alzheimer's Disease Demonstration on caregiver burden and depression. *Health Serv Res* 34:669–689.

56. Mittelman MS, Ferris SH, Shulman E, Steinberg G, Ambinder A, et al. (1995) A comprehensive support program: effect on depression in spouse-caregivers of AD patients. *Gerontologist* 35:792–802.

57. Mittelman MS, Ferris SH, Shulman E, Steinberg G, Levin B (1996) A family intervention to delay nursing home placement of patients with Alzheimer's disease. *JAMA* 276:1725–1731.

58. Mittelman MS, Haley WE, Clay OJ, Roth DL (2006) Improving caregiver well-being delays nursing home placement of patients with Alzheimer disease. *Neurology* 67:1592–1599.

59. Belle SH, Czaja SJ, Schulz R, Zhang S, Burgio LD, et al. (2003) Using a new taxonomy to combine the uncombinable: integrating results across diverse interventions. *Psychol Aging* 18:396–405.

60. Gitlin LN, Belle SH, Burgio LD, Czaja SJ, Mahoney D, et al. (2003) Effect of multicomponent interventions on caregiver burden and depression: the REACH multisite initiative at 6-month follow-up. *Psychol Aging* 18:361–374.

61. Gitlin LN, Winter L, Corcoran M, Dennis MP, Schinfeld S, et al. (2003) Effects of the home environmental skill-building program on the caregiver-care recipient dyad: 6-month outcomes from the Philadelphia REACH Initiative. *Gerontologist* 43:532–546.

62. Belle SH, Burgio L, Burns R, Coon D, Czaja SJ, et al. (2006) Enhancing the quality of life of dementia caregivers from different ethnic or racial groups: a randomized, controlled trial. *Ann Intern Med* 145: 727–738.

63. Whitlatch CJ, Judge K, Zarit SH, Femia E (2006) Dyadic intervention for family caregivers and care receivers in early-stage dementia. *Gerontologist* 46:688–694.

64. Callahan CM, Hendrie HC, Tierney WM (1995) Documentation and evaluation of cognitive impairment in elderly primary care patients. *Ann Intern Med* 122:422–429.

65. Ganguli M, Rodriguez E, Mulsant B, Richards S, Pandav R, et al. (2004) Detection and management of cognitive impairment in primary care: the Steel Valley Seniors Survey. *J Am Geriatr Soc* 52: 1668–1675.

66. Gitlin LN, Corcoran M, Winter L, Boyce A, Hauck WW (2001) A randomized, controlled trial of a home environmental intervention: effect on efficacy and upset in caregivers and on daily function of persons with dementia. *Gerontologist* 41:4–14.

67. Teri L, Gibbons LE, McCurry SM, Logsdon RG, Buchner DM, et al. (2003) Exercise plus behavioral management in patients with Alzheimer disease: a randomized controlled trial. *JAMA* 290:2015–2022.

68. Gaugler JE, Jarrott SE, Zarit SH, Stephens MA, Townsend A, et al. (2003) Respite for dementia caregivers: the effects of adult day service use on caregiving hours and care demands. *Int Psychogeriatr* 15: 37–58.

69. Graff MJ, Adang EM, Vernooij-Dassen MJ, Dekker J, Jonsson L, et al. (2008) Community occupational therapy for older patients with dementia and their care givers: cost effectiveness study. *Bmj* 336: 134–138.

70. Gitlin LN, Winter L, Dennis MP, Hodgson N, Hauck WW (2010) A biobehavioral home-based intervention and the well-being of patients with dementia and their caregivers: the COPE randomized trial. *JAMA* 304:983–991.

71. O'Neil ME, Freeman M, Christensen V, Telerant R, Addleman A, et al. (2011). A Systematic Evidence Review of Non-pharmacological Interventions for Behavioral Symptoms of Dementia. Washington, DC.

72. Boustani M, Sachs G, Callahan CM (2007) Can primary care meet the biopsychosocial needs of older adults with dementia? *J Gen Intern Med* 22:1625–1627.

73. Jencks SF, Cuerdon T, Burwen DR, Fleming B, Houck PM, et al. (2000) Quality of medical care delivered to Medicare beneficiaries: a profile at state and national levels. *JAMA* 284:1670–1676.

74. Iliffe S, Mitchley S, Gould M, Haines A (1994) Evaluation of the use of brief screening instruments for dementia, depression and problem drinking among elderly people in general practice. *Br J Gen Pract* 44: 503–507.

75. Downs M, Turner S, Bryans M, Wilcock J, Keady J, et al. (2006) Effectiveness of educational interventions in improving detection and management of dementia in primary care: cluster randomised controlled study. *BMJ* 332:692–696.

76. Waldorff FB, Almind G, Makela M, Moller S, Waldemar G (2003) Implementation of a clinical dementia guideline. A controlled study on the effect of a multifaceted strategy. *Scand J Prim Health Care* 21: 142–147.

77. Donath C, Grassel E, Grossfeld-Schmitz M, Menn P, Lauterberg J, et al. (2010) Effects of general prac-titioner training and family support services on the care of home-dwelling dementia patients – results of a controlled cluster-randomized study. *BMC Health Serv Res* 10:314.

78. Challis D, von Abendorff R, Brown P, Chesterman J, Hughes J (2002) Care management, dementia care and specialist mental health services: an evaluation. *Int J Geriatr Psychiatry* 17:315–325.

79. Callahan CM, Boustani MA, Unverzagt FW, Austrom MG, Damush TM, et al. (2006) Effectiveness of collaborative care for older adults with Alzheimer disease in primary care: a randomized controlled trial. *JAMA* 295:2148–2157.

80. Chodosh J, Berry E, Lee M, Connor K, DeMonte R, et al. (2006) Effect of a dementia care management intervention on primary care provider knowledge, attitudes, and perceptions of quality of care. *J Am Geriatr Soc* 54:311–317.

81. Vickrey BG, Mittman BS, Connor KI, Pearson ML, Della Penna RD, et al. (2006) The effect of a disease management intervention on quality and outcomes of dementia care: a randomized, controlled trial. *Ann Intern Med* 145:713–726.

82. Graff MJ, Vernooij-Dassen MJ, Thijssen M, Dekker J, Hoefnagels WH, et al. (2006) Community based occupational therapy for patients with dementia and their care givers: randomised controlled trial. *BMJ* 333:1196.

83. Graff MJ, Vernooij-Dassen MJ, Thijssen M, Dekker J, Hoefnagels WH, et al. (2007) Effects of community occupational therapy on quality of life, mood, and health status in dementia patients and their caregivers: a randomized controlled trial. *J Gerontol A Biol Sci Med Sci* 62:1002–1009.

84. Gitlin LN, Winter L, Burke J, Chernett N, Dennis MP, et al. (2008) Tailored activities to manage neu-ropsychiatric behaviors in persons with dementia and reduce caregiver burden: a randomized pilot study. *Am J Geriatr Psychiatry* 16:229–239.

85. Callahan CM, Arling G, Tu W, Rosenman MB, Counsell SR, et al. (2012) Transitions in care for older adults with and without dementia. *J Am Geriatr Soc* 60:813–820.

86. Grumbach K, Bodenheimer T (2002) A primary care home for Americans: putting the house in order. *JAMA* 288:889–893.

87. Callahan CM, Boustani M, Sachs GA, Hendrie HC (2009) Integrating care for older adults with cognitive impairment. *Curr Alzheimer Res* 6:368–374.

88. Boustani MA, Sachs GA, Alder CA, Munger S, Schubert CC, et al. (2011) Implementing innovative models of dementia care: the Healthy Aging Brain Center. *Aging Ment Health* 15:13–22.

89. Callahan CM, Boustani MA, Weiner M, Beck RA, Livin LR, et al. (2011) Implementing dementia care models in primary care settings: the Aging Brain Care Medical Home. *Aging Ment Health* 15:5–12.

90. Wenge NS, Roth CP, Shekelle P; the ACOVE Investigators (2007) Introduction to the assessing care of vulnerable elders-3 quality indicator measurement set. *J Am Geriatr Soc* 55(s2):S247–S252.

91. Hort J, O'Brien JT, Gainotti G, Pirttila T, Popescu BO, et al. (2010) EFNS guidelines for the diagnosis and management of Alzheimer's disease. *Eur J Neurol* 17:1236–1248.

92. Vroomen JM, Van Mierlo LD, van de Ven PM, Bosmasn JE, van den Dungen P, et al. (2012) Comparing Dutch Case management care models for people with dementia and their caregivers: the design of the COMPAS study. *MBMC Health Ser Res* 12:132–142.

Section 2

Service models

Chapter 3

Services for people with young onset dementia

Raymond T.C.M. Koopmans and Denise Thompson

Department of Primary and Community Care, Centre for Family Medicine, Geriatric Care and Public Health, Radboud University Nijmegen, Medical Centre, The Netherlands

With contributions of:

Adrienne Withall[a] and Meredith Gresham[b] (Australia)

[a]School of Public Health and Community Medicine, Kensington Campus, University of New South Wales, Australia
[b]HammondCare Foundation, Australia

David Conn[a] and Tiffany Chow[b] (Canada)

[a]Department of Psychiatry, University of Toronto, Canada
[b]Department of Medicine, Geriatric Psychiatry Division, University of Toronto, Canada

Florence Pasquier[a] and Florence Lébert[b] (France)

[a]Praticien-Hospitalier en Neurologie au Centre, Hospitalier et Universitaire de Lille, France
[b]Centre national de référence des malades Alzheimer jeunes, Université Lille Nord de France, France

Christian Bakker[a] and Marjolein de Vugt[b] (The Netherlands)

[a]Radboud University Nijmegen, The Netherlands
[b]School for Mental Health and Neuroscience, Alzheimer Centrum Limburg, Maastricht University, The Netherlands

Tor Rosness[a] and Aud Johannessen[b] (Norway)

[a]Norwegian Centre for Dementia Research, Department of Geriatric Medicine, Ullevaal University Hospital, Norway
[b]Aldring og Helse, Nasjonalt Kompetansesenter, Norway

Yung-Jen Yang (Taiwan)

Tsao-Tun Psychiatric Centre, Taiwan

Denise Rettenmaier (USA)

Ambulatory Care Clinic, USA

Designing and Delivering Dementia Services, First Edition. Edited by Hugo de Waal, Constantine Lyketsos, David Ames, and John O'Brien.
© 2013 John Wiley & Sons, Ltd. Published 2013 by John Wiley & Sons, Ltd.

Introduction

Young onset dementia (YOD) refers to the onset of dementia before the age of 65. The term 'pre-senile dementia' as used in the published literature until about 10 years ago, is no longer favoured [1]. Terms like 'young onset dementia', 'younger onset dementia' and 'younger people with dementia' are now commonly used. The term 'early onset dementia' is still used in current literature. There is some debate whether this term should be preferred over using YOD. Some state that the term 'early onset dementia' refers to the early stages of the dementia process, while others reserve this term for people in which the onset of dementia was before the age of 45. People who suffer from dementia see themselves as 'young', so from a person-centred point of view, this term is preferred. We therefore use YOD in this chapter.

Figures on the prevalence of YOD are scarce. In 2003, Harvey and colleagues published an often-cited study on the prevalence of dementia in people under the age of 65 of a large catchment area in the UK covering 567,500 people [2]. The prevalence in those aged 30–64 was 54.0 per 100,000, for those aged 45–64 years, it was 98.1–118.00 per 100,000. From the age of 35 onwards, the prevalence of dementia approximately doubled with each 5-year increase of age.

A Japanese study investigated the prevalence of YOD by sending a questionnaire to a variety of medical institutions [3]. They then asked some additional information about the type of dementia. They found an estimated prevalence of 42.3 cases per 100,000. The most frequently diagnosed type was vascular dementia (42.5%), followed by Alzheimer's disease (25.6%), dementia caused by head trauma (7.1%), dementia with Lewy bodies/Parkinson's dementia (6.2%), fronto-temporal dementia (FTD) (2.6%) and other causes (16%).

A report commissioned by the Alzheimer's Society of Canada estimated that in 2010, there were more than 500,000 people living with dementia in Canada [4]. The report suggests that approximately 71,000 of these individuals are under 65.

However, a recent study from Australia yielded a much higher prevalence of 68.2/100,000, with the rates equating to approximately 1/750 population at risk for those aged 45–64 and 1/1500 for those aged 30–64 [5]. Alcohol-related dementia was the most common type (21%), followed by Alzheimer's disease (17%), unspecified dementia (13%), dementia secondary to other medical illness (including HD, MS, HIV/AIDs, epilepsy and CJD: 17%) and fronto-temporal dementia (including Pick's disease, semantic dementia and progressive non-fluent aphasia: 12%).

There have been a series of convenience samples which all lend support to the view that Alzheimer disease, dementia with Lewy bodies and vascular cognitive impairment comprise a smaller portion of cases in younger patients than in the older populations, with a relatively higher prevalence of FTD and alcohol-related dementia in patients with YOD [1]. However, the younger the onset of the dementia, the more likely it is that the patient has a genetic or metabolic disease. Kelley et al. published a retrospective medical chart observational study of all individuals with cognitive decline between the ages of 17–45 years at the Mayo Clinic, Rochester, MN, in the USA, over a 10-year inclusion period [6]. They identified 235 cases. Causes varied, with neurodegenerative aetiologies accounting for 31.1% of the cohort; Alzheimer's disease was uncommon. Autoimmune or inflammatory causes accounted for 21.3%. At last follow-up, 44 patients (18.7%) had an unknown aetiology, despite exhaustive evaluation.

Because YOD can differ strongly from late onset dementia (LOD) in aetiology and course of disease, people with YOD and their caregivers have specific needs. In a short e-survey held in 2011 among the 98 Alzheimer Disease Associations, with 31% response after a 2- and 4-week reminder, 40% of the countries reported having specific services for people with YOD. Specific services for YOD caregivers exist in 50% of the responding countries and 17% report having specific YOD long term-care facilities. Countries with specific services are mostly western countries but also other countries, for example India.

In this chapter, we address the specific needs of people with YOD and what is necessary for good service delivery. Further, we report on services for YOD from countries from all continents.

What is necessary for good service delivery?

The evidence for good service delivery arises mostly out of the practical experience of professionals, carers and people with YOD themselves. A large proportion of the literature consists of stories, biographies, autobiographies and testimonies, which are a vital source of experiential information, an important guide for practice and a resource for evaluations. There are few examples of programmes that have been systematically evaluated, but there are nevertheless a number of common themes in the literature around what constitutes good practice.

Diagnosis

Difficulty with diagnosis is one of the most pressing problems for people with YOD and their family members. A lack of awareness of the existence of dementia in younger people both among the general public and on the part of the general practitioners to whom people usually first present; the relative infrequency of dementia in people under 65 when compared with causes, such as depression, anxiety and other illnesses; the prominence of behavioural change early in the presentation, as well as the drawn out nature of the diagnostic process with younger clients, all contribute to significant delays in diagnosis for this group [7,8].

Early diagnosis is crucial in YOD. Importantly, some dementias, such as alcohol-related dementia, normal pressure hydrocephalus and HIV-related dementia, are reversible and/or preventable [8]. Additionally, some of the dementias that present more commonly in young people have a relatively rapid disease progression (e.g. CJD and motor neurone disease with dementia). Often by the time the diagnosis is made, the person with dementia is unable to understand the implications and/or significant strains have occurred within their family relationships [8]. Delay in diagnosis means that referrals to support and care services are also delayed, and this can have a profound emotional impact on the person with YOD and their family. The delay can also have serious consequences for putting in place legal arrangements, such as wills and powers of attorney.

It is imperative that awareness and an understanding of the importance of early diagnosis is raised among general practitioners, since they represent the first health professional consulted by most people with YOD [8,9]. Specialists, such as geriatricians, neurologists and psychiatrists, also need additional knowledge about diagnostic methods for this group.

Information

The provision of information, both what people are told and the way they are told, is another issue of pressing importance. Carers have been critical of the methods of disclosure used by some clinicians and of the limitations of the information available. Carers complained about being passed from consultant to consultant. They had not received enough information, practical help, support or counselling. The burden of responsibility for finding out about available help was left with the carers and their families [10].

Differences

In the literature, there is a wide-ranging discussion on how developing dementia at a younger age differs from LOD. Two of the main differences are that, unlike older people, people with YOD could still be bringing up children and are likely still to be supporting a family financially.

Demotion, early retirement and diminished retirement income are more likely among those of workforce age, as are mortgages, significant levels of debt and a lack of legal planning. Younger people are more likely to be physically fit, and the unexpected nature of dementia at such an early age is more likely to lead to relationship breakdown. Carers of people with YOD have been found to have greater levels of psychological distress and carer responsibility [11,12], and this burden appears to extend to their children [13].

The main reason for these differences is the stage of life at which the disease occurs. People aged in their 40s and 50s, and even in their 60s, could normally expect years of productive activity ahead of them. Instead, with the onset of dementia, they have to radically revise their expectations of life and what they can accomplish.

Children and family responsibilities

One of the chief ways in which the impact of YOD can differ from the impact of LOD is the presence of dependent children. Children can have strong reactions if their parent is behaving in an unusual manner [14]. Research has found that children can come into conflict with the affected parent (more often with a father than with a mother), and the younger the parent the more likely this seems to occur [6]. It is not often realised that in the case of YOD, some caregiving is likely to be performed by young children [10].

Very little has been written about the experiences and needs of the children of people with YOD [15]. However, it is known that those children are sometimes very young, not only because the disease can develop in people who are comparatively young, but also because of the growing tendency to postpone childbirth. They may feel shame about their parent's unusual behaviour, anxiety about difficulties in their parents' relationship, fear of and grief for the losses the parent is going through, loneliness because the healthy parent has to focus more attention on the YOD parent, and worry about the chances of themselves getting dementia in the future.

Employment

Employment can be a significant and unique issue for people with YOD, with most LODs occurring after the conventional retirement age. The workplace is often the place where signs of dementia are first noticed and a lack of understanding by employers can lead to discrimination. Yet people usually prefer to remain in the workforce as long as possible. Moreover, sickness or disability benefits might be difficult to access, and retirement income might not be immediately available because the person is too young. Carers, too, can find employment difficult because of inflexible workplace practices.

Maslow suggested that what was needed was to raise awareness of YOD among employers and human resources personnel, and to disseminate information about ways in which workplaces could accommodate people with YOD and about the legal requirements for workplace accommodation [16].

Services, specific and otherwise

The need for appropriate age-specific services for people with YOD is a recurring theme in the literature [17]. Mainstream dementia services are usually problematic for people with YOD [14]. In contrast to older people, they are likely to be physically fitter, more likely to be sexually active, to have different interests and to identify more closely with staff. This can create particular difficulties for staff, who can find these clients confronting, and for the integration of younger and older clients in the same service [8].

Tyson said that appropriate provision of respite and day care for people with YOD should acknowledge that the needs of younger people are different from those of older people and provide separate premises designated specifically for people with YOD [18]. The review also said that those consulted in the study were in favour of more home support so that the younger person could be cared for longer in their own home.

However, there are difficulties with the use of age as a criterion for receiving services [19]. Using age as a criterion fails to account for differences within and similarities across age groups and requiring clients to leave a service when they turn 65 disrupts continuity of care. Services specifically for younger people could be taken to imply that older people do not have the same needs as those under 65 and may imply that people of different generations do not socialise with each other. Many of the issues raised in the context of YOD-specific services are also highly relevant for older people, for example, the overemphasis on the later stages of the disease, problems accessing services, the need to incorporate a multidisciplinary approach and inadequate care and assessment [20].

People with YOD benefit from both specialist and generalist services. Age-appropriate services are often stressed as the way to develop good practice for YOD but people need other services that are not necessarily age specific. Mainstream services tend to be already well-established and based on recognised expertise. Research has reported that it does not particularly matter in terms of effectiveness whether domiciliary care for people with dementia is organised on a specialist or a generic basis [17]. What matters most is the extent to which the service conforms to quality standards for dementia care.

Person-centred services

The need for person-centred services is echoed throughout the literature, with people with YOD and their families being actively involved in the decision-making. Staff can contribute to maintaining people's personhood by using the experience and knowledge of people with YOD themselves [21].

Services should be underpinned by both person- and family-centred practice. There is a special need in the case of YOD, because of the particular stage in life, to understand the effect of the disease on the family members' functioning and roles, as well as on the person with dementia. However, to date, there are very few intervention strategies that target both the carer and the person with dementia as a dyad [22].

Multidisciplinary services

People with YOD do not readily fit into any of the conventional health service categories. They often fall within the age limits of adult mental health but require the expertise found within older persons' mental health services. Depending on their geographical location, they might be seen by a geriatrician, neurologist, old age psychiatrist or within a memory clinic, where they can benefit from a multidisciplinary approach.

A suite of service options, including counselling and information, needs to be offered to people at the point of diagnosis [18]. This kind of holistic approach is more likely to take into account the more varied social circle of people of pre-retirement age, including children still living at home and a spouse and friends who are still employed.

Carers

The research literature is still unclear about whether or not there are any differences between caring for someone with YOD and caring for someone with later-onset dementia. However, there is general agreement that YOD carers do experience specific problems related to their phase in life and that, for that reason, it is likely that YOD has an even greater impact on the person and their family than later onset dementia [23]. Work-related problems, financial problems, problems with children, diagnostic uncertainty and delays in referral occur less often in the case of LOD [24]. Moreover, YOD has a different clinical manifestation from LOD, being more often characterised by neuropsychiatric symptoms and self-awareness, which is partly due to the higher prevalence of FTD.

Overall, the consensus in the literature is that the burden for carers of people with YOD is greater than for carers of people who develop dementia later in life. At least one research study has found significantly higher levels of stress among carers of people with YOD than among carers of older people [12]. Other research has found that having to cope constantly with challenging behaviours is a major cause of carer stress, and there is evidence of higher levels of depression in spouses of people with FTD [25].

Behavioural disturbances have been found to be more worrying in YOD than in late-onset dementia, partly because of the person's greater strength and physical ability, and partly because of the higher prevalence of FTD among people with YOD. One study found that the needs of FTD carers were significantly higher than those of the carers of people with Alzheimer's, due to the younger onset of FTD, the characteristics typical of FTD, difficulties with access to services, information and support, and financial problems [26]. The study also found that women carers were more likely than men to report disruptive symptoms associated with FTD, and other studies have found that husbands caring for their wives report less emotional distress than wives caring for their husbands [6,26].

Alt and Beatty identified a number of requirements of those caring for people with YOD. They needed more intensive help and support than older carers throughout the whole duration of their caregiving [27]. Companionship and support from carers in a similar situation was also important (because they may have lost their earlier friends or no longer felt comfortable with them), as was assistance that supported and strengthened the relationship with their partner. Service providers needed to be aware that carers aged under 50 may have to place the person with YOD into residential care sooner rather than later. There was also a need for workers from ethno-specific organisations to assist carers from non-English-speaking communities to access relevant services.

Respite

What people with YOD require of respite services can strain traditional models, which may be designed around fairly sedentary activities. Younger people often express a preference for activities that involve exercise. They do not identify themselves as being aged, and they need staff who understand their particular life stage. Research has found that carers are reluctant to use respite care, despite their need for a break, because in their view, the services are inappropriate [18]. They believe that their loved one feels isolated because they do not fit in with the older clients. They also feel that their relative would deteriorate in an unfamiliar environment and that they might have problems resettling at home. Suggested improvements involve models that collaborate with both the carer and the person with YOD and that view respite not only as a service for the carer, but also as an opportunity for younger people to get together and participate in activities that give them self-esteem and a sense of capability [18]. It is important for services to work with carers to familiarise them with what they can offer so that they might be willing to take up the service.

International perspectives

In this paragraph, a short overview is given of services for people with YOD in Australia, Canada, France, the Netherlands, Norway, Taiwan and the USA.

Australia

While dementia generally has achieved significant public awareness through the work of advocacy groups over the last two decades, recognition of YOD in Australia is only just emerging. Under-recognised by health practitioners, the accurate diagnosis of younger onset dementia is often a slow process. This situation is compounded by the perception among the general public and many health professionals that dementia is a disease of old age. Frequently, there is an atypical presentation, and diagnostic expertise can be particularly difficult to find for people living outside major metro-politan centres. From the perspective of the person living with younger onset dementia, there is stigma associated with having an 'old person's disease', and advocacy groups report that younger people with dementia resulting from specific diseases, including multiple sclerosis and Parkinson's disease, do not identify with having dementia.

YOD services are, in general, ad hoc. In Australia, various levels of government take responsibil-ity for differing policy and programme areas. At the present time, there is no coordinated policy to shape YOD services or to place them in the context of existing service delivery structures. Current policy divides service streams by age: for clients over 65 years, long-term community and residen-tial care is a Commonwealth (federal) responsibility, with responsibility for the person under 65 requiring long-term care falling to State or Territory disability services. While each stream has its expertise and advantages, the young person with dementia frequently 'falls between the cracks'. For example, a diagnosis of dementia usually assumes inability to learn new skills and as such precludes these people from rehabilitative and restorative care normally afforded in the disability sector.

Compared internationally, Australia has a small population spread over vast areas, with most living in coastal regions. Finding enough people living with YOD in a geographically similar area to offer financially justifiable specialised services is difficult. Many community services, including adult day centres, are willing to accommodate these clients where possible but find the needs of this group difficult to meet. Aged care models are characterised by slower, sedentary activity and are unable to meet the needs of the younger person. Service providers are frequently concerned about mixing younger, physically robust people with dementia with older and frailer clients, espe-cially in respite and residential settings. Anecdotally, staff report feeling inadequate to meet the needs of younger people living with dementia, especially regarding their life stage, family, relation-ship, financial and employment issues.

Young people with dementia are typically accommodated in residential aged care late in the disease process when other forms of accommodation, including care at home, are unable to meet 24-hour care requirements. At the time of writing, we are aware of only one specialist YOD resi-dential service in Australia.

Despite operational difficulty and lack of a policy context services for the young person with dementia and their families are emerging. The Australian Alzheimer's Associations have spear-headed patient and family information services, and specialised community, day and residential services have developed through the interest and willingness of individual service providers.

Canada

Large Canadian cities have a wide range of services for individuals with dementia, including memory clinics, psychogeriatric services, inpatient units, long-term care homes, homecare and respite services, community outreach and support groups, as well as day centres. Most of these services do not differentiate between individuals above or below the age of 65. In fact, there are very few services that cater specifically for individuals with YOD. Baycrest Centre in Toronto has provided some innovative programmes related to FTD, including a community day programme that specialises in helping individuals with FTD and their caregivers. The programme opened in 2006 after the need for a special service was identified. It was integrated into a long-standing Community Day Programme, which originated in 1959 and serves moderately to severely cognitively impaired seniors. The programme was developed in partnership with the Baycrest Ross Memory Clinic utilising a collaborative model of care with the goal of meeting the diverse needs of the clients and their families. The programme includes an interdisciplinary team consisting of nursing, social work, recreation and programme/personal support workers. Clients and their families receive a combination of health and wellness support, case management, counselling, education and support in accessing other services. Grinberg and Phillips describe this programme and emphasise that the supports required by FTD clients and their families are somewhat unique [28]. Another innovative Canadian initiative focusing on FTD is in the form of a new website for teenagers and their parent caregivers entitled 'When Dementia is in the House'. This website has been developed by Dr Tiffany Chow and colleagues. Dr Chow developed this when she became aware that the children of these patients had no resources dedicated to their education and support. This online resource is hosted and managed by the Canadian Dementia Knowledge Transfer Network (CDKTN) and can be accessed at http://lifeandminds.ca/whendementiaisinthehouse/. In addition, Marziali and Climans have described the feasibility of an Internet-based videoconferencing support group for spousal caregivers of patients with FTD [29]. All of the participants were very positive about being able to access support using this approach.

France

In France, medico-social aids differ according to age of patients: before 60, they come under the law for disabled adults, whereas at 60 years and over, they come under the regulation for the elderly (Ministry of Solidarities and Social Cohesion). Most services for people with dementia are only available for patients over 60 (day care, nursing homes with specialised units and corresponding allowance). To enter a day care or a nursing home before the age of 60, a special dispensation is needed, delivered by the 'Conseils Généraux' (General Councils of France, i.e. the legislative bodies of the departments of France). There are 100 such departments (including overseas), each having its own policy regarding the dispensation. Overall, individualised home-care allocations for disabled people younger than 60 are greater than the customised allocation for older people, but the financial aids for the younger cannot be used to cover the cost of institutionalisation, whereas the financial assistance for older people can. One objective of the French Alzheimer plan 2008–2012 was to list the services available for and the needs of patients with YOD and their family. In 2010–2011, a national survey was conducted by the National Reference Centre for YOD (NRC-YOD) and the Fondation Médéric Alzheimer in all accommodations possibly receiving patients with YOD to establish how many patients with Alzheimer's disease or associated disorders (ADAD) younger than 60 (estimated to be about 5000 in France) were currently living in such places. The response rate was 77%. Of these, nearly 15,000 accommodations (8%) declared receiving patients with YOD; of the 2700 patients younger than 60 with dementia, most had a psychotic disease, Down syndrome, stroke, brain injury, alcoholism or mental or cognitive disability. Of these, 150 residents suffered from ADAD, all living in a nursing home for the elderly (with a dispensation), and 30 were temporarily hospitalised on a psychiatric unit because of severe behavioural problems.

The low rate of institutionalisation (<5%) in patients with ADAD younger than 60 was supported by a study of 110 caregivers of patients with YOD, followed up at the Lille Memory Clinic, which showed that 8% entered an institution before 60 years old (9% went to day care and 22% to respite care before institutionalisation) and 20% before 65 years. Before 60, the majority of patients suffered from FTD or presented with a frontal lobe syndrome and severe behavioural problems, whereas after 60, the majority of patients had Alzheimer's disease.

A survey in the various settings showed the limitations professional carers in nursing homes for the elderly experienced. They all expressed their need for specific training and support, but agreed that the living together of patients of various ages was usually not a problem, because most patients entered at a severe stage. Most of the staff in residential care for disabled adults considered that this place was not appropriate for patients with YOD and that living together with psychotic patients was difficult, but they wanted to keep and offer the best care to the residents with Down syndrome suffering from dementia.

Regional networks of services from home to nursing homes, including access to the new services created by the Alzheimer plan (e.g. special units for acute behavioural disorders and respite care) are being established, with medical support provided by the memory resources and research centres coordinated by the NRC-YOD.

The Netherlands

In the Netherlands, it is increasingly recognised that people with YOD and their families have specific needs. However, services for YOD are still rather scarce in the Netherlands and there are often difficulties in meeting these complex needs. Regions differ in the availability and quality of specific care and in the development of new YOD services. As a consequence, access and nearness of suitable services differ for individuals throughout the country. This inconsistency in care is probably related to financial–economic factors and to a lack of systematic knowledge of the specific needs of this group.

Notwithstanding the unavailability of systematic knowledge of care needs in YOD, a national task force on YOD presented a 'national YOD care programme' in 2004, based on best practices. The objectives of this national care programme were to improve quality of care in YOD and to strive for social and financial economic acknowledgement. The special care needs of this group were recognised by the Dutch government in 2006 with the introduction of an extra financial compensation for YOD services and adaptation of recommendations for building regulations for more spacious care facilities. These policy developments stimulated care organisations to start or improve dedicated services for YOD, for example by offering specific daytime activities, creating special care units in the nursing home and improving team expertise by staff training. Several nursing homes started to implement the 'national YOD care programme' in their organisation. To date, about 25 care organisations offer specialised care for people with YOD. Most care homes have YOD specialised units where people with YOD live together, or have day-care centres. Most of them offer outreach care and advise or support groups for spouses and children. The service provision in the units and day-care centres differs from that provided in dementia special care units for people with LOD. There is more emphasis on hobbies, creating artwork, woodcarving, fitness, walking, and so on.

To ensure quality of care for these patients and their families, a quality mark was established. The quality indicators for this mark have been derived from the 'national YOD care programme'. The Florence 'Centre for Specialised Care in YOD' in The Hague was one of the first to receive the quality mark. Other organisations have since then followed, indicating that quality of care for this special group is continuously improving in the Netherlands.

Norway

Several studies, including young patients with FTD and young onset Alzheimer's disease (YO-AD) and their carers have been carried out in Norway. Establishing a correct diagnosis as soon as possible is vital. This alleviates the burden both for the patient and the carer. In Norway, there is not a specific designated clinical service, which diagnoses young patients with dementia. This can cause a long delay in establishing a correct dementia diagnosis [30]. The healthcare system is divided between hospitals and local authority care. The recommendations mention how and by whom these patients should be examined in the specialist service, but diagnosing dementia in young patients usually occurs at memory clinics, psychogeriatric, geriatric or neurological outpatient clinics. There is a need for better collaboration between different disciplines within the hospitals and outpatient clinics to increase the competence of the medical staff, so that they can diagnose these patients at an early stage of the disorder. The current lack of collaboration makes it difficult to reach out with information about the existing services that have been adapted for younger persons with dementia and their carers.

Patients with an FTD diagnosis were often offered nursing-home placement, either involving short-term or long-term stays, and the predominance of personality changes may be the prevailing reason for this [30]. The family carers of FTD patients tended to be less satisfied with the provision of support they had received from the specialist health service compared with the carers of late onset AD patients and were in need of both more and different forms of support [31].

We observed a reduction in depression in carers when the patients received domiciliary nursing care [32]. There are only two nursing homes in Norway, which are specifically designed for younger patients with dementia and only one of these offers day care. We could not discern any beneficial effect of the day-care centres, which may be ascribed to the fact that the staff of these facilities did not have the skills and knowledge to care for these younger patients with dementia sufficiently. There are currently only four day-care centres in Norway that cater specifically for younger patients with dementia.

Support groups for carers and for younger people with dementia have been set up at some hospitals in urban areas, but guidelines on how to support these families are still lacking. A study by Johannessen and Möller showed that healthcare services should focus on providing younger persons with dementia with the means to maintain contact with society and that their views should not be overlooked [33]. There is a need for guidelines to help families face the challenge of a dementia diagnosis and to maintain their quality of life throughout the entire process of the disorder. Hopefully, the new Collaboration Act (2008–2009) and the revised Dementia Plan 2015 (2011) will contribute to a better service in a country with many small cities and large rural areas.

Taiwan

The societies in the Asia-Pacific area are experiencing rapid ageing in the coming decades and Taiwan is one of the leading countries as evidenced by the highest ageing index. Dementia and related issues did not attract adequate attention until just ten years ago when the Taiwan Alzheimer's Disease Association (TADA) was established. However, despite the rapid growth of research in dementia, development of a caring system, promotion of service models, issuing of regulations and legislations, systematic and holistic treatment, and caring networks are still lacking and not widespread. In addition, most of the services mainly aim at people with so-called common dementia, that is people who are 65 years or older. Hence, people with YOD are usually neglected.

Due to the inadequate expertise and low sensitivity to cognitive symptoms in local practitioners (including family physicians, neurologists and even psychiatrists), most YOD people receive the diagnosis at a relatively late stage. A small local study also indicated that misdiagnosis (especially depression) delayed confirmation of diagnosis and subsequent referral to specialists, and it identified that active and timely interventions were commonly lacking.

Most people with YOD are cared for together with 'common' patients with dementia in the routine caring system and settings, and there are very few specialised care facilities. The first YOD-supportive group was established in 2004 in Taipei. Despite the fact that some experimental studies and trials investigating care models have been attempted, there is sadly still no official consensus, treatment guidelines or a nationwide epidemiological study on YOD in Taiwan.

A nationwide epidemiological survey on dementia is underway and special attention will be given to YOD. An initiative by the Taiwanese Society of Geriatric Psychiatry (TSGP) started in 2011, aiming at formulating appropriate treatment recommendations for local practitioners. Some empirically effective care models and services will be further integrated in the current 'routine' care setting. For instance, a previous highly effective care model integrating patients with YOD (and their caregivers) with patients and caregivers with 'common' dementia will be examined and extended. Because of the outdated social welfare regulations and laws, some services do not cover patients with YOD, simply due to age limits. Local interest groups have urged the legislators to amend or draft regulations and laws for those with YOD. The public interest groups (e.g. TADA) have identified the higher needs of patients and families with YOD and plan to involve mass media in propagating relevant information about YOD. The issues particularly important for people with YOD, that is impact of the illness, needs of patients and carers, and the need for resources, form the initial focus of the media campaign.

Like many countries around the world, YOD is just gaining attention in Taiwan. Regional cooperation and collaboration are necessary for success.

USA

Access to mental health and other services (e.g. neurology) in the USA may be quite limited depending on the person's location and resources, which can limit recognition and diagnosis. The very fact that these changes are happening to a younger person can mean that it is difficult for the individual and the people around them to admit that the primary change is cognitive loss progressing to dementia with loss of function and result in a delay of diagnosis and referral for evaluation. Once a decision to seek help is made, help may be difficult to obtain, even for a younger patient.

In the United States, access to mental health services and provision of care are often directly related to financial resources. Mental health services are usually provided with private health insurance, and the length or amount of mental health services depends on the type of insurance. For those with managed healthcare plans, the length or amount of mental health services may be limited, which may impact the ability to properly assess and diagnose the patient with YOD.

As YOD patients progress and become more dependent, issues of ongoing care become more crucial. They may require the support of their spouses, children, siblings or elderly parents. Depending on their circumstances and financial situation, care may continue to be provided at home with community assistance, privately hired care or adult day-care programmes. Unsafe behaviour or wandering may require transfer to an institutional setting.

For seniors, government Medicare and Medicaid programmes can provide payment for adult day-care programmes and skilled nursing facilities if private resources cannot. However, for YOD patients, declaration of disability is usually required for government aid and that may be difficult to obtain. Long-term care insurance can provide care for elders in a skilled nursing setting but may not be useful for the YOD patient. Financial support for those in the YOD patients' age group can be very limited.

When a patient exceeds the ability to be cared for at home, even with supportive services, such as adult day care, and does not yet meet skilled nursing requirements, the 'in-between' option is privately funded assisted living or admission into a residential care facility. With a diagnosis of dementia, it would be expected that the patient would be admitted to an assisted living dementia special care unit or other type of group home. Access to age-appropriate activities can be very limited at every level, from adult day care to assisted living facilities and nursing homes. The predominance of frailer elders in these programmes can make caring for the younger, more physically capable demented patient challenging. The emotionality associated with YOD can be exceptionally draining, for patients and their loved ones, affecting every aspect of their life.

In conclusion

In sum, it can be said that, while there is still too little awareness of younger onset dementia, the situation is changing. There is growing interest by policy makers, service providers and researchers, and it is possible for people with YOD and their families to see themselves as an identifiable group, with particular needs and specific requirements for service provision. That does not translate directly into adequate and appropriate services, but it is a step in the right direction. However, there is still a need for more research specifically aimed at people with YOD. Many areas are understudied, such as non-Alzheimer types of YOD, palliative care for YOD, the course of YOD in community dwelling, as well as institutionalised people, prevalence of neuropsychiatric symptoms and differences with LOD, psychotropic drug use, and so on. Services specifically designed for YOD are in their infancy, and in developing countries, there seems to be a total lack of services. This is a great challenge for organisations such as Alzheimer's Disease International and the International Psychogeriatric Association.

References

1. Rossor MN, Fox NC, Mummery CJ, Schott JM, Warren JD (2010 August) The diagnosis of young-onset dementia. *Lancet Neurol* 9(8):793–806.
2. Harvey RJ, Skelton-Robinson M, Rossor MN (2003 September) The prevalence and causes of dementia in people under the age of 65 years. *J Neurol Neurosurg Psychiatry* 74(9):1206–1209.
3. Ikejima C, Yasuno F, Mizukami K, Sasaki M, Tanimukai S, Asada T (2009 Aug) Prevalence and causes of early-onset dementia in Japan: a population-based study. *Stroke* 40(8):2709–2714.
4. Alzheimer Society of Canada (2010) Rising Tide: The Impact of Dementia on Canadian Society: Alzheimer's Society of Canada. Report by the Alzheimer Society of Canada.
5. Withall A, Draper B (2009) What is the burden of younger onset dementia in Australia? In: *International Psychogeriatrics*. New York: Springer, pp. 245–259. Presented at International Psychogeriatric Association 14th International Congress: Path to Prevention, Montreal, Canada, September 1–5.
6. Kelley BJ, Boeve BF, Josephs KA (2008 November) Young-onset dementia: demographic and etiologic characteristics of 235 patients. *Arch Neurol* 65(11):1502–1508.
7. Luscombe G, Brodaty H, Freeth S (1998 May) Younger people with dementia: diagnostic issues, effects on carers and use of services. *Int J Geriatr Psychiatry* 13(5):323–330.
8. Chemali Z, Withall A, Daffner KR (2010 March) The plight of caring for young patients with frontotemporal dementia. *Am J Alzheimers Dis Other Demen* 25(2):109–115.
9. Maslow K (2006) Early Onset Dementia: A National Challenge, A Future Crisis. Available at: http://www.alz.org/national/documents/report_earlyonset_full.pdf (last accessed on 20 February 2013).
10. Williams T, Dearden AM, Cameron IA (2001) From pillar to post – a study of younger people with dementia. *Psychiatr Bull* 25:384–387.
11. Arai A, Matsumoto T, Ikeda M, Aria Y (2007) Do family caregivers perceive more difficulty when they look after patients with early onset dementia compared to those with late onset dementia? *Int J Geriatr Psychiatry* 22:1255–1261.
12. Freyne A, Kidd N, Coen R, Lawlor BA (1999 September) Burden in carers of dementia patients: higher levels in carers of younger sufferers. *Int J Geriatr Psychiatry* 14(9):784–788.
13. Svanberg E, Stott J, Spector A (2010) 'Just helping': children living with a parent with young onset dementia. *Aging Ment Health* 14:740–751.
14. Health N (2011) The NSW Dementia Services Framework 2010–2015. Available at: http://www.health.nsw.gov.au/policies/gl/2011/GL2011_004.html (last accessed on 20 February 2013).
15. Gelman CR, Greer C (2011 February) Young children in early-onset Alzheimer's disease families: research gaps and emerging service needs. *Am J Alzheimers Dis Other Demen* 26(1):29–35.
16. Withall A, Draper B (2010) Alcohol-related dementia: a common diagnosis in younger persons. *Alzheimer's and Dementia* 6:s188–s189.

17. Challis D, Clarkson P, Hughes J, Chester H, Davies S, Sutcliffe C, Xie C, et al. (2010) Community Support Services for People with Dementia: The Relative Costs and Benefits of Specialist and Generic Domiciliary Care Services. Available at: http://www.nursing.manchester.ac.uk/pssru/research/ servicearrangementsandintegration/communitysupportservicesforpeoplewithdementia/dpm245-3.pdf (last accessed on 21 February 2013).

18. Tyson M (2007) Exploring the Needs of Younger People with Dementia in Australia. Available at: http://www.alzheimers.org.au/common/files/NAT/20101027-Nat-YOD-Exploring-needs-Australia.pdf (last accessed on 20 February 2013).

19. Moore K, Renehan E (2011) Evaluation of the Linking Lives Pilot: Supporting younger people with dementia Victoria: National Ageing Research Institute, for Alzheimer's Australia.

20. Beattie AM, Daker-White G, Gilliard J, Means R (2002 August) Younger people in dementia care: a review of service needs, service provision and models of good practice. *Aging Ment Health* 6(3):205–212.

21. Chaston D (2010 February–March) Younger adults with dementia: a strategy to promote awareness and transform perceptions. *Contemp Nurse* 34(2):221–229.

22. Clare L, Kinsella G, Logsdon R (2011) Building resilience in mild cognitive impairment and early-stage dementia: innovative approaches to intervention and outcome evaluation. In: Resnick B (ed.), *Resilience in Aging: Concepts, Research, and Outcomes*. New York: Springer, pp. 245–259.

23. van Vliet D, de Vugt ME, Bakker C, Koopmans RT, Verhey FR (2010 November) Impact of early onset dementia on caregivers: a review. *Int J Geriatr Psychiatry* 25(11):1091–1100.

24. Bakker C, de Vugt ME, Vernooij-Dassen M, van Vliet D, Verhey FR, Koopmans RT (2010 December) Needs in early onset dementia: a qualitative case from the NeedYD study. *Am J Alzheimers Dis Other Demen* 25(8):634–640.

25. Kaiser S, Panygeres P (2007) The psychosocial impact of young onset dementia on spouses. *Am J Alzheimers Dis Other Demen* 21:398–402.

26. Nicolaou P, Egan N, Gasson N, Kane R (2010) Identifying needs, burden, and distress of carers of people with frontotemporal dementia compared to Alzheimer's disease. *Dementia* 9:215–235.

27. Consulting AB (2007) Appropriate HACC Service Models for People with Younger Onset Dementia & People with Dementia and Behaviours of Concern: Issues for Aboriginal and Torres Strait Islander People and People from Culturally and Linguistically Diverse Backgrounds. Available at: http://www.adhc .nsw.gov.au/__data/assets/file/0003/228162/12_AltBeatty_Dementia_Models_Report.pdf (last accessed on 21 February 2013).

28. Grinberg A, Phillips D (2009) The impact of a community day program on the lives of patients with frontotemporal dementia and their caregivers. *Can Rev Alzheimers Dis Other Demen* 12:17–22.

29. Marziali E, Climans R (2009) New technology to connect Frontotemporal Dementia spousal caregivers online. *Can Rev Alzheimers Dis Other Demen* 12:23–26.

30. Rosness TA, Haugen PK, Passant U, Engedal K (2008 August) Frontotemporal dementia: a clinically complex diagnosis. *Int J Geriatr Psychiatry* 23(8):837–842.

31. Rosness TA, Haugen PK, Engedal K (2008 July) Support to family carers of patients with frontotemporal dementia. *Aging Ment Health* 12(4):462–466.

32. Rosness TA, Mjorud M, Engedal K (2011 April) Quality of life and depression in carers of patients with early onset dementia. *Aging Ment Health* 15(3):299–306.

33. Johannessen A, Möller A (2011) Experiences of persons with early-onset dementia in everyday life: a qualitative study. *Dementia* December, 1–15.

Chapter 4

Services for people with incipient dementia

Nicola T. Lautenschlager[a,b] and Alexander F. Kurz[c]

[a]Academic Unit for Psychiatry of Old Age, Department of Psychiatry, The University of Melbourne, St. George's Campus, St. Vincent's Hospital, Australia
[b]School of Psychiatry and Clinical Neurosciences and WA Centre for Health & Ageing, The University of Western Australia, Australia
[c]Department of Psychiatry and Psychotherapy, Klinikum rechts der Isar, Technische Universität München, Germany

Introduction

Deterioration of intellectual ability and psychosocial competence in late life that culminates in disability and dependence has become a paramount public health problem as a consequence of increased population longevity [1]. The most prevalent underlying brain pathologies are progressive neurodegenerative diseases; they often occur in combination with vascular changes [2,3]. Regarding clinical manifestations, initial asymptomatic stages are followed by subjective cognitive complaints [4], prodromal dementia, including mild cognitive impairment [5], and eventually by full-blown dementia. Increasing public concern about cognitive decline in old age and the prospect of treatments that delay neurodegeneration are driving the call for early diagnosis. In asymptomatic individuals with a family history of monogenic Alzheimer's disease (AD) or fronto-temporal dementia (FTD), an increased individual risk of developing dementia can be determined by predictive testing for known mutations many years or even decades before the onset of symptoms. In future, the feasibility of pre-clinical diagnosis may be enhanced by novel non-genetic laboratory or imaging techniques, which identify relevant features of ongoing neurodegeneration [6]. At the stage of prodromal dementia, when minor symptoms are present, evidence of the underlying brain pathology can be gained from combinations of neuropsychological tests, laboratory measurements and brain imaging [7]. In this chapter, the term 'incipient dementia' is meant to encompass both asymptomatic or pre-clinical and prodromal stages of the underlying brain pathology. Earlier diagnosis of dementia is associated with better opportunities for successful coping and disease management by patients, family carers and physicians, but also allows more time for people to deal with mental decline and progressive disability [8]. Therefore, once individuals have been assigned an increased risk of dementia, they should be offered counselling, as well as the best available preventative and therapeutic interventions. We discuss the needs of people with incipient dementia and the types of services that may be provided to meet these needs.

Designing and Delivering Dementia Services, First Edition. Edited by Hugo de Waal, Constantine Lyketsos, David Ames, and John O'Brien.
© 2013 John Wiley & Sons, Ltd. Published 2013 by John Wiley & Sons, Ltd.

Needs of people with incipient dementia

Asymptomatic risk states

Two forms of asymptomatic risk states need to be distinguished because they differ with regard to frequency, diagnostic implications and practical consequences. The first refers to individuals who are genetically determined to develop dementia but have little brain pathology. In these rare cases, the family history and the demonstration of a deterministic gene mutation in a first-degree relative may initiate predictive genetic testing. Since known mutations for AD [9] and FTD [10] have an autosomal dominant mode of transmission and an almost complete penetrance, a positive test has not only implications for the tested individual, but also for their offspring.

A second form of pre-clinical risk states, which is much more frequent than the former, includes older adults where a progressive neurodegeneration is ongoing in the absence of deterministic mutations but still can be compensated for and therefore does not become manifest in overt symptoms. However, subtle decline in performance and increased effort associated with usual tasks may be recognised by affected individuals and may trigger the quest for diagnostic evaluation. These early stages of neurodegeneration cannot be identified by current diagnostic procedures. This may change, however, when refined laboratory tests and imaging methods that detect specific features of neurodegeneration, such as abnormal protein accumulation, aberrant enzyme activities or loss of neurons and synapses, become available [6]. Predictive genetic tests, as well as diagnostic procedures that identify pre-symptomatic stages of neurodegeneration, should be conducted in a setting of appropriate counselling and psychological support that covers the purpose of testing, the meaning of positive or negative results, the implications for the patient and their family, the financial and legal consequences, and the available options for prevention and treatment [11].

Prodromal dementia

Prodromal dementia often goes through the early clinical stage of subjective memory complaints without objective impairment to then move into a phase with emerging observable and measurable decline of functioning. This second phase would fall into the categories of 'cognitive impairment, no dementia' (CIND) or 'mild cognitive impairment' (MCI). The former represents a broad category that includes various underlying causes; the latter, especially the subform 'amnestic MCI', was originally used to describe individuals at increased risk to develop AD [12,13]. More recently, attempts have been made to identify the presence of AD pathology in such individuals, more specifically using biomarkers: in such cases, the term 'prodromal AD' is deemed more appropriate [14].

Neuropsychological testing in patients with MCI may not only reveal problems with memory, but also subtle impairment of executive function, information processing speed or visuospatial ability. Executive dysfunction is more closely associated with impairment of activities of daily living than with memory impairment [15]. Complex activities of daily living can be already impaired at the clinical stage of MCI [16,17]. Certain behavioural and psychological symptoms (BPS) are frequent, particularly depression, apathy, anxiety and irritability. These emotional changes are found in 1/3 to 2/3 of subjects [18–20]. Moreover, MCI can have adverse effects on social life in terms of isolation [21] or disruption of affectional expression and communication [22]. Because of its negative impact on cognitive functioning, practical skills, mood and interpersonal relationships, prodromal dementia is a significant threat to quality of life [23].

The prodromal phase of the behavioural variant of FTD typically presents initially with changes of personality and behaviour in areas such as motivation, emotional control, social awareness, behavioural inhibition and behavioural flexibility [24]. Language variants of FTD often show early reduction of verbal output, impaired naming and irregular word reading [25]. Neurocognitive test results regarding memory and executive functioning may not be specific at early stages of the disease. Prodromes of dementia with Lewy bodies and Parkinson's disease are less well studied. For emerging Parkinson's disease dementia, executive dysfunction has been reported as an early clinical sign [26].

On clinical grounds and at cross-sectional examination, prodromal dementia may be indistinguishable from conditions of cognitive, functional and behavioural impairment, which are caused by non-progressive or reversible disorders. Therefore, the early diagnosis of a disease that will lead to dementia requires that evidence can be provided for the specific ongoing pathological process and for the deterioration from a previous level of memory, attention, executive function or visuospatial ability [7]. Established indicators for the pathology of AD include determination of amyloid β and tau proteins in the cerebrospinal fluid (CSF), magnetic resonance imaging (MRI) and positron emission tomography (PET). These measures have been evaluated with regard to their potential for early diagnosis in several recent prospective studies, which involved participants with amnestic or amnestic multiple domain MCI and used progression to a clinical diagnosis of AD as outcome [27,28]. These investigations have shown that the neurobiological indicators for AD pathology achieve reasonable sensitivity, whereas specificity is low, and that combining indicators provides only minor gains in accuracy over using one single method. Importantly, the patient-relevant positive and negative predictive values of the neurobiological indicators (i.e. the probability of having the disease if the test is positive and the probability of not having the disease if the test is negative) [29] and hence the rate of false negative and false positive predictions in individuals with MCI are not satisfactory, even in a memory clinic setting where the prevalence of AD is high. Given the imprecision of current prognostic indicators, considering the dramatic consequences of the diagnosis for the individual and their families, and in view of the limited treatment options (see the next section), utmost caution should be exercised when establishing and disclosing the diagnosis of AD at the stage of MCI. In the case of diagnostic indicators showing abnormal values, it appears wise to emphasise diagnostic uncertainty and to conduct follow-up examinations in order to verify or exclude cognitive, functional or behavioural deterioration. For neurodegenerative disorders other than AD, no CSF or imaging diagnostic indicators are currently available for use in clinical practice [30,31].

Services for asymptomatic individuals at increased risk of dementia

Asymptomatic individuals with increased risk of developing dementia as determined by genetic tests or by early diagnostic indicators of neurodegeneration require interventions that prevent or delay the onset of symptoms, taking advantage of a long exposure time. Several strategies may be applied, aimed at modifiable risk factors for cognitive decline and AD, including treatment of vascular risk factors, applying potentially neuroprotective agents, and strengthening brain reserve.

Medical treatment of vascular risk factors

Vascular risk factors, including hypertension, dyslipidemia, hyperhomocysteinemia and diabetes, are among the most robustly established factors that predispose to cognitive decline and AD [32]. The potential of interventions that aim at preventing intellectual deterioration by modifying such factors in cognitively unaffected older individuals has been investigated in a number of prospective, randomised controlled trials (RCTs). Treatment of hypertension was evaluated in six trials, including individuals aged ≥ 60 years with normal cognition at baseline using stroke or coronary events as primary outcome and cognitive decline or incidence of dementia as secondary end points.

Regarding reduction of cognitive decline, two studies were positive and two were negative. In terms of lowering the incidence of dementia one study was positive and one was negative. Thus, the evidence for prevention of cognitive decline or dementia by lowering blood pressure in late life remains inconclusive [33]. Interventions targeted at other vascular risk factors, including use of statins, lowering plasma homocysteine, managing diabetes mellitus, or combinations of pharmacological and non-pharmacological strategies had no demonstrable impact on cognitive decline or on the incidence of dementia when used in older adults [34].

Neuroprotective agents

Supplementation of folic acid, vitamins B6 and B12 [35] or vitamins C and E and beta carotene [36] was compared with placebo in women aged ≥65 years with pre-existing cardiovascular disease or cardiovascular risk factors over more than 5 years. Neither regimen was associated with a lower rate of cognitive decline. Treatment with ginkgo biloba at a dose of 240 mg per day over 6 years had no impact on the rate of cognitive decline in cognitively healthy older individuals and did not reduce the incidence of dementia or AD [37]. Several other herbal preparations have interesting neuroprotective, antioxidant and anti-apoptotic properties, including cannabinoids, curcumin, resveratrol and ginsenosides [38]. However, no long-term trials have been conducted to determine the ability of such preparations to reduce cognitive decline in cognitively unaffected individuals.

Nutritional supplementation

The Mediterranean-type diet refers to an eating pattern which is rich in fish, vegetables, fruits, cereals and unsaturated fatty acids, but low in dairy products, meat and saturated fatty acids, and includes moderate use of red wine, usually with meals. Several prospective observational studies have examined the relationship between adherence to this nutritional style and cognitive decline, most of which were conducted on the same cohort of multiethnic Medicare beneficiaries in northern Manhattan. In the New York studies, higher adherence to a Mediterranean-type diet was associated with a lower risk of developing MCI during a mean follow-up period of 4–5 years in participants who were cognitively healthy at baseline [39]. In contrast, in a population-based study in France on cognitively healthy older adults, higher adherence to Mediterranean-type diet was associated with a slower decline on the Mini Mental State Examination within an average observation interval of 5 years but not on other cognitive tests. In that study, nutritional style was also not associated with the risk of incident dementia [40]. Thus, the evidence on the cognitive effects of the Mediterranean diet remains inconclusive. Omega-3 polyunsaturated fatty acids, particularly eicosapentaenoic acid (EPA) and docosahexaenoic acid (DHA), the principal natural source of which is fatty fish, have been assigned antioxidative, anti-inflammatory and membrane function-enhancing properties. Combinations of EPA and DHA were compared with placebo oil in two RCTs involving cognitively healthy elderly using cognitive performance as an outcome. In a Dutch study, which had a duration of 26 weeks, no effect on any cognitive domain was observed [41]. Likewise, in a longer-term study conducted in England and Wales over 2 years, no difference in cognitive function between active treatment and placebo was detected [42].

Strengthening brain reserve

Retrospective studies have consistently found an association between a cognitively enriched lifestyle and reduced risk of dementia [43]. It has been speculated that this relationship is mediated by compensatory mechanisms, including enhancement of structural or functional reserve [44]. Furthermore, several RCTs have demonstrated that cognitive exercise training can enhance cognitive abilities in healthy older adults [45–47] and may help maintain functional ability [48], although the specificity of training effects have been called into question [49]. However, no studies have been conducted to show that cognitive exercise can prevent or delay the onset of cognitive impairment in individuals at risk [50,51].

Physical activity

Regular physical activity is universally acknowledged as part of a healthy lifestyle at any age. Guidelines recommend at least 30 minutes of moderate physical activity on most days of the week. Epidemiological studies have consistently reported health benefits and reduced mortality [52]. Next to reducing the risk of cardiovascular disease and diabetes, there is also evidence that physical activity can contribute to reducing the risk of cerebrovascular disease [53–55]. A recent meta-analysis of RCTs of non-demented participants of various age groups with normal cognition, mild cognitive impairment or other medical conditions demonstrated that physical activity is associated with modest improvement in cognitive performance in the areas of attention, processing speed, executive function and memory [56]. While a number of longitudinal studies have provided evidence that regular physical activity is associated with a reduced risk for cognitive decline, dementia in general, vascular dementia and AD [40,57,58], no RCT has demonstrated yet that a physical activity intervention can reduce the incidence of dementia compared with a control group.

There are numerous hypotheses how physical activity could protect the ageing brain, including improved vascular health and cerebral blood flow, reduced impact of stress, inflammation and oxidation, enhancement of neurogenesis and synaptogenesis through factors, such as the brain-derived neurotrophic factor (BDNF), with many derived from animal research, but increasingly also from trials with humans [59]. A recent RCT with 120 sedentary cognitively healthy older adults showed that 12 months of supervised aerobic exercise 3 days per week increased the volume of the hippocampus (measured with MRI) by 2% compared with a control group. The authors compare this 2% volume increase with reversing age-related loss of volume by 1–2 years [60]. There are ongoing discussions on which types of exercise, duration and intensity are the best for protecting brain health with currently support for aerobic exercise with a dose–response relationship [61]. Others point out that the biggest differences are found between sedentary people and those who do some physical activity [62], but more research is needed.

Services for people with prodromal dementia

Interventions for individuals with prodromal dementia have three major objectives:

1. to reduce cognitive, functional and behavioural problems
2. to support coping with these symptoms
3. to prevent or at least delay the progression to dementia.

A number of well-designed clinical trials have been conducted to explore the potential of cognition-focused interventions, psychotherapy, pharmacological treatments, medical foods, physical activity and assistive technologies for reaching these aims,

Cognitive interventions

Treatment strategies belonging to this group have been inconsistently labelled as cognitive stimulation, cognitive training or cognitive rehabilitation. Cognitive stimulation refers to activities aimed at general enhancement of cognitive and social functions. Cognitive training usually involves structured practice on tasks relevant to specific cognitive domains, such as memory, attention or executive function. Cognitive rehabilitation is an individualised approach focusing on the development of strategies to improve the management of day-to-day difficulties. During recent years, a few RCTs have evaluated cognitive interventions in people with MCI. In the majority of studies, moderate effects on memory performance and on global measures of cognitive ability were achieved. Computer-based exercises involving multiple cognitive domains had larger effects than unimodal memory training strategies. The latter may have limited effects and generalisability to overall cognitive functioning because they rely on the ability appropriately to apply newly acquired strategies. Moreover, high-volume exercises appear to result in greater benefit than lower amounts of training [63]. The clinical relevance of these findings has been questioned in several respects. The duration of effects is unknown since most trials were short and follow-up was lacking. Also, the specificity of effects is unclear because active control groups appear to do as well as those receiving training [49]. Furthermore, no convincing impact has been demonstrated for cognitive interventions on the ability of participants to carry out day-to-day tasks [64,65]. No long-term studies have been conducted to date to demonstrate whether cognitive interventions can slow cognitive decline and delay the onset of dementia in people with MCI.

Psychological therapy

Most interventions have been designed primarily aiming at enhancing cognitive or functional performance: only a few help people deal with these impairments and focus on emotional, practical and interpersonal needs. A specific form of group psychotherapy combines principles of cognitive behavioural therapy, psycho-education and memory rehabilitation: the programme consists of 10 weekly sessions of 2 hours and focuses on the acquisition of knowledge and skills to enhance coping with symptoms and their consequences. Cognitive–behavioural strategies were adjusted to the cognitive capacities of participants by shortening instructions and using written notes. The programme was compared with a waiting-list control group in a non-randomised study involving 93 patients with mild MCI of any type who were accompanied by their significant others. The intervention was associated with improved acceptance of the condition and improved marital harmony [66].

Pharmacological treatments

Cholinesterase inhibitors have been evaluated in patients with MCI in eight RCTs (three trials on donepezil, two trials on galantamine and two trials on rivastigmine) of which five were published [67]. Patient populations were characterised as having an amnestic form of MCI; treatment periods ranged from 4 to 36 months. In a 24-week trial of donepezil involving 270 patients with MCI, measures of episodic memory and global function did not show any significant treatment effects [68]. In a longer-term trial, the primary endpoint was the development of probable or possible AD at 36 months. Donepezil treatment was associated with lower progression during the first 12 months of the trial, but not thereafter [69]. In a 48-week trial, a small but statistically significant advantage of donepezil over placebo was observed on cognitive ability (less than 1 point on the modified Alzheimer's Disease Assessment Scale), but there was no difference on a measure of general severity [70]. In a 4-month study on a small patient sample galantamine treatment was associated with minor improvements on a computerised cognitive test battery and on functional abilities of daily living [71]. In two 24-month trials on much larger patient samples, however, galantamine failed significantly to modify progression to dementia [72]. In a 48-month trial of rivastigmine, there were no statistically significant differences between the actively treated group and the placebo group regarding the amount of cognitive change from baseline to end point or the rate of progression to

AD-type dementia [73]. There are no published studies on the use of memantine in subjects with MCI [74]. A 12-month trial of piracetam at high doses showed no statistically significant differences between active treatment and primary or secondary outcome variables [75]. The Ginkgo Evaluation of Memory (GEM) Study included 482 elderly subjects with MCI diagnosed according to revised consensus criteria [5]. In this subgroup, active treatment with 240 mg/d ginkgo biloba neither reduced the amount of cognitive decline nor lowered incidence of dementia or AD, compared with placebo [37]. The time to diagnosis of AD was also not delayed by treatment with rofecoxib over up to 4 years [76].Vitamin E did not provide any benefit with regard to delaying progression from amnestic MCI to dementia within a follow-up period of 3 years [69]. To explain the lack of efficacy of drug treatments that were tried in subjects with MCI, thus far, several arguments have been put forward including aetiological and hence prognostic heterogeneity of the condition, lack of decline in placebo groups, short study duration and poor sensitivity of outcome measures [75]. With regard to cholinesterase inhibitors, another possible reason is the absence of a cholinergic deficit in Alzheimer's disease at the prodromal stage [77].

Medical foods

The rationale for using 'medical' foods in people with incipient dementia is that the preservation of neuronal function may require more specific nutrients than can be delivered by modifying a normal diet [78]. Two medical food preparations have been developed for AD and tested in patients. Tricaprylin is a triglyceride composed of glycerin and caprylic acid that elevates serum ketone bodies as an alternative source of energy for the brain in the presence of impaired glucose utilisation as present in AD. In a short-term RCT involving152 subjects with mild to moderate AD, tricaprylin was associated with temporary improvements in cognitive ability and global functioning relative to placebo [79]. A multi-nutrient preparation containing omega-3 fatty acids (EPA and DHA), phospholipids, choline, uridine monophosphate, several vitamins, selenium and folic acid was tested in a RCT involving 225 patients with mild AD over 12 weeks. Actively treated patients showed a statistically significant improvement of episodic memory but not on other tests or with regard to global performance [80]. No study has been conducted to date to determine whether medical foods can delay the progression from MCI to dementia.

Physical activity

Compared with cognitively unimpaired people, the evidence of the benefits of physical activity for the brain is much sparser when it comes to MCI or prodromal dementia. In 2008, an Australian RCT with 170 participants with subjective cognitive complaints with or without MCI demonstrated significant cognitive benefits after a 6-month home-based physical activity intervention focusing on walking, compared with a control group. Interestingly, the cognitive benefit was still measurable 12 months after completion of the supervised intervention [81]. In 2010, Baker and colleagues demonstrated in an RCT with 33 sedentary participants with amnestic MCI, comparing a 6-month intervention of supervised aerobic exercise with a flexibility exercise control group, a gender-specific effect with women showing improved executive functions as well as biological factors (increased glucose disposal, reduced fasting plasma levels of insulin, cortisol and brain-derived neurotrophic factor). Men showed improvement in the Trails B test and had increased plasma levels of insulin-like growth factor 1 [82]. The same authors suggested that older adults with impaired glucose tolerance and normal cognition could be considered at increased risk of AD since they had a similar FDG PET(fludeoxyglucose F 18-positron emission tomography) pattern as patients with AD [83]. In a small RCT in 2010, they demonstrated that this at-risk population can improve executive functions as well as biological parameters with a physical activity intervention [84]. Not all

RCTs with MCI reported positive results, but several more are currently underway, so more evidence should be available in the near future. To our knowledge, no long-term study has been conducted to determine whether physical activity delays the progression from a prodromal stage to frank dementia. Since physical activity has several health benefits, it has been suggested to recommend it to individuals diagnosed with MCI, pointing out the overall health benefits, but acknowledging the current limitations of evidence regarding the potential protective effect on cognition [13].

Assistive technologies

The use of assistive technologies in older adults with prodromal dementia relies on the assumption that performance on a task results from the interaction between cognitive ability and available support: declining intellectual ability can be offset by socio-technical support. Such technologies may be particularly important for the growing group of older cognitively impaired people who are living alone.

Assistive technologies for cognition have been evaluated mostly in single-case or small-scale non-randomised studies that typically involved patients with traumatic brain injury [85]. Results suggest that organisation and planning can be assisted by interactive prompting devices, time management can be enhanced by reminders, and episodic memory is supported by technology for the storage and display of information. The largest trial evaluating assistive technology for cognition was a randomised control crossover study involving 143 participants with problems in memory, planning, organisation or attention [86]. The device tested was a pager worn on a wristband that alerted the wearer to a message reminding of a task to be carried out. Times and tasks were individually programmed following approval by the participants and were fed into a computer system which transmitted the messages to the pager. More than 80% of those who completed the 16-week trial were significantly more successful in carrying out everyday activities in comparison with their baseline ability. While pagers represent outdated technology, modern mobile phones are ubiquitously used as memory aids and have large potential for people with cognitive impairment. Phones with customised patient-friendly software can support mnemonic functioning in individuals with mild degrees of impairment and absence of severe executive deficits, particularly when healthcare workers or family members are available to programme the device [87,88]. The use of assistive technology in dementia in general is discussed in more detail in chapter 17 of this book.

Co-ordination of services and case management

Individuals with MCI and more recently with prodromal AD are mostly diagnosed in the setting of research trials or academic memory clinics. With the expected increase of incidence and prevalence of these conditions due to increasing life expectancy, this approach will need to broaden. In a recent survey of Dutch memory clinics, it was demonstrated that over a period of 11 years, the proportion of cases identified as having non-dementia cognitive impairment rose from 10% to 24% and that memory clinics tended to be increasingly part of regional care approaches outside university centres [89]. The need for non-academic services has been recognised, and models for primary care-based memory clinics and video-telemedicine for rural areas are being trialled [90,91]. Ideally, broader access to memory clinics should be combined with an efficient referral system to academic centres, where available, to provide access to specialist diagnostic assessments and participation in research.

This chapter aimed to highlight the needs of individuals either in the asymptomatic or in the pre-dementia phase of a dementing illness. An increasing number of publications highlight the symptoms and social implications of pre-dementia syndromes, so this evidence should be used to develop and pilot better services. Most likely, a combination of various models could offer flexible approaches depending on infrastructure and type of population. Ideally, such a model should move seamlessly from assessment, diagnosis and disclosure of diagnosis to a variety of management approaches depending on the individual needs and preferences of the patient and family. Such services should explore non-pharmacological and pharmacological management of cognitive and non-cognitive symptoms, participation in research, practical advice on financial and longer-term planning (including advanced directives) [92,93], work situation, living situation [94], driving [95,96], using aids including assistive technologies, psychological therapy, support for family, and so on. Recent literature has highlighted that preferences regarding participation in care planning may differ between patients and family members and can be impacted by impaired capacity and anosognosia [97,98]. It should be investigated whether case management as is frequently being used in psychiatric and aged care services might also be a useful approach for patients with MCI or prodromal AD. New funding models of services should be considered if memory clinics are to offer wider support to primary care than just assessment and treatment.

Summary and conclusions

Services should optimally support primary care, long before dementia evolves. At the asymptomatic stage, pathologies that ultimately lead to dementia can presently be identified in very rare instances by demonstrating a genetic disposition. In future, novel techniques may become available that may reveal characteristic neurobiological features of brain diseases before they become clinically manifest. Patients who are diagnosed at the pre-clinical stage require interventions that prevent or delay the onset of symptoms. Strategies that could be applied include treatment of vascular risk factors, administration of neuroprotective agents, nutritional supplementation and strengthening brain reserve by cognitive or physical activity. However, studies carried out thus far provide insufficient evidence that the onset of full-blown dementia can be prevented by any of these approaches. The prodromal stage of the most frequent cause of dementia, Alzheimer's disease, can be identified using neuropsychological tests in conjunction with laboratory or imaging procedures that demonstrate abnormal protein accumulation and neuronal damage. For patients diagnosed at that stage, interventions are needed to reduce cognitive, functional and behavioural problems, to enhance coping with impairment, and to prevent or delay progression to dementia. Pharmacological treatments, including cholinesterase inhibitors, ginkgo biloba, piracetam and vitamin E, were ineffective in RCTs. Cognition-focused interventions and physical activity were shown to provide modest symptomatic improvements, but no long-term studies have been conducted using progression to dementia as outcome. The role of medical foods and the value of assistive technologies are unclear. At the pre-symptomatic stage, prevention of cognitive decline is currently not possible. At the prodromal stage, cognition-focused interventions and physical activity have modest symptomatic effects, but more RCTs are needed to investigate their potential for delaying the onset of dementia.

In conclusion, establishing targeted services for people with incipient dementia will be crucial to support as optimally as possible the increasing number of older adults and their families who may for many years live with the knowledge that they are at risk of future progression of cognitive impairment. These services need to be established beyond highly specialised academic memory clinics, and care models must be developed, which are cost-effective, culturally appropriate, well integrated with primary care and accessible to patients wherever they may live.

References

1. Larson EB (2010) Prospects for delaying the rising tide of worldwide, late-life dementias. *Int Psychogeriatr* 22:1196–1202.

2. Matthews FE, Brayne C, Lowe J, McKeith I, Wharton SB, Ince P (2009) Epidemiological pathology of dementia: attributable-risks at death in the Medical Research Council Cognitive Function and Ageing Study. *PLoS Med* 6(11):e1000180.

3. Stephan BC, Matthews FE, Hunter S, Savva GM, Bond J, McKeith IG, et al. (2011 September 22) Neuropathological profile of mild cognitive impairment from a population perspective. *Alzheimer Dis Assoc Disord* 26(3):205–212.

4. Reisberg B, Prichep L, Mosconi L, John ER, Glodzik-Sobanska L, Boksay I, et al. (2008) The pre-mild cognitive impairment, subjective cognitive impairment stage of Alzheimer's disease. *Alzheimers Demen* 4:S98–S108.

5. Winblad B, Palmer K, Kivipelto M, Jelic V, Fratiglioni L (2004) Mild cognitive impairment: beyond controversies, towards a consensus. *J Int Med* 256:181–182.

6. Sperling R (2011) The potential of functional MRI as a biomarker in early Alzheimer's disease. *Neurobiol Aging* 32:S37–S43.

7. Albert MS, DeKosky ST, Dickson D, Dubois B, Feldman HH, Fox NC, et al. (2011) The diagnosis of mild cognitive impairment due to Alzheimer's disease: recommendations from the National Institute on Aging and Alzheimer's Association workgroup. *Alzheimers Demen* 7(3):270–279.

8. Larson EB, Shadlen MF, Wang L, McCormick WC, Bowen JD, Teri L, et al. (2004) Survival after initial diagnosis of Alzheimer disease. *Ann Intern Med* 140:501–509.

9. Atkins ER, Panegyres PK (2011) The clinical utility of gene testing for Alzheimer's disease. *Neurol Int* 3(e1):1–2.

10. Quaid KA (2011) Genetic counseling for frontotemporal dementias. *J Mol Neurosci* 45:706–709.

11. Arribas-Ayllon M (2011) The ethics of disclosing genetic diagnosis for Alzheimer's disease: do we need a new paradigm? *Br Med Bull* 100:7–21.

12. Plassman BL, Langa KM, Fisher GG, Heeringa SG, Wier DR, Ofstedal MB, et al. (2008) Prevalence of cognitive impairment without dementia in the United States. *Ann Intern Med* 148:427–434.

13. Petersen RC (2011) Mild cognitive impairment. *N Engl J Med* 364:2227–2234.

14. Dubois B, Feldman HH, Jacova C, Cummings JL, DeKosky ST, Barberger-Gateau P, et al. (2010) Revising the definition of Alzheimer's disease: a new lexicon. *Lancet Neurol* 9:1118–1127.

15. Royall DR, Lauterbach EC, Kaufer D, Malloy P, Coburn KL, Black KJ (2007) The cognitive correlates of functional status: a review from the Committee on Research of the American Neuropsychiatric Association. *J Neuropsychiatry Clin Neurosci* 19:249–265.

16. Perneczky R, Pohl C, Sorg C, Hartmann J, Komossa K, Alexopoulos P, et al. (2006) Complex activities of daily living in mild cognitive impairment: conceptual and diagnostic issues. *Age Ageing* 35:240–245.

17. Gold DA (2012 November 4) An examination of instrumental activities of daily living assessment in older adults and mild cognitive impairment. *J Clin Exp Neuropsychol* 34(4):11–34.

18. Apostolova LG, Cummings JL (2008) Neuropsychiatric manifestations of mild cognitive impairment: a systematic review of the literature. *Dement Geriatr Cogn Disord* 25:115–126.

19. Monastero R, Mangialasche F, Camarda C, Ercolani S, Camarda R (2009) A systematic review of neuropsychiatric symptoms in mild cognitive impairment. *J Alzheimers Dis* 18:11–30.

20. Rozzini L, Vicini-Chilovi B, Conti M, Delrio I, Borroni B, Trabucchi M, et al. (2008) Neuropsychiatric symptoms in amnestic and nonamnestic mild cognitive impairment. *Dement Geriatr Cogn Disord* 25:32–36.

21. Joosten-Weyn Banningh L, Vernooij-Dassen M, Olde Rikkert M, Teunisse JP (2007) Mild cognitive impairment: coping with an uncertain label. *Int J Geriatr Psychiatry* 23:148–154.

22. Davies HD, Newkirk LA, Pitts CB, Couglin CA, Sridhar SB, McKenzie-Zeiss L, et al. (2010) The impact of dementia and mild memory impairment (MMI) on intimacy and sexuality in spousal relationships. *Int Psychogeriatr* 22:618–628.

23. Steeman E, Cierckx de Casterlé B, Godderis J, Grypdonck M (2006) Living with early-stage dementia: a review of qualitative studies. *J Adv Nurs* 54:722–738.

24. Wittenberg D, Possin KL, Rascovsky K, Rankin KP, Miller BL, Kramer JH (2008) The early neuropsychological and behavioral characteristics of frontotemporal dementia. *Neuropsychol Rev* 18:91–102.

25. Hallam BJ, Silverberg DD, LaMarre AK, Mackenzie IRA, Feldman HH (2008) Clinical presentation of prodromal frontotemporal dementia. *Am J Alzheimers Dis Other Demen* 22:456–467.

26. Tröster AI (2008) Neuropsychological characteristics of dementia with Lewy bodies and Parkinson's disease with dementia: differentiation, early detection, and implications for 'mild cognitive impairment' and biomarkers. *Neuropsychol Rev* 18:103–119.
27. Hansson O, Zetterberg H, Buchhave P, Londos E, Blennow K, Minthon L (2006) Association between CSF biomarkers and incipient Alzheimer's disease in patients with mild cognitive impairment: a follow-up study. *Lancet Neurol* 5:228–234.
28. Mattson N, Zetterberg H, Hansson O, Andeasen N, Parnetti L, Jonsson M, et al. (2009) CSF biomarkers and incipient Alzheimer disease in patients with mild cognitive impairment. *JAMA* 302:385–393.
29. Warner J (2004) Clinicians' guide to evaluating diagnosic and screening tests in psychiatry. *Adv Psychiatr Treatm* 10:446–454.
30. Bian H, Van Swieten JC, Leight S, Massimo L, Wood E, Moore MFO, et al. (2008) CSF biomarkers in frontotemporal lobar degeneration with known pathology. *Neurology* 70:1827–1835.
31. Hu WT, Chen-Plotkin A, Grossman M, Arnold SE, Clark CM, McCluskey L, et al. (2010) Novel CSF biomarkers for frontotemporal lobar degenerations. *Neurology* 75:2079–2086.
32. Williams JW, Plassman BL, Burke J, Holsinger T, Benjamin S (2010) *Preventing Alzheimer's Disease and Cognitive Decline*. Rockville, MD: Agency for Healthcare Research and Quality.
33. Daviglus ML, Plassman BL, Pirzada A, Bell CC, Bowen PE, Burke JR, et al. (2011) Risk factors and preventive interventions for Alzheimer disease. State of the science. *Arch Neurol* 68:1185–1190.
34. Lighthart SA, Moll-van-Charante EP, van Gool WA, Richard E (2010) Treatment of cardiaovascular risk factors to prevent cognitive decline and dementia: a systematic review. *Vasc Health Risk Manag* 6:775–785.
35. Kang JH, Cook N, Manson J, Buring JE, Albert CM, Grodstein F (2008) A trial of B vitamins and cognitive function among women at high risk of cardiovascular disease. *Am J Clin Nutr* 88:1602–1610.
36. Kang JH, Cook NR, Manson JAE, Buring JE, Albert CM, Grodstein F (2009) Vitamin E, vitamin C, beta carotene, and cognitive function among women with or t risk of cardiovascular disease: the Women's Antioxidant and Cardiovascular Study. *Circulation* 119:2772–2780.
37. DeKosky ST, Williamson JD, Fitzpatrick AL, Kronmal RA, Ives DG, Saxton JA, et al. (2008) Ginkgo biloba for prevention of dementia. A randomized controlled trial. *JAMA* 300:2253–2262.
38. Howes MJR, Perry E (2011) The role of phytochemicals in the tretment and prevention of dementia. *Drugs Agomg* 28:439–468.
39. Scarmeas N, Stern Y, Mayeux R, Manly J, Schupf N, Luchsinger JA (2009) Mediterranean diet and mild cognitive impairment. *Arch Neurol* 66:216–225.
40. Sofi F, Macchi C, Abbate R, Gensini GF, Casini A (2010) Effectiveness of the mediterranean diet: can it help delay or prevent Alzheimer's disease? *J Alzheimers Dis* 20:795–801.
41. Van de Rest O, Geleijnse JM, Kok FJ, Van Staveren WA, Dullemeijer C, Olde Rikkert MGM, et al. (2008) Effect of fish oil on cognitive performance in older subjects. A randomized, controlled trial. *Nerology* 71(6):430–438.
42. Dangour AD, Allen E, Elbourne D, Fasey N, Fletcher AE, Hardy P, et al. (2010) Effect of 2-y n-3 long-chain polyunsaturated fatty acid supplementation on cognitive function in older people: a randomized, double-blind, controlled trial. *Am J Clin Nutr* 91:1725–1732.
43. Valenzuela M, Brayne C, Sachdev P, Wilcock G, Matthews F (2011) Cognitive lifestyle and long-term risk of dementia and survival after diagnosis in a multicenter population-based cohort. *Am J Epidemiol* 173:1004–1012.
44. Valenzuela MJ, Matthews FE, Brayne C, Ince P, Halliday G, Kril JJ, et al. (2011 November 2) Multiple biological pathways link cognitive lifestyle to protection from dementia. *Biol Psychiatry* 71:783–791.
45. Ball K, Berch DB, Helmers KF, Jobe JB, Leveck MD, Marsiske M, et al. (2002) Effects of cognitive training interventions with older adults: a randomized controlled trial. *JAMA* 288:2271–2281.
46. Oswald WD, Gunzelmann T, Rupprecht R, Hagen B (2006) Differential effects of single versus combined cognitive and physical training with older adults: the SimA study in a 5-year perspective. *Eur J Ageing* 3:179–192.
47. Gates N, Valenzuela M (2010) Cognitive exercise and its role in cognitive function in older adults. *Curr Psychiatry Rep* 12:20–27.
48. Willis SL, Tennstedt SL, Marsiske M, Ball K, Elias J, Mann-Koepke K, et al. (2006) Long-term effects of cognitive training on everyday functional outcomes in older adults. *JAMA* 296:2805–2814.

49. Martin M, Clare L, Altgassen AM, Cameron MH, Zehnder F (2011) Cognition-based interventions for healthy older people and people with mild cognitive impairment. *Cochrane Database Syst Rev* (1): CD006220.

50. Papp KV, Walsh SJ, Snyder PJ (2009) Immediate and delayed effects of cognitive interventions in healthy elderly: a review of current literature and future directions. *Alzheimers Demen* 5:50–60.

51. Valenzuela M, Sachdev P (2009) Can cognitive exercise prevent the onset of dementia? Systematic review of randomized trials with longitudinal follow-up. *Am J Geriatr Psychiatry* 17:179–187.

52. MacAuley D (1994) A history of physical activity, health and medicine. *J R Soc Med* 87:32–35.

53. Warburton DE, Nicol CW, Bredin SS (2006) Health benefits of physical activity: the evidence. *CMAJ* 174:801–809.

54. Lee CD, Folsom AR, Blair SN (2003) Physical activity and stroke risk: a meta-analysis. *Stroke* 34: 2475–2481.

55. Williamson DF, Vinicor F, Bowman BA (2004) Primary prevention of type 2 diabetes mellitus by lifestyle intervention: implications for health policy. *Ann Intern Med* 140:951–957.

56. Smith PF, Blumenthal JA, Hoffman BM, Cooper H, Strauman TA, Welsh-Bohmer K, et al. (2010) Aerobic exercise and neurocognitive performance: a meta-analytic review of randomized controlled trials. *Psychosomat Med* 72:239–252.

57. Hamer M, Chida Y (2009) Physical activity and risk of neurodegenerative disease: a systematic review of prospective evidence. *Pschol Med* 39:3–11.

58. Aarsland D, Sardahaee FS, Anderssen S, Ballard C (2010) Is physical activitiy a potential preventive factor for vascular dementia? A systematic review. *Aging Ment Health* 14:386–395.

59. Lautenschlager NT, Cox K, Cyarto EV (2012) The influence of exercise on brain aging and dementia. *Biochim Biophys Acta* 1822:474–481.

60. Erickson KI, Voss MW, Prakash RS, Basak C, Szabo A, Chaddock L, et al. (2011) Exercise training increases size of hippocampus und improves memory. *PNAS* 108:3017–3022.

61. Van Gelder BM, Tijhuis MA, Kalmijn S, Giampaoli S, Nissinen A, Kromhout D (2004) Physical activity in relation to cognitive decline in elderly men: the FINE Study. *Neurology* 63:2316–2321.

62. Middleton LE, Barnes DE, Lui LY, Yaffe K (2010) Physical activity over the lifecourse and its association with cognitive performance and impairment in old age. *J Am Geriatr Soc* 58:1322–1326.

63. Gates NJ, Sachdev PS, Fatarone-Singh MA, Valenzuela M (2011) Cognitive and memory training in adults at risk of dementia: a systematic review. *BMC Geriatr* 11:55.

64. Kurz AF, Lautenschlager NT (2011) The clinical significance of cognition-focused interventions for cognitively impaired older adults. *Int Psychogeriatr* July 11:1–12.

65. Stott J, Spector A (2011) A review of the effectiveness of memory interventions in mild cognitive impairment (MCI). *Int Psychogeriatr* 23:526–538.

66. Joosten-Weyn Banningh LWA, Prins JB, Vernooij-Dassen MJFJ, Wijnen HH, Olde Rikkert MGM, Kessels RPC (2010 July 20) Group therapy for patients with mild cognitive impairment and their significant others: results of a waiting-list controlled trial. *Gerontology* 57:444–454.

67. Raschetti R, Albanese E, Vanacore N, Maggini M (2007) Cholinesterase inhibitors in mild cognitive impairment: a systematic review of randomised trials. *PLoS Med* 4:1818–1828.

68. Salloway S, Ferris S, Kluger A, Goldman R, Griesing T, Kumar D, et al. (2004) Efficacy of donepezil in mild cognitive impairment: a randomized placebo-controlled trial. *Neurology* 63:651–657.

69. Petersen RC, Thomas MG, Grundman M, Bennett D, Doody R, Ferris S, et al. (2005) Vitamin E and donepezil for the treatment of mild cognitive impairment. *N Engl J Med* 352:2379–2388.

70. Doody RS, Ferris SH, Salloway S, Sun Y, Goldman R, Watkins WE, et al. (2009 May 5) Donepezil treatment of patients with MCI. A 48-week randomized, placebo-controlled trial. *Neurology* 72(18): 1555–1561.

71. Koontz J, Baskys A (2005) Effects of galantamine on working memory and global functioning in patients with mild cognitive impairment: a double-blind placebo-controlled study. *Am J Alzheimers Dis Other Demen* 20:295–302.

72. Winblad B, Gauthier S, Scinto L, Feldman H, Wilcock GK, Truyen L, et al. (2008) Safety and efficacy of galantamine in subjects with mild cognitive impairment. *Neurology* 70:2024–2035.

73. Feldman HH, Rerris S, Winblad B, Sfikas N, Mancione L, He Y, et al. (2007) Effect of rivastigmine on delay to diagnosis of Alzheimer's disease from mild cognitive impairment: the InDDEx study. *Lancet Neurol* 6:501–512.

74. Schneider LS, Dagerman KS, Higgins JP, McShane R (2011) Lack of evidence for the efficacy of memantine in mild Alzheimer's disease. *Arch Neurol* 68:991–998.

75. Jelic V, Kivipelto M, Winblad B (2006) Clinical trials in mild cognitive impairment: lessons for the future. *J Neurol Neurosurg Psychiatry* 77:429–438.

76. Thal LJ, Ferris SH, Kirby L, Block GA, Lines CR, Yuen E, et al. (2005) A randomized, double-blind, study of rofexocib in patients with mild cognitive impairment. *Neuropsychopharmacology* 30:1204–1215.

77. Mufson EJ, Counts SE, Perez SE, Ginsberg SD (2008) Cholinergic system during the progression of Alzheimer's disease: therapeutic implications. *Exp Rev Neurother* 8:1703–1718.

78. Shah RC (2011) Medical foods for Alzheimer's disease. *Drugs Aging* 28:421–428.

79. Henderson ST, Vogel JT, Barr LJ, Garvin F, Jones JJ, Costantini LC (2009) Study of the ketogenic agent AC-1202 in mild to moderate Alzheimer's disease: a randomized, double-blind, placebo-controlled, multicenter trial. *Nutr Metab (Lond)* 6):31.

80. Scheltens P, Kamphuis PJ, Verhey FR, Olde Rikkert MG, Wurtman RJ, Wilkinson D, et al. (2010) Efficacy of a medical food in mild Alzheimer's disease: a randomized, controlled trial. *Alzheimers Dement* 6:1–10.

81. Lautenschlager NT, Cox KL, Flicker L, Foster JK, Van Bockxmeer FM, Xiao J, et al. (2008) Effects of physical activity on cognitive function in older adults at risk for Alzheimer disease. A randomized trial. *JAMA* 300:1027–1037.

82. Baker LD, Frank LL, Foster-Schubert K, Green PS, Wilkinson CW, McTiernan A, et al. (2010) Effects of aerobic exercise on mild cognitive impairment. A controlled trial. *Arch Neurol* 67:71–79.

83. Baker LD, Cross DJ, Minoshima S, Belongia D, Watson GS, Craft S (2011) Insulin resistance and Alzheimer-like reductions in regional cerebral glucose metabolism for cognitively normal adults with prediabetes or early type II diabetes. *Arch Neurol* 68:51–57.

84. Baker LD, Frank LL, Foster-Schubert K, Green PS, Wilkinson CW, McTiernan A, et al. (2010) Aerobic exercise improves cognition for older adults with glucose intolerance, a risk factor for Alzheimer's disease. *J Alzheimers Dis* 22:569–579.

85. Gillespie A, Best C, O'Neill B (2012) Cognitive function and assistive technology for cognition: a systematic review. *J Int Neuropsychol Soc* 18:1–19.

86. Wilson BA, Emslie HC, Quirk K, Evans JJ (2001) Reducing everyday memory and planning problems by means of a paging system: a randomised control crossover study. *J Neurol Neurosurg Psychiatry* 70:477–482.

87. Stapleton S, Adams M, Atterton L (2008) A mobile phone as a memory aid for individuals with traumatic brain injury: a preliminary investigation. *Brain Injury* 21:401–411.

88. Svoboda E, Richards B (2009) Compensating for anterograde amnesia; A new training mehtod that capitalizes on emerging smartphone technologies. *J Int Neuropsychol Soc* 15:629–638.

89. Ramakers IH, Verhey FR (2011) Development of memory clinics in the Netherlands: 1998 to 2009. *Aging Ment Health* 15:34–39.

90. Lee L, Hillier LM, Stolee P, Heckman G, Gagnon M, McAiney CA, et al. (2010) Enhancing dementia care: a primary care-based memory clinic. *J Am Geriatr Soc* 58:2197–2204.

91. Barton C, Morris R, Rothlind J, Yaffe K (2011) Video-telemedicine in a memory disorders clinic: evaluation and management of rural elders with cognitive impairment. *Telemed J E Health* 17:789–793.

92. Okonkwo OC, Wadley VG, Griffith HR, Belue K, Lanza S, Zamrini EY, et al. (2008) Awareness of deficits in financial abilities in patients with mild cognitive impairment: going beyond self-information discrepancy. *Am J Geriatr Psychiatry* 16:650–658.

93. Triebel KL, Martin H, Griffith HR, Marceaux J, Okonkwo OC, Harrell L, et al. (2009) Declining financial capacity in mild cognitive impairment: a 1-year longitudinal study. *Neurology* 73:928–934.

94. Garand L, Dew MA, Lingler J, DeKosky ST (2011) Incidence and predictors of advance care planning among persons with mild cognitive impairment. *Am J Geriatr Psychiatry* 19:712–720.

95. Frittelli C, Berghetti D, Iudice G, Bonanni E, maestri M, Tognoni G, et al. (2009) Effects of Alzheimer's disease and mild cognitive impairment on driving ability: a controlled clinical study by simulated driving test. *Int J Geriatr Psychiatry* 24:232–238.

96. Wadley VG, Okonkwo O, Crowe M, Vance DE, Elgin JM, Ball KK, et al. (2009) Mild cognitive impairment and everyday function: an investigation of driving performance. *J Geriatr Psychiatry Neurol* 22:87–94.
97. Okonkwo OC, Griffith HR, Copeland JN, Belue K, Lanza S, Zamrini EY, et al. (2009) Medical decision-making capacity in mild cognitive impairment: a 3-year longitudinal study. *Neurology* 71:1474–1480.
98. Hamann J, Bronner J, Margull J, Mendel R, Diehl-Schmid J, Bähner M, et al. (2011) Patient participation in medical and social decisions in Alzheimer's disease. *J Am Geriatr Soc* 59:2045–2052.

Chapter 5

Services for people with mild dementia

Roy W. Jones

The RICE Centre, Royal United Hospital, UK

Introduction

Receiving a diagnosis of dementia is a highly significant event for the person with dementia and their family and loved ones. There is a significant stigma surrounding dementia, and many people still question the value of an early diagnosis given the paucity and limited effectiveness of current drug treatments, although many studies confirm that patients with Alzheimer's disease (AD) do better if they are receiving specific drug treatment than those who are not.

The Dementia Action Alliance in England issued the National Dementia Declaration in October 2010 (http://wwww.dementiaaction.org.uk) for people with dementia:

- I have personal choice.
- I know services are designed for me.
- I have support that helps me live.
- I know how to get what I need.
- I find the environment enabling and supportive.
- I feel I belong and am valued.
- I know there is research which is going on which will bring me a better life.

The declaration stated that there should be good quality early diagnosis for everyone. This may be provided by rapid and competent specialist assessment, together with sensitive communication, treatment, care, support and capacity.

There have been significant advances in the way in which people with dementia are cared for. A growing body of experience, knowledge and awareness of the rights and needs of people with dementia has led to these advances. Nevertheless, there is still considerable variability not only across the different countries of the world but even within a given country. Such variability may depend on the nature of the medical system and the existence or not of a close-knit family structure: in some countries, most people with dementia remain within their family, whereas in others they are more likely to be managed within an institution, such as a nursing home. The greatest need is to ensure that there are locally appropriate services that deal with both the medical and non-medical aspects of AD and other types of dementia. A number of approaches appear to depend more on the enthusiasm of the therapists than the nature of the therapy, and such approaches are less clearly generalisable, even within the country where it has been developed.

Designing and Delivering Dementia Services, First Edition. Edited by Hugo de Waal, Constantine Lyketsos, David Ames, and John O'Brien.
© 2013 John Wiley & Sons, Ltd. Published 2013 by John Wiley & Sons, Ltd.

The present chapter will describe some of the relevant service areas that are of particular importance to people with mild dementia at the time of, or soon after, they have been diagnosed. It will try and avoid discussing in detail areas such as management of behavioural issues that tend to be more of a problem in moderate or severe dementia and will therefore be covered in more detail in Chapters 6 and 7 in this book.

Dementia care is usually provided by a number of different agencies, and the UK is a good example of this. It involves the National Health Service and the social care system, together with privately funded services and those provided by voluntary organisations and family caregivers. The care may be provided in a range of different settings that will vary from one part of the country to another. Inevitably, there is a danger that such a system is too fragmented and people either do not get into the system to receive the appropriate help they and their families need or they may fall into gaps in the service. It is important, therefore, to try and ensure that the system of care being provided in a local area is integrated as far as possible, that the different parts of the system talk to each other and that there are easy cross-referral systems. Such complexity also makes it more difficult for a national or government policy to increase the quality of care through regulation: in the UK, the separation of health and social care has been a particularly divisive force. Increasingly, health and social care services are now seeking to work more closely together and to use coterminous boundaries for their area of activity, and this will undoubtedly improve the overall level of service provision.

Whilst national standards and inspection processes are necessary, it is also important to promote plurality of providers, to have adequate levels of flexibility in the system and to ensure that there is some choice for users.

The definition of mild dementia

In general clinical settings, the clinician's main goal is to make a diagnosis of dementia and to try and define the subtype, most commonly AD. The severity of the dementia – mild, moderate, moderately severe or severe – is less commonly specified or formally assessed. Assessment of severity is usually only formally undertaken using standardised scales in research settings and in particular when considering patients for inclusion in clinical trials. In clinical settings, most often, cognitive function is used as the main marker of severity, supplemented by an impression of overall functioning as may emerge from taking the history, including corroborative history.

The Mini-Mental State Examination [1] remains the most widely used relatively short assessment of memory and cognition with a maximum score of 30. In an early comprehensive review [2], three levels of severity of cognitive impairment were suggested: 24–30 = no cognitive impairment; 18–23 = mild to moderate impairment, and 17 or below = severe impairment. However, intelligent patients may have a significant problem even though scoring 24 or above. In contrast, patients with marked language impairment or limited education may score poorly, suggesting that they are more severely affected than they are. In current clinical trials of potential drugs for mild AD, a MMSE cut-off of around 20 is increasingly selected as an inclusion criterion.

The severity of dementia has been most clearly characterised through two global rating scales that were originally developed in the 1980s. Such an assessment of global functioning allows a single subjective integrated judgement of the patient's symptoms and performance by an experienced clinician. Although these have mainly been applied in research settings, the principle of an overall global assessment is in fact how every clinician ultimately makes a judgement about a patient's level of dementia, and this cannot be done by the use of any single cognitive or other type of assessment. Although dementia does not necessarily progress in an orderly, linear way, these assessments are helpful in deciding whether a patient has mild, moderate or severe dementia.

The Clinical Dementia Rating Scale (CDR) was first described in 1982 [3]. Six domains are assessed: memory, orientation, judgement and problem-solving, community activities, home and hobbies, and personal care. It has a 5-point scale with 0 for no impairment, 0.5 for questionable or very mild dementia, and 1, 2, and 3 for mild, moderate and severe dementia, respectively. CDR-1 represents mild dementia where the person has moderate memory loss, especially for recent events and this interferes with daily activities. The person also has moderate difficulty solving problems, cannot function independently at community affairs, and has difficulty with daily activities and hobbies, especially complex ones. The CDR has become the most widely used global severity rating scale for clinical trials in AD, mainly because the scale was further developed within each domain [4].

The Global Deterioration Scale (GDS) was also described in 1982 and has equally stood the test of time [5]. It takes less time than the CDR to complete. It divides the disease into seven stages based on the amount of cognitive decline, where 1 = normal and 7 = very severe cognitive decline (late dementia). It is most useful for the assessment of AD because of the emphasis on memory. Stage 4 (the stage of moderate cognitive decline) equates to mild dementia. This stage includes difficulty with concentration and reduced memory for recent events. Travelling alone, especially in unfamiliar places, becomes more difficult as does handling money. Complex tasks are particularly problematic. Denial may become the subject's main defence mechanism, and they may also begin to withdraw from family and friends because socialisation becomes more difficult.

The GDS has often been combined with the Functional Assessment Staging Tool (FAST), which looks more at the level of functioning and performance of activities of daily living than cognition [6]. Mild dementia is represented on the FAST both by stage 3 (early dementia with noticeable deficits in demanding situations) and stage 4 (mild dementia where the person requires assistance with complex tasks, such as finance or planning social occasions).

People with mild dementia will usually retain insight. Problems are more likely to occur with complex instrumental activities of daily living rather than with basic activities. They are also better placed than people with more advanced dementia to be actively involved in decisions that affect them and to understand and benefit from strategies for coping with memory and other cognitive problems.

Memory clinics and other specialist services for dementia diagnosis and assessment

Memory clinics

Specialist services for people with memory problems and mild dementia have a relatively short history and have tended to develop separately from other provisions for people with dementia, such as psychogeriatric services [7]. The memory clinic model began to develop in the USA in the mid-1970s to serve as an outpatient diagnostic, advice and treatment service for people with mild dementia. They began partly as a result of the frustration felt by the families of people with dementia because many physicians appeared to be reluctant to diagnose dementia, especially in those who appeared to have reasonable social skills and moderate everyday abilities. The term 'memory clinic' allowed the clinic to focus on memory-related problems, which were usually one of the first areas where problems were noted and avoided the term 'dementia clinic', which would potentially be unattractive and stigmatising [8]. The clinics were generally established by experienced and research-active specialists from a range of disciplines (particularly geriatric medicine, neurology and psychiatry) and allowed a focus on a group of disorders that had largely been ignored in terms of obtaining an accurate diagnosis and developing specific and effective management and treatment strategies.

In the 1980s and 1990s, there was a steady increase in the number of memory clinics in the USA, and they also developed in other countries, including in the UK, where the number increased from 20 in 1993 to 102 in 2002 [9,10]. The growth in memory clinics was apparently stimulated by the licensing of cholinesterase inhibitor drugs for AD and the development of services for early onset dementia. Most of the newer clinics had been set up within NHS old age psychiatry services and tended to be smaller and with less of an academic focus than the older clinics.

There is no precise definition of what constitutes a memory clinic and the speciality of the clinician leading the clinic varies both within countries and between countries. The early clinics in the UK usually had a strong research focus in contrast to the later clinics that developed following the licensing of cholinesterase inhibitors. The recent Prime Minister's challenge on dementia has emphasised that consent to participate in research must again become a focus of attention, and this will be one of the conditions of accreditation for memory services [11]. Another feature that seems to be important is that the clinic should have a multi-disciplinary focus or, if not, provide ready access to other relevant specialties. A multidisciplinary approach to the diagnosis of dementia has been shown to have more effect on the quality of life (QoL) of the patient and carer [12] and is also cost-effective in comparison with assessment as usual [13]. Other studies support the cost-effectiveness of memory clinics [14]. Referrals to memory clinics are usually from general practitioners, but some clinics also take self-referrals [15].

There is no doubt that memory clinics encourage earlier detection of dementia [16]. Patients, caregivers and general practitioners have positive opinions about the assessments, investigation and diagnosis, but improvements could focus on the clarity of diagnostic information and advice to relatives [16,17]. The benefits of memory clinics for post-diagnosis treatment and coordination of care are less clear cut. A 1-year study following diagnosis of dementia in nine Dutch memory clinics assigned patients post-diagnosis to either the memory clinic or the general practitioner. While quality of life of the patients was numerically higher and the caregiver burden lower in those followed up in the memory clinic, there were no significant differences between the two groups [18].

In the UK, the National Institute for Health and Clinical Excellence (NICE) has identified the key components of a memory assessment service to be the early identification and referral of people with a possible diagnosis of dementia and the development of a high-quality service for dementia assessment, diagnosis and management [19]. It includes recommendations from their Dementia Clinical Guideline [20] that memory assessment services should be the single point of referral for all people with a possible diagnosis of dementia and include a full range of assessment, diagnostic, therapeutic and rehabilitation services to accommodate the needs of people with different types and severities of dementia and the needs of their carers and families. It should also ensure an integrated approach with local healthcare, social care and voluntary organisations [20].

Other specialist services

Although many people with memory problems or dementia are now referred to memory assessment services, such patients will also present to specialists in routine outpatient clinics such as care of the elderly, neurology and psychiatry (particularly old age psychiatry). It is important that patients with mild dementia presenting in this way are given similar access to information, advice and treatment opportunities as those presenting to memory clinics. Referral on to the memory clinic or other services according to the local management pathway is recommended.

A comparison between patients referred to a memory clinic and those referred to traditional old age psychiatry services did demonstrate differences [21]. Memory clinic patients were significantly younger and had a wider range of diagnoses. Those diagnosed with dementia were found to be approximately 2 years earlier in the course of the disease compared with old age psychiatry patients. This does suggest that patients with mild dementia are more likely to be referred to a memory clinic.

The learning disability specialist services also have an important role to play. Learning disability (LD) is a term used almost exclusively in the UK to cover the ICD-10 categories for mental retardation (F70-79) in people of all ages. People with Down's syndrome are at particular risk of developing AD and at an earlier age than the general population [22], while the prevalence of dementia in people with LD without Down's syndrome is around two to three times that expected in people over 65 [23]. In this population, the diagnosis relies mainly on history and observation, as cognitive testing is more difficult and requires specific instruments [20]. It is more difficult to assess the severity of dementia in patients with LD where the dementia is often recognised as a change in behaviour rather than in cognition or function. Nevertheless, it is important for the specialist LD team to be aware of this and to offer advice (including potentially discussion of the diagnosis [20]) and help to the individual and their family and carers).

The role of primary care in diagnosis and assessment

There has been a widespread reticence among primary care doctors to make the diagnosis of dementia, and primary care diagnosis cannot be relied on according to a consultation exercise involving eight EU states (the Netherlands, Belgium, the UK, Spain, Italy, Portugal, France and Ireland) [24]. This generates a culture of 'concealment, minimisation or ignoring of early signs and symptoms'. Yet diagnosis is the gateway to care [25]: without it, neither drug nor non-drug treatment can be given.

Diagnosing in primary care is perceived as a problem in many countries, resulting in delayed recognition and adverse outcomes for patients and their carers [26]. Improving early detection has been recognised as an area for development in the English National Dementia Strategy [27]; subsequent to this, there has been increasing discussion about whether primary care physicians (PCPs) can do more to diagnose people with dementia and, if so, what help can be provided to overcome some of the difficulties. Attempts have been made to educate and improve the abilities and confidence of people working within primary care in order to make adequate provision for people with dementia in their practice, but this has met with limited success [26]. From a primary care perspective, another problem is that the numbers seen by any one PCP are generally insufficient to provide the necessary experience and confidence in accurate diagnosis and management. In a demographically average area in the UK, the PCP might currently diagnose one to two patients per year and have 12–15 patients with dementia in a total list of 2000 patients [28].

One suggestion has been to modify the terminology and talk about 'recognition' rather than 'diagnosis' [26]. A two-step process has also been suggested, whereby the PCP detects cognitive impairment and loss of function, but the actual diagnosis and sub-typing is confirmed by a specialist [29]. This could potentially work well, but relies on good communication between the PCP and the specialist and easy access to the latter. It also relies on educational initiatives by local specialists to increase the confidence of PCPs and to ensure that they understand and accept the rationale for early diagnosis. Referral pathways may also be preferable to simple guidelines [26].

One attempt in Gnosall in the UK has been to develop a combined approach with the specialist team working within primary care and using the practice health visitor as the key liaison figure [30]. There is a monthly half-day session by a specialist old-age psychiatrist, with the availability of support and telephone expertise from a specialist between times.

Specialist versus non-specialist diagnosis: Getting the balance right

The UK enjoys a comprehensive Primary Health Care service within the National Health Service, yet this system often seems to fail people with dementia and their families: it may fail to recognise dementia and often feels poorly equipped to deal with the needs of individuals and families dealing with dementia. On the other hand, the number of people with dementia, some 800,000 currently in the UK, is an enormous challenge if it is to be dealt with purely by secondary health care. AD and other dementias are long-term conditions yet they are primarily managed in the UK by old-age psychiatrists. In the early stages, this is not necessarily appropriate, and there are other challenges: older people with dementia often have medical co-morbidities that complicate the management of the dementia and vice versa. Some of these can be managed in primary care, whereas others may need specialist input. These difficulties are by no means restricted to developed countries like the UK and the USA, but will also be a challenge in the future for less affluent countries [31].

It is challenging for PCPs to make a diagnosis of dementia in people in the early stages of the disease. On the other hand, it will be increasingly difficult to restrict diagnosing to specialists in view of the large numbers of people developing dementia in the coming years. A three-tier system has been suggested [32]:

1. a memory clinic within primary care, provided on a monthly basis by a specialist
2. a secondary (district) memory service that could provide support to the primary care service as well as initiating treatment
3. a tertiary (regional) memory service that can help with complex or unusual problems.

As discussed in the Memory Clinics section above, NICE in the UK has suggested that a memory assessment service should be the single point of referral for all people with a possible diagnosis of dementia although the location of such services could be within primary care [20]. It is difficult to see how specialists could provide a routine memory assessment service within all primary care locations, in line with the Gnosall model described earlier [30]. However, it is essential that there is closer working between Primary and Secondary Care, and while the diagnosis may be better made by specialists, follow-up care can be provided successfully in either Secondary or Primary Care [18]. If adequate education and support are provided to the Primary Care Team, this will also allow the specialist Memory Assessment Services to concentrate on accurate diagnosis as well as being a focus for research. It is wrong, however, to try and make the diagnosis of early dementia exclusively a primary care activity since making the diagnosis is difficult, particularly when trying to identify the subtype, and this is important when deciding on appropriate treatment and advice including information about the prognosis.

Discussing the diagnosis

Being diagnosed with dementia is a very significant event for the individual, as well as for friends and family. It is also challenging for the professionals who make the diagnosis. The diagnosis may be met with anxiety, distress and even disbelief, not only from the individual concerned but also from those around them. It is important for professionals to be aware of the impact they may have, depending on how they share information and deal with any questions or concerns. Discussing the diagnosis and its potential ramifications takes time and should not be rushed, despite the inevitable pressures on a clinician's time.

Most people with mild dementia want to know their diagnosis [33] and all practitioners should assume that it will be discussed with the person with dementia, unless there are clear reasons not to do so [20]. In the past, it was common to use the patient's relatives and carers as a proxy when discussing diagnosis, treatment and prognosis, but this is usually inappropriate, particularly for people with mild dementia: the person with dementia should routinely be asked if they wish to know the diagnosis and with whom this should be shared [33]. It has been suggested that reluctance by professionals to give the diagnosis to the patient may reflect the 'malignant social psychology' of Kitwood [34], where infantilisation, disempowerment and objectification may occur, even though this may not be intentionally malicious but rather reflective of limitations in skills in such circumstances. In a qualitative study, looking at diagnostic disclosure in dementia [35], most patients and carers reported that the disclosure had been a confirmation of their assumptions. A minority of patients and carers felt threatened and shocked by the diagnosis because they had not expected it. It is important, therefore, to know what expectations there are about the diagnosis before such a discussion begins. Disclosure can generally be carried out without causing stress to the patient or carer, and it facilitates guidance [35]. It also appears to help carers to start to adapt to their altered role and should take place before starting medical treatment and care because of the positive effect it has on both patients and carers.

Post-diagnosis information

Following a diagnosis of dementia, it is recommended [20] that health and social care professionals provide (preferably written) information, unless the person clearly indicates to the contrary and this should cover:

* the signs and symptoms of dementia
* the course and prognosis of the condition
* treatments
* local care and support services
* sources of financial and legal advice and advocacy
* medico-legal issues, including driving
* other local information sources such as libraries and voluntary organisations.

Some of these issues will now be considered in more detail, together with some general issues about safety.

Legal issues and autonomy

The advantages of an early diagnosis for someone with dementia is that it is possible to discuss and deal with issues relating to the later stages of the disease at a point when the person still has capacity and autonomy. Autonomy is increasingly compromised as dementia progresses, but a diagnosis of dementia is not synonymous with a lack of capacity. Autonomy must be respected as far as possible and remaining abilities and human rights recognised. Human rights legislation in Europe is covered by the *Convention for the Protection of Human Rights and Fundamental Freedoms (Council of Europe 2003)*, and throughout this convention, there is an implicit respect for autonomy. Nevertheless, it may be difficult at times when strict adherence to the rights of a person with dementia may interfere with the rights of other people, such as family caregivers.

Legal and financial issues

It is important to encourage the person with mild dementia to consider future legal and financial issues, to put in place any necessary safeguards and to make the necessary decisions at a time when capacity is still sufficiently intact, as this is likely to erode. Capacity is a legal concept and it is necessary to be aware of national legislation and guidance on assessment of capacity and other issues, such as advanced directives. The legal framework and terminology for these issues will clearly vary from country to country, and that provided here is a general guide based on the UK legislative framework.

Capacity to deal with financial affairs

A power of attorney allows one person to give another person the authority to act on their behalf and in their name in relation to issues surrounding financial affairs and property. Such a power of attorney is not usually suitable for a person with dementia since it ceases to be effective when a person becomes mentally incapacitated.

What is required is a so-called enduring or durable power of attorney, which either continues or comes into effect after an individual has become mentally incapable. It is critical that the person completing such a power of attorney has the capacity to understand it at the time they sign the relevant forms, and this is why it is important to encourage someone with mild dementia to consider this at an early stage. In England and Wales, the Mental Health Capacity Act 2005 created a new type of Power of Attorney, known as a Lasting Power of Attorney, which can deal both with the person's property and affairs but also with issues of personal welfare.

Capacity to make a will

Testamentary capacity describes the level of understanding needed when preparing a will at the time of signing. The capacity to make a will is likely to be greater than that needed to sign a power of attorney, especially if the details of the will are complex or if the person is changing a previously completed will. Again, it is important to encourage a person with mild dementia to consider this at a time when they are still able to understand what is involved.

Specialists and PCPs are likely to be asked from time to time to comment on whether a person has testamentary capacity and it is important to make a record of any examination or findings that contributed to the advice that was given.

Advanced decisions, advanced directives and living wills

These allow someone to specify particular types of treatment that they would not wish to be given should they lack the mental capacity to decide. There is the opportunity for a person with mild dementia to make such decisions, in writing and signed and witnessed, so that as their disease progresses, it is clear to everyone how they want to be treated.

Driving

Driving safety is a very important issue and can cause great difficulty to the person with dementia and the family. There are clearly potential repercussions for the community should the person's driving lead to an accident.

Driving is a complex task, and it is important that the driver can make sense of and respond to whatever they see and anticipate and react appropriately to the actions of other road users, as well as following road signs, and remember where they are going. Some people with dementia will choose to stop driving because they have lost confidence and are unsure of their ability. They will need support from the people around them when making this decision. Sometimes a carer may be resistant to this, particularly if they are dependent on the patient as driver. On the other hand, concern about a person's driving is sometimes the reason for the family to contact a doctor, yet they may find it difficult to raise the issue with the individual concerned.

It is therefore important to discuss driving with anyone with mild dementia and useful to provide written information [36]. In most countries, there will be specific rules concerning the continuation of driving and the national driving licensing authority will usually have medical assessors who can offer advice to both the person with dementia and their family and physicians. In the UK, for example, the individual is expected to notify the national licensing authority that they have a significant memory problem or dementia [37]. Such a notification may be difficult for someone with significant memory and cognitive problems, in which case it may be necessary for the family or the doctor to carry this out, but it should wherever possible be done with the agreement of the patient and with regard to any relevant rules about confidentiality. A formal driving assessment, including a road test, may sometimes be helpful [36].

While it may still be safe for someone to continue driving, it is inevitable that a time will come when this is not the case. It is advisable, therefore, to discuss this with the patient and their family and to prepare the way for a time when they have to stop. It may be useful advice to reduce risk by limiting driving to shorter drives at quieter times of the day on familiar roads. Driving at night may be particularly difficult for an older driver with dementia if they also have reduced visual acuity.

Safety issues

People with dementia are more prone to accidents and injuries, and issues concerning safety are frequently raised by family members, especially if he or she lives alone. Once again, it is important to strike a balance between protecting someone and allowing them continuing independence. Many services will have access to specialist occupational therapists to assess risks and advice on ways to mitigate against them.

It is helpful to give advice about issues such as kitchen safety, the provision of smoke and gas detectors, and looking at the home from the point of view of safety, particularly with regard to issues such as falls. Sometimes, this presents an opportunity to consider relocation to simpler accommodation on a single level or possibly closer to family members. Provision of safety rails or a stairlift and other such aids may be helpful and these issues are dealt with in more detail in Chapter 17 of this book. It is usually better to consider changes in accommodation at an early stage so that there is the opportunity to adapt to a new environment.

A person with dementia is more likely to lose their way outside the home. Although this is less likely in someone with mild dementia, carrying an identification bracelet may be helpful.

Interventions for cognitive symptoms and maintenance of function

Pharmacological interventions

Current drug treatments for AD are symptomatic. The only drugs licensed for use in mild dementia are the acetylcholinesterase inhibitors (ChEIs) donepezil, galantamine and rivastigmine. The N-methyl-D-aspartate antagonist memantine is only licensed for moderate to severe AD, although it is clear that in some countries, such as the USA, it is often used in mild AD, almost always in combination with a ChEI.

Recommendations about the way these drugs are used in different countries do vary. In the UK, NICE [38] recommends that only specialists in the care of patients with dementia (i.e. psychiatrists, neurologists and geriatricians) should initiate treatment. Treatment should only be continued when it is considered to be having a worthwhile effect on cognition, global, functional or behavioural symptoms. Patients should be reviewed regularly by an appropriate specialist unless there are locally agreed protocols for shared care. It is important to take into account physical, sensory, communication or learning disabilities that might affect assessment and to be mindful of the need to secure equity of access to treatment for people from different ethnic groups and different cultural backgrounds.

Although NICE has been clear that these drugs should only be initiated by specialists, there is increasing pressure to consider initiating by PCPs without necessarily taking specialist advice. This is potentially dangerous since this decision is predicated on a correct diagnosis of AD, which is not easy in primary care, as previously discussed and treatment initiation should be accompanied by advice about the diagnosis and other information.

Specific drug treatment for dementia is currently focussed mainly on AD, although one drug (rivastigmine) is also licensed for the treatment of dementia in Parkinson's disease. They are also regarded as useful for people with dementia with Lewy bodies.

Non-pharmacological interventions

Many psychosocial interventions can be helpful and non-drug interventions are worth trying, particularly when symptoms are neither causing distress nor placing a person at risk to themselves or others (in those situations medication may be the first consideration) [39].

Maintenance of cognitive function

There has been poor consistency in the application and availability of psychological therapies in dementia services. Such approaches have often been advocated more as a result of the enthusiasm of those introducing the therapy rather than being based on evidence and have either lacked systematic evaluation or general acceptance. Rigorous evaluation of non-pharmacological interventions is not easy and still at a relatively early stage of development [20].

Three major approaches with a cognitive focus have been described [40]:

1. *Cognitive stimulation*: a range of activities and discussions, usually in a group setting, aimed at enjoyment and general enhancement of cognitive and social function. Its roots can be traced back to Reality Orientation (RO), which was developed in the late 1950s as a response to confusion and disorientation in older patients in hospital units in the USA [41]. RO involved the engagement of nursing assistants in a hopeful, therapeutic process, but later became associated with a rigid confrontational approach to people with dementia, which led to criticism [42,43]. It has therefore fallen out of favour and has been little practised or researched outside of a few countries (notably Italy) since the 1990s [44]. A recent Cochrane review concluded that there was consistent evidence that cognitive stimulation benefits people with mild to moderate dementia over and above any medication effects. Future research should look at longer-term programmes and their clinical significance.
2. *Cognitive training*: specific training exercises designed for particular cognitive functions, such as memory, attention or problem solving. It includes practice and repetition, may be individual or group based and can involve pencil and paper or computer-assisted sessions. A Cochrane review in 2003 found no evidence for the efficacy of cognitive training although there were indicators of some modest, non-significant effects in various cognitive domains [45]. Further research from randomised controlled trials would be helpful.
3. *Cognitive rehabilitation (CR)*: an individualised approach with a therapist to identify personally relevant goals and to devise strategies to achieve these. The emphasis is on improving performance in everyday life by building on a person's strengths and finding ways of compensating for

impairments. The 2003 Cochrane review also reviewed CR but found insufficient evidence to evaluate it [45]. There is clearly a need for more effective and beneficial interventions, and some areas of cognition are relatively spared in early AD (e.g. procedural memory for skills and actions, semantic knowledge and implicit memory [46]). It should therefore be possible to use this capability to deliver beneficial interventions. A single-blind randomised controlled pilot study of the clinical efficacy of goal-oriented CR found that CR produced significant improvements in rating of goal performance and satisfaction in the treatment groups. The behavioural changes in the CR group were also supported by functional MRI changes in a subset of participants [47]. These promising findings will hopefully be confirmed by a larger study of CR that is currently in progress.

The 2006 NICE-SCIE Dementia guideline in the UK concluded that there is reasonable evidence to support the use of cognitive stimulation approaches for people with mild to moderate dementia [20]. This should be commissioned and provided by a range of health and social care staff with appropriate training and supervision and offered irrespective of any drug prescribed for the treatment of cognitive symptoms of dementia, since one study showed that cognitive stimulation appeared to add to the effects of donepezil in both mild and moderate AD [48].

Cognitive training has generally not been associated with benefits beyond the particular tasks that formed part of the training. At present, there is insufficient evidence to evaluate fully the effects of cognitive rehabilitation on cognitive function. Further research on these approaches is necessary.

Interventions for non-cognitive symptoms

Almost everyone with dementia will at some point develop one or more non-cognitive symptoms in the form of behavioural and psychological symptoms (BPSD) [49]. The most common problems are affective syndromes (depression, anxiety and irritability), apathy, agitation, aggression, psychosis (delusions and hallucinations) and sleep disorders. Depression and anxiety are especially common in mild dementia, when the person may have considerable insight. These problems can also be distressing for the family.

Good practice recommendations, such as the NICE-SCIE Dementia Guideline [20], recommend non-pharmacological interventions as the first line approach for BPSD and emphasise the importance of assessing pain and other medical conditions, which can often precipitate the development of these problems. Pharmacological treatment should be used sparingly, although antidepressants and anti-anxiety medication can sometimes be helpful, as can short-term treatment (4 weeks) for sleep disturbance with a hypnotic if sleep hygiene measures have failed [50].

Although behavioural changes are seen throughout the course of dementia, they tend to be more problematic in the later stages, but the principles of management are similar, irrespective of the stage. The management of these difficult problems are discussed in more detail in Chapters 6 and 7 in this book.

References

1. Folstein MF, Folstein SE, McHugh PR (1975) 'Mini Mental State': a practical method for grading the cognitive state of patients for the clinician. *J Psychiatr Res* 12:189–198.
2. Tombaugh TN, McIntyre NJ (1992) The Mini-Mental State Examination: a comprehensive review. *J Am Geriatr Soc* 40:922–935.

3. Hughes CP, Berg L, Danziger WL, Coben LA, Martin RL (1982) A new clinical scale for the staging of dementia. *Br J Psychiatry* 140:566–572.

4. Morris JC (1993) The Clinical Dementia Rating (CDR): current version and scoring rules. *Neurology* 43:2412–2414.

5. Reisberg B, Ferris SH, de Leon MJ, Crook T (1982) The global deterioration scale for assessment of primary degenerative dementia. *Am J Psychiatry* 139:1136–1139.

6. Reisberg B (1988) Functional Assessment Staging (FAST). *Psychopharmacol Bull* 24:653–659.

7. Lindesay J, Morris JC (1999) Introduction. In: Wilcock GK, Bucks RS, Rockwood K (eds), *Diagnosis and Management of Dementia: A Manual for Memory Disorders Teams*. Oxford: Oxford University Press, pp. 1–9.

8. Fraser M (1992) Memory clinics and memory training. In: Arie T (ed.), *Recent Advances in Psychogeriatrics*, Vol. 2. London: Churchill Livingstone, pp. 105–115.

9. Wright N, Lindesay J (1995) A survey of memory clinics in the British Isles. *Int J Geriatr Psychiatry* 10:379–385.

10. Van Diepen E, Lindesay J, Marudkar M, Wilcock G (2002) The second Leicester survey of memory clinics in the British Isles. *Int J Geriatr Psychiatry* 17:41–47.

11. Hughes J, Davies S, Walport M, Pickup S, Carruthers I, Rippon A (2012) The Prime Minister's Challenge on Dementia. Delivering Major Improvements in Dementia Care and Research by 2015: A Report on Progress. Available at: https://www.wp.dh.gov.uk/dementiachallenge/files/2012/11/The-Prime-Ministers -Challenge-on-Dementia-Delivering-major-improvements-in-dementia-care-and-research-by-2015-A -report-of-progress.pdf (last accessed on 20 February 2013).

12. Wolfs CA, Kessels A, Dirksen CD, Severens JL, Verhey FR (2008) Integrated multidisciplinary diagnostic approach for dementia care: randomised controlled trial. *Br J Psychiatry* 192(4):300–305.

13. Wolfs CA, Dirksen CD, Kessels A, Severens JL, Verhey FR (2009) Economic evaluation of an integrated diagnostic approach for psychogeriatric patients: results of a randomized controlled trial. *Arch Gen Psychiatry* 66(3):313–323.

14. Geldmacher DS (2002) Cost-effective recognition and diagnosis of dementia. *Semin Neurol* 22:63–70.

15. Mullins J, Fitch F (2000) Diagnosis by request: a self-referral memory clinic. *J Dement Care* 8(2):30–32.

16. Jolley D, Moniz-Cook E (2009) Memory clinics in context. *Indian J Psychiatry* 51(Suppl 1):S70–S76.

17. Van Hout HP, Vernooji-Dassen MJ, Hoefnagels WH, Grol RP (2001) Measuring the opinions of memory clinic users: patients, relatives and general practitioners. *Int J Geriatr Psychiatry* 16:846–851.

18. Meeuwsen EJ, Melis RJF, Van Der Aa GCHM, et al. (2012) Effectiveness of dementia follow-up care by memory clinics or general practitioners: randomised controlled trial. *BMJ* 344:e3086.

19. NICE (2012) Specifying a memory assessment service for the early identification and care of people with dementia. Available at: http://www.nice.org.uk/usingguidance/commissioningguides/memoryassessmentservice/ SpecifyingAMemoryAssessmentService.jsp (last accessed on 20 February 2013).

20. NICE-SCIE (2006, amended March 2011) The NICE-SCIE guideline on supporting people with dementia and their carers in health and social care (Clinical Guideline 42). Available at: http://www.nice.org.uk/ CG042 (last accessed on 20 February 2013).

21. Luce A, McKeith I, Swann A, Daniel S, O'Brien J (2001) How do memory clinics compare with traditional old age psychiatry services? *Int J Geriatr Psychiatry* 16:837–845.

22. Holland AJ, Hon J, Huppert FA, et al. (1998) Population-based study of the prevalence and presentation of dementia in adults with Down's syndrome. *Br J Psychiatry* 172:493–498.

23. Cooper SA (1997) High prevalence of dementia among people with learning disabilities not attributable to Down's syndrome. *Psychol Med* 27:609–616.

24. Vernooij-Dassen MJFJ, Moniz-Cook ED, Woods RT, et al. (2005) Factors affecting the timely recognition and diagnosis of dementia across Europe: from awareness to stigma. *Int J Geriatr Psychiatry* 20(4): 377–386.

25. Knapp M, Comas-Herrera A, Somani A, Banerjee S (2007) Dementia: international comparisons (National Audit Office report). Available at: http://www.nao.org.uk//idoc.ashx?docId=3f7e8831-0aa3-4fa7-98ef -222c4dc07156&version=-1 (last accessed on 20 February 2013).

26. Koch T, Iliffe S; the EVIDEM-ED project (2010) Rapid appraisal of barriers to the diagnosis and management of patients with dementia in Primary Care; a systematic review. *BMC Fam Pract* 11:52.

27. Department of Health (2009) Living well with dementia: a national dementia strategy. Available at: ttp://www.dh.gov.uk/en/Publicationsandstatistics/Publications/PublicationsPolicyAndGuidance/DH_094058 (last accessed on 21 February 2013).
28. Iliffe S, Robinson L, Brayne C, et al. (2009) Primary care and dementia: 1. Diagnosis, screening and disclosure. *Int J Geriatr Psychiatry* 24:895–901.
29. Waldemar G, Phung KT, Burns A, et al. (2007) Access to diagnostic evaluation and treatment for dementia in Europe. *Int J Geriatr Psychiatry* 22:47–54.
30. Greaves I, Jolley D (2010) National Dementia Strategy: well intentioned – but how well founded and how well directed? *Br J Gen Pract* 60:193–198.
31. Ferri CP, Prince M, Brayne C, et al. (2005) Global prevalence of dementia: a Delphi consensus study. *Lancet* 366:2112–2117.
32. Jolley D, Greaves I, Greaves N, et al. (2010) Three tiers for a comprehensive regional memory service. *J Dement Care* 18:26–29.
33. Pinner G, Bouman WP (2003) What should we tell people about dementia? *Adv Psychiatr Treat* 9:335–341.
34. Kitwood T (1990) The dialectics of dementia: with particular reference to Alzheimer's disease. *Aging Soc* 10:177–196.
35. Derksen E, Vernooij-Dassen M, Gillissen F, Olde Rikkert M, Scheltens P (2006) Impact of diagnostic disclosure in dementia on patients and carers: qualitative case series analysis. *Aging Ment Health* 10(5):525–531.
36. Alzheimer Society Driving and Dementia. Available at: https://www.alzheimers.org.uk/factsheet/439 (last accessed on 20 February 2013).
37. Drivers Medical Group, DVLA, Swansea UK At a glance guide to the current medical standards of fitness to drive. Available at: http://www.dft.gov.uk/dvla/medical/ataglance.aspx (last accessed on 20 February 2013).
38. NICE (2011) Donepezil, galantamine, rivastigmine, and memantine for the treatment of Alzheimer's disease. Available at: http://guidance.nice.org.uk/TA217 (last accessed on 20 February 2013).
39. Burns A, Iliffe S (2009) Alzheimer's disease. *BMJ* 338:b158.
40. Clare L, Woods RT (2004) Cognitive training and cognitive rehabilitation for people with early-stage Alzheimer's disease. *Neuropsychol Rehabil* 14:385–401.
41. Taulbee LR, Folsom JC (1966) Realty orientation for geriatric patients. *Hosp Community Psychiatry* 17:133–135.
42. Powell-Proctor L, Miller E (1982) Reality orientation: a critical appraisal. *Br J Psychiatry* 140:457–463.
43. Dietch JT, Hewett LJ, Jones S (1989) Adverse effects of reality orientation. *JAGS* 37:974–976.
44. Woods B, Aguirre E, Spector AE, Orrell M (2012) Cognitive stimulation to improve cognitive functioning in people with dementia. *Cochrane Database Syst Rev* (2):CD005562.
45. Clare L, Woods R (2003) Cognitive rehabilitation and cognitive training for early-stage Alzheimer's disease and vascular dementia. *Cochrane Database Syst Rev* (4):CD003260.
46. Fernandez-Ballesteros R, Zamarron MD, Tarraga L, Moya R, Iniguez J (2003) Cognitive plasticity in healthy, mild cognitive impairment (MCI), subjects and Alzheimer's disease patients: a research project in Spain. *Eur Psychol* 8:148–159.
47. Clare L, Linden DE, Woods RT, et al. (2010) Goal-oriented cognitive rehabilitation for people with early-stage Alzheimer's disease: a single-blind randomized controlled trial of clinical efficacy. *Am J Geriatr Psych* 18:928–939.
48. Chapman SB, Weiner MF, Rackley A, et al. (2004) Effect of cognitive-communication stimulation for Alzheimer's disease patients treated with donepezil. *J Speech Lang Hear Res* 47:1149–1163.
49. Steinberg M, Shao H, Zandi P, et al. (2008) Point 5-year period prevalence of neuropsychiatric symptoms in dementia: the Cache County Study. *Int J Geriatr Psychiatry* 23:170–177.
50. Alzheimer's Society (2012) Optimising treatment and care for people with behavioural and psychological symptoms of dementia: a best practice guide for health and social care professionals. Alzheimer's Society. Available at: http://www.alzheimers.org.uk/bpsdguide (last accessed on 20 February 2013).

Chapter 6

Services for people with moderate dementia

Laura M. Struble[a], Janet Kavanagh[b] and Mary Blazek[c]

[a]University of Michigan School of Nursing and the Department of Psychiatry, University of Michigan Medical School, USA
[b]Project Development and Administration, Program for Positive Aging, Department of Psychiatry, University of Michigan Medical School, USA
[c]Department of Psychiatry, Geriatric Psychiatry Section, University of Michigan Medical School, USA

Introduction

As dementia progresses from the mild to the moderate stage, the frustrations and challenges of cognitive impairment are compounded by loss of functional independence and an increase in behavioural symptoms. Over the disease course, the severity of symptoms increases, resulting in a corresponding need for additional time, energy and assistance from caregivers and highlighting the interdependent nature of the caregiver–care recipient dyad. Despite major research efforts into dementia care, service delivery for people with dementia and their caregivers remains patchy, fragmented and reactive [1,2]. Service recipients often underutilise or are unaware of the full range of services available [3]. Perhaps the most challenging feature in the moderate stage is the ever-changing picture of the person with dementia: patients will have varying needs across the domains of cognition, function and behaviour as the disease progresses. This *moving target* quality requires frequent assessment and reassessment if appropriate services are to be delivered. A more holistic psychosocial model is more helpful than a traditional medical model, and optimal care requires a multidisciplinary approach, including involvement of people with dementia and their caregivers, in determining needs and planning for services.

Moderate dementia defined

During the mild stages of dementia, deficits may only be evident on careful clinical interview. In contrast, people with moderate dementia can no longer manage without some assistance. Patients experience a major transition from a manageable disease to one that is demanding and distressing. In moderate dementia, cognitive abilities decline, functional autonomy is lost and behavioural symptoms become increasingly problematic. Co-morbid medical conditions, such as cardiovascular disease, pulmonary disorders, arthritis, and diminution of vision and hearing are common, and affect care planning, communication methods, benefits and risks of treatments, and adherence to treatment [4]. Malnutrition and movement disorders become more prevalent as well.

Designing and Delivering Dementia Services, First Edition. Edited by Hugo de Waal, Constantine Lyketsos, David Ames, and John O'Brien.
© 2013 John Wiley & Sons, Ltd. Published 2013 by John Wiley & Sons, Ltd.

People with moderate dementia frequently display disorientation to time or place. They do retain knowledge of major facts regarding themselves and others, and invariably know their own names and those of their spouse and children. As they progress into moderately severe dementia, they are largely unaware of recent events and experiences in their own lives and start to confuse family relationships and the names of family members, including their own spouse. Short- and long-term memory declines, aphasia advances, and judgment and problem solving recedes to basic levels. They now require full-time supervision [5].

People with moderate dementia can be independent in the performance of most activities of daily living (ADL s), but may still require assistance with tasks, for example choosing appropriate clothing. In the moderate-severe stage, gradually increasing assistance with dressing, bathing and hygiene, feeding and toileting are required. Both urinary and faecal incontinence become more common [6]. Additionally, nutritional status and mobility are affected and require careful consideration when providing services. People with dementia who are malnourished often experience more cognitive and functional decline and have an increase in behavioural symptoms [7]. Problems with gait and abnormal movements (including bradykinesia, Parkinsonism, rigidity, multifocal myoclonus and tendency to fall) are also more prevalent, are dependent on the type of dementia and significantly impact the person's ability to function [8,9].

Neuropsychiatric symptoms are extremely common in the middle stages of dementia, with prevalence rates estimated between 61% and 88% [10]. As dementia progresses and aphasia increases, people with dementia express their emotions nonverbally and behaviourally. There is a wide range of behaviours that are superimposed on cognitive deficits, including:

- agitation (e.g. aggressive and physically nonaggressive behaviours, pacing, rummaging, wandering and verbal agitation)
- psychiatric symptoms (e.g. delusions and hallucinations)
- personality changes
- inappropriate sexual behaviour and other forms of disinhibition
- mood disturbance (e.g. apathy, depression, euphoria and emotional lability)
- neuro-vegetative changes (e.g. appetite changes and sleep disturbance) [11,12].

Various factors influence behavioural symptoms, including ethnicity, premorbid personality, social milieu and physical environment [9,13,14]. In addition, frequency, intensity and type of behavioural symptoms vary, dependent upon the specific type of dementia. For example, people with Lewy body dementia experience a higher incidence of hallucinations while people with vascular dementia commonly express more depressive symptomatology and emotional lability [15].

Moderate dementia can be operationally defined using scores from the Clinical Dementia Rating Scale (CDR). The CDR is a global assessment instrument to stage dementia severity; it is widely used in clinical settings and demonstrates high validity and reliability [16,17]. This scale assesses six domains: memory, orientation, judgment and problem-solving, function in community affairs, home and hobbies, and personal care. A score of 2 (of a maximum of 3) categorises those in the moderate stage of dementia. Other well-established psychometric indications of mid-stage or moderate dementia include stages 5 and 6 on both the Global Deterioration Scale (GDS) and the Functional Assessment Staging (FAST).

Table 6.1 describes the stages of dementia, behavioural symptoms and time spent in caregiving activities. It should be noted that many scales were developed primarily for individuals with Alzheimer's dementia (AD). However, people suffering from vascular dementia or dementias of other aetiologies (e.g. Lewy body, Parkinson's and fronto-temporal) have demonstrated limitations in ADLs equal to or greater than those with classic AD [18]. Therefore, they will have equivalent or greater need for supportive services.

Table 6.1 Description of clinical staging, behavioural symptoms, caregiver supervision and setting for dementia

	Mild	**Moderate**	**Severe**
Staging			
Clinical Dementia Rating Scale (CDR)[a]	1	2	3
Functional Assessment Staging (FAST)[b]	4	5–6	7
MMSE[c]	30–21	20–11	10–0
Clock Drawing Test (CDT)[d]	0.5–1.5	2	3
Functional abilities [b, e]	Impaired IADLs: Financial and legal affairs Fitness to drive Meal preparation and shopping	Impaired IADLs > ADLs Needs more assistance with eating Gradually lost ability to ambulate independently	Total dependence for dressing, feeding, bathing and ambulation
Behavioural symptoms [f, g]	1 – Apathy and agitation 2 – Irritability and disinhibition 3 – Anxiety 4 – Euphoria 5 – Aberrant motor behaviour, depression, delusions and hallucinations	1 – Apathy 2 – Aberrant motor behaviour 3 – Depression 4 – Anxiety 5 – Agitation 6 – Delusions 7 – Irritability 8 – Hallucinations 9 – Disinhibition 10 – Euphoria	1 – Apathy 2 – Agitation 3 – Aberrant motor behaviour 4 – Depression 5 – Anxiety 6 – Delusions and disinhibition 7 – Hallucinations and euphoria
Caregiver supervision [h, i]	Minor supervision 1–10 hours per week	Increased caregiver support 4 to >10 hours	24-hour supervision
Physical environments	Home and assisted living	Home, dementia assisted living, nursing home	Home, dementia assisted living, nursing home, hospice

[a]Morris (1993) [17].
[b]Reisberg (1988) [5].
[c]Folstein et al. (1975) [23].
[d]Sunderland et al. (1989) [24].
[e]Galasko et al. (1997) [28].
[f]Mega et al. (1996) [13].
[g]Gauthier (2002) [98]
[h]Feldman and Woodward. (2005) [9].
[i]Georges et al. (2008) [52].

Assessing the need for services

Ideally patients are evaluated during the mild stage of their disease, with groundwork laid in anticipation of the inevitable need for increased support and supervision. Unfortunately, it is not uncommon for a person to present for initial evaluation when the disease has already progressed to the moderate
stage. In either case, people with moderate dementia will require ongoing assessment and continual
reassessment in order to respond to changing needs for services and multiple transitions in care.

In order to determine the type and extent of services required, assessment of the person with
dementia should include three domains: cognitive, functional (including nutritional and mobility
assessment) and behavioural. The assessment process pinpoints the areas of services required and
provides a baseline for comparison as the disease progresses. Co-morbidities in people with dementia should also be assessed throughout the course of the disease, especially if sudden changes in
cognitive or behavioural symptoms occur [19]. In a large post-mortem study, co-morbid conditions
were found that would have affected the clinical management of the person with dementia, had
they been known ante mortem [20]. Depression, falls, mobility issues and malnutrition are very
common complications and should be evaluated as well. Comprehensive assessment should include
the individual's primary caregivers' and support systems. The impact of caregiving responsibilities
for people in moderate dementia is tremendous. As the person with dementia becomes more dependent, family caregivers often experience significant psychological and physical illness, with accompanying high levels of anxiety and depression, and they too will need support [21,22].

Cognitive assessment

Once an initial diagnosis of dementia has been made, brief screening tools can be used to establish
a baseline of cognitive function, both in anticipation of future decline and to devise interventions.
The Mini-Mental State Examination (MMSE) is a widely used instrument for assessing general
cognitive impairment [23]. The MMSE can be used to track cognitive changes over time, and to
evaluate orientation, memory and language functions. It has age and education specific normative
scores, and has been translated into a number of different languages. The moderate stages of dementia correlate with MMSE scores ranging between 11 and 20 out of a total score of 30. The MMSE,
however, has been found to be influenced by patients' levels of education and literacy, as well as
their age, culture and ethnicity and recently problems have surfaced regarding patent-related costs
of usage. The Clock Drawing Test (CDT) complements the MMSE by measuring visual-constructional
executive functions, and is relatively free of educational and cultural bias [24]. Scoring is based on
the patient's ability to draw a clock and set the hands at a specific time. The Schulman method of
scoring the CDT corresponds with the severity of global impairment [25]. There are six categories
(ranging from perfect clock = 1 through to no reasonable representation of a clock = 6). A score
≥ 3 on the CDT reflects significant cognitive deficit in the middle stages of dementia.

Functional assessment

Functional abilities are influenced by physical capacity, cognitive abilities, physical environment
and social support. The use of standardised scales provides a common language for patients, informal caregivers and health professionals to determine service needs across settings. Multiple
performance-based and observational instruments have been developed. Function is frequently
gauged in terms of ADLs. Basic self-maintenance skills can be assessed using the Katz Index of
Independence in Activities of Daily Living [26]. This scale assesses bathing, dressing, transferring,
toileting, continence and feeding. It can be repeated to determine changing needs. The Instrumental
Activities of Daily Living Scale (IADL) evaluates more complex physical functioning that is

dependent on memory, abstract judgment, attention and language [27]. The IADL measures a person's ability to use a telephone, shop, prepare a meal, keep house, do laundry, administer medications, use transportation and manage money. Periodic assessments will help determine the need for more support.

The Modified Alzheimer's Disease Cooperative Study-Activities of Daily Living Inventory (ADCS-ADL) is a validated caregiver-rated scale that assesses both IADLs and ADLs [28]. This instrument is used specifically to assess those with dementia in the moderate stage. The ADCS-ADL has been used primarily in clinical drug trials to identify progression of functional decline. In the middle stages of dementia, IADL skills are typically lost earlier than basic ADLs. Galasko demonstrated that both IADLs and ADLs were lost in a hierarchical manner, with tasks that depend on short-term memory lost before overlearned activities [29]. The loss of ability to perform IADLs and ADLs leads to a need for increased levels of care, but is not solely related to cognitive ability. Common aspects of ageing, such as vision and hearing loss, and physical decline in gait, strength and mobility can also negatively affect the person's functional capabilities.

Nutritional assessment

People with dementia are considered to be at high risk of weight loss and malnutrition, risk factors that are associated with institutionalisation [30]. People in the middle stages of dementia initially require assistance with cooking and shopping, but as the disease progresses, they may experience an increase in apathy, functional impairment, agnosia and dysphagia affecting their nutritional status. Since most nutritional problems are reversible, regular follow-up of people at risk of malnutrition with appropriate and efficient services can delay weight loss [31]. The Mini Nutritional Assessment tool has been used in clinical research and international studies, and has been used in a variety of settings [32,33]. A shortened version of the tool screens six domains and measures body mass index [34].

Mobility assessment

One of the hallmarks of middle stage dementia is the loss of mobility, which in turn leads to wider functional disability and an increased need for personal assistance from caregivers and the use of assistive devices. Failure to treat reversible functional loss adversely affects the health status and quality of life of people with dementia and their informal caregivers [35,36]. Some of the functional losses related to mobility are reversible [37]. In one study, Slaughter et al. found that over 50% of walking disability in people with middle stage dementia may be modifiable with supportive devices and physical therapy services [38]. The Get Up and Go Test is a performance-based measure of ambulation, balance, and gait that can be performed anywhere [39,40].

Behavioural and psychological assessment

Often, behavioural disturbances rather than cognitive impairment, prompt people to seek help. It is well documented that disruptive behaviours may lead to caregiver stress and early institutionalisation [41–43]. Behavioural changes occur from the early stages of dementia onwards, but some occur more frequently in the middle stages of dementia, such as wandering, purposeless activities and inappropriate activities [44]. The Neuropsychiatric Inventory (NPI) is a behavioural scale widely used in clinical trials and observational studies [45]. It is administered through a caregiver interview and rates the presence or absence of 12 symptom types: delusions, hallucinations, agitation, depression, anxiety, euphoria, apathy, disinhibition, irritability, aberrant motor behaviours, night-time disturbances and eating disorders.

Depressive symptoms are some of the most frequent neuropsychiatric symptoms that accompany dementia [46]. The importance of assessment and treatment of depression is emphasised because of its association with poor outcomes [21]. Additionally, there may be a link between depressive symptoms and physical aggression [47]. The Geriatric Depression Scale-Short Form is a widely used 15-item self-report screening instrument, but as language skills deteriorate, it becomes less effective [48]. The Cornell Scale for Depression in Dementia may be a more accurate predictor of depression in people in the middle stages of dementia [49]. Some people with dementia and depression present with unexplained somatic symptoms and may deny sadness or loss of pleasure. Consequently, the use of both clinical judgment, as well as interviewer-rated depression scales, are recommended in order accurately to assess depression in people with dementia [50].

Caregiver assessment

As the person with moderate dementia becomes increasingly dependent, the caregiver gradually adjusts and compensates. The two individuals function as a dyad and the well-being of the care recipient cannot be assessed without a simultaneous assessment of the caregiver [51]. Caregivers identify behavioural difficulties and assistance with ADLs as most problematic [52]. The most consistently used measure is the Zarit Burden Interview (ZBI), a 22-item self-administered questionnaire that assesses burden associated with functional/behavioural impairments and home care context. The items measure common areas of concern, such as health, finances, social life and interpersonal relations [53]. Three dimensions of burden have been described: effect on the social and personal life of caregivers, psychological burden, and feelings of guilt. Spouses and children frequently perceive burden differently. Spouse caregivers emphasise the deterioration of their personal and social life, while children are more likely to express guilt that they are not doing enough for their parents [54]. The ZBI score has shown a stronger correlation between depressive mood of caregivers and behaviour problems of care recipients than between the recipient's cognitive and functional status [55]. Another caregiver assessment tool is the 12-item Caregiver Strain Index (CSI) [56]. The CSI helps to identify families with caregiving concerns who may benefit from more in-depth assessment and follow-up.

Goals and desired outcomes of services

The principal goals of services for moderate dementia are:

- the optimisation of physical health, cognition, activity and well-being
- the detection and treatment of behavioural and psychological symptoms of dementia (BPSD)
- the provision of information and long-term support to caregivers [57].

Traditionally, these goals have focused on aspects external to the patient, such as safety and hygiene. Indeed, the majority of care required is basic and task oriented, but more recently goals have expanded to include maintenance of personhood.

Kitwood's social–psychological theory of 'personhood in dementia' asserts that although a degeneration of cognitive functioning occurs due to disease progression, individuals do not disintegrate from a psychological and emotional point of view [58]. Younger and Martin described good dementia care as 'that which enables the person to feel supported, valued and socially confident'. They proposed 'a shift in the culture of care' advocating meaningful activity, which must take place on recreational, interpersonal and therapeutic levels, with reminiscence and stimulation as part of the process [59].

Bamford and Bruce described the overall aim of community care for patients with dementia as having access to normal activities and patterns of life in ways that maximise choice and control. They distinguished two types of community-care outcomes for patients with dementia: quality-of-life outcomes and service-process outcomes.

Quality-of-life outcomes include:

- access to social contact and company
- a sense of social integration
- access to meaningful activity and stimulation
- maximising a sense of autonomy
- maintaining a sense of personal identity
- feeling safe and secure and feeling financially secure
- being personally clean and comfortable
- living in a clean and comfortable environment.

Service process outcomes include:

- having a say in services
- feeling valued and respected
- being treated as an individual
- being able to relate to other service users [60].

Because caregivers experience significant stress that may affect their own health, the goals of caregiver support and reduction of caregiver burden are strongly emphasised. Services that help caregivers include:

- support to continue caring for the person in their own home for as long as practical
- maintenance of a caring relationship between caregiver and patient with dementia
- provision of fulfilment and satisfaction in the caring role [61].

Avoidance of premature institutionalisation or nursing home placement is an overarching goal for services for people with dementia anywhere in the world, for financial reasons as well as other factors:

- Nursing home entry is associated with rapid declines in health, increased mortality and emotional challenges for families [62].
- The psychosocial effects of nursing home placement include increased stress and confusion while adapting to a new environment.
- Caregivers can feel increased guilt with fear that their relatives are not receiving adequate care, leading to conflicts with nursing home staff.
- Nursing home placement does not decrease caregiver distress [63].

Although delay in nursing home placement is desired, the decision should be supported when it becomes ultimately necessary.

Approaches for services in moderate dementia

Although there are considerable variations in services, all face the same challenges of fragmentation, disjointed care and high costs. The economic impact of dementia, particularly for people in the middle and late stages of the disease, is enormous and a major contributor to overall cost in health care. Furthermore, it is projected that 43% of people with dementia will need a high level of care and supervision [64]. This burden has a great impact on how healthcare systems organise services and finance care.

Primary care providers are usually the first point of contact, but primary care practitioners cannot provide the necessary care services alone. Current clinical guidelines for best-practice management of dementia are extensive and include:

• appropriate treatment of co-morbid medical conditions
• optimisation of physical health
• development and implementation of an ongoing treatment plan
• use of cholinesterase inhibitors and memantine
• treatment of behavioural problems and mood disorders with both pharmacologic and non-pharmacologic interventions
• referral to specialists and social service agencies or support organisations [4,19,65,66].

The diverse and individual nature of dementia and the caregiving experience requires a carefully tailored, individualised approach to services and is therefore best delivered using a multidisciplinary approach. Coordination of care is invaluable, and there is evidence that access to case management services results in an increased uptake of community services [67,68].

A collaborative framework has been shown to improve quality of care for people with dementia and their caregivers [57,69]. Optimally, this would include well-educated primary care teams who focus on continuing care needs, with regular assessments, medical health maintenance, treatments for behavioural and psychological symptoms of dementia, and use of community support services. An example of this type of approach is the UK-based Croydon Memory Service Model, which utilises a multi-agency approach to provide specialised assessment and care [70]. This model includes joint ownership by health services, social services and the voluntary sector. An ideal model would consist of a collaboration between general practitioners and specialised memory clinics or specialists (e.g. geriatricians, neurologists and psychiatrists) to create a tailored programme for individualised care [19,71]. To achieve such optimal care advanced education for general practitioners is needed, combined with structural changes, such as increased visit time, appropriate funding and availability of interdisciplinary teams. To prevent and ameliorate behavioural and physical crises, rapid and expedited access to outpatient psychiatric care and rapid response home care visits are recommended [72].

The process of service delivery is also important. There has been a paradigm shift from providing formal services *for* people with dementia to working *with* people and their caregivers [73]. Particularly in the early and middle stages of the disease, people with dementia are able to provide accurate and valid reports of their experience with services [60,74]. Nolan and colleagues developed a 'Senses Framework' that is based on the belief that all parties involved in dementia care should experience relationships that promote a sense of security, belonging, continuity, purpose, achievement and significance [75]. This led to the development of *'The authentic partnership'*, which emphasised that early establishment of a strong partnership between people with dementia, family caregivers and professionals is likely to provide a better sense of the wishes and desires of the person with dementia, even as the disease progresses [73].

Integrated models of care for older adults

Well-known models which fully integrate services for older adults include:

• Programme of All-inclusive Care for Elderly People (PACE) [76]
• Systeme de Soins Integres pour Personnes Agees (SIPA) [77]

- the Programme of Research to Integrate Services for the Maintenance of Autonomy (PRISMA) [78].

These three successful models of care have common characteristics (note: they are not specific for people with dementia) [49]:

- umbrella organisational structure
- case-managed, multidisciplinary teams to evaluate, plan and provide patient needs
- organised provider networks joined together by standardised referral procedures
- services agreement
- financial incentives.

Internationally, the Netherlands is the only country to develop a separate nursing home medical discipline. This specialty developed a continuum of medical care ('The Dutch Model'), where family physicians serve the community, the nursing home physician provides care for the institutionalised older adults and the clinical geriatrician and other medical specialists care for older adults who are hospitalised [79].

The Dutch large-scale residential and nursing home facilities were designed by Herman Hertzberger more than 35 years ago. The original 520-bed care home utilised a 'village within the community' concept of care [80]. There are a broad range of institutional and outreaching care functions that makes the Dutch Model unique, including day care, rehabilitation, residential care, supervised group living, specialised dementia care, stroke care and nursing care, all at one site. This model provides a multidisciplinary, cyclically evaluated systematic approach to dementia care [81]. It is an exemplar system that provides smooth transitions of care across settings.

These examples exhibit the qualities of best-practice dementia care by focusing on maintenance of function, prevention of acute exacerbation of disease, prevention of disease, and cure or palliative care for acute conditions. The various components are integrated and are therefore best able to encompass medical, social, rehabilitative and personal care services, while ensuring services adjust to the functional and cognitive decline and link services for pharmacology and psychosocial treatments.

Caregiver service recommendations

The benefits of caregiver interventions emphasise once again the intertwined nature of the patient caregiver dyad. Interventions that have been demonstrated to be helpful to caregivers include:

- psycho-education
- structured presentation of information regarding disease and caregiving issues
- cognitive behavioural therapy and counselling
- case management
- general support
- respite care [82].

Caregiver interventions have immediate positive effects on caregiver burden, caregiver depression and subjective well-being, ability and knowledge sufficient to take care of a person with dementia, and improved care recipient symptoms [19]. Such efforts also delay institutionalisation of the person with dementia [83]. Psycho-educational interventions have the broadest effects, but only if caregivers actively participate. The longer the duration of the intervention, the stronger the positive effects will be. Service providers must tailor interventions to the specific needs of the individual caregiver, as most interventions have been demonstrated to have domain specific outcomes [3,19,82].

Existence of a service is not sufficient to ensure adequate care: informal caregivers often do not take advantage of available services. Reasons for non-use of services include perceived lack of need, resistance to accepting help and lack of knowledge of available services. Denial of need for services can occur despite the caregiver's reported low levels of satisfaction with the caregiving role, resentment and overload. This may reflect caregiver stoicism or negative expectations of services offered. Caregivers appear more likely to accept services if the person with dementia has physical disabilities [3].

Services provided in the community

It has been shown that if patients and caregivers use community-based services early on (such as home-based personal care, help with chores, adult day care and respite care) institutionalisation may be delayed [83]. Two studies demonstrated that home-based counselling for family caregivers [84] or behavioural management interventions [85] lowered caregiver stress and improved quality of life for the person with dementia. Home-based occupational therapy and physical therapy can improve daily functioning and reduce caregiver burden [86]. Traditional support groups and psycho-educational programmes, which focus on caregiver stress and coping, can lower reactions to behavioural problems, as well as reduce the frequency of problematic behaviours [87]. Online resources are increasingly making various kinds of information accessible, including generic dementia education and support or guidance on financial and legal issues. External memory prompts (e.g. reminders to take medications), Internet-based multimedia systems (e.g. simplified TV or computer systems to increase user friendliness), and monitoring of health and safety (e.g. wandering global positioning systems, alarms, smart home technology) are all technologies that show promise in supporting people with dementia and caregivers. Table 6.2 provides a description of the types of services available across settings, and this topic is further addressed in detail in Chapter 17 of this book.

Long-term residential and nursing home care

Internationally, there is a wide range of philosophical and operational definitions of housing options, including assisted living, senior homes, special care units and nursing homes, all with wide variations in environments and services offered. Services that may be offered in institutional settings include:

- long-term care
- rehabilitation
- respite care
- generic and specialist medical and psychiatric care
- palliative and hospice care.

Most management and service principles are similar to community settings, with one exception: long-term care focuses more on the physical environmental design for people with dementia and provides a 'prosthetic' environment. Such settings use specially designed structural elements (e.g. walls and windows), finishes (e.g. lighting and grab bars) and flexible components (e.g. activity supplies) to support patient deficits and maximise on their abilities. Person-centred programming

Table 6.2 Types of services available for dementia care

Resources	Service descriptions
Health care	
Primary/geriatric medical providers	Education about dementia
	Coordination of care with specialist and services
	Treatment of co-morbid conditions
	Optimise health
	Treat acute conditions, prevent delirium
Neurology	Diagnosis of dementia and treatment
Psychiatry	Non-pharmacological and pharmacological treatments for neuropsychiatric symptoms
	Counselling for the person with dementia and family caregiver, suicide prevention
Dementia care manager: advanced practice nurse, nurse or social worker who is embedded in healthcare systems or community agencies	Assessment, treatment, education/support and safety
Ophthalmologist	Maximise vision, glasses, early treatment of eye diseases
Audiologist	Maximise hearing, hearing aids
Speech therapist	Diagnosis and treat swallowing difficulties, provide communication strategies
Physical therapist	Improve mobility, prevent falls, assistive devices
Occupational therapist	Enhance function, engage in meaningful activities
Visiting nurses/psychiatric visiting nurses	Provide safety evaluation, education, disease management and medication management
Social work	Person with dementia and caregiver counselling support and education services
Dieticians	Maximise hydration and nutritional status
Dentists	Prevent and treat dental disease and maximise oral hygiene
Podiatry home or clinic based	Foot care services
Alternative and complementary medicine: acupuncturists, homeopathic, naturopathic, chiropractic and massage therapist	Broad range of treatments to promote health and well-being
In-home services	
Personal care	Provides personal hygiene, meal preparation, running errands and walking/exercise
Housekeeping/home repair	Household chores, meal preparation, keeping house in good repair
Daytime activities	
Adult day care	Social activities, exercise, respite
Senior centre programs	Social activities, exercise, education
Volunteer services	Social activities, respite
Activity therapist	Provides meaningful activities to improve function
Community services	
Meals on wheels	Main meal provided, social encounter
Area agency on aging	Administers programs for the elderly funded by the state and federal governments.
Alzheimer's association	Education and support services
Legal assistance	Advice and representation on benefits and legal matters

(Continued)

Table 6.2 (*Continued*)

Resources	Service descriptions
Technology services	Lifeline alert/emergency response team, appointment and medication reminders, global tracking devices, communication technologies and smart house technologies (e.g. smoke and motion sensors and stove shut off valves)
Financial assistance	Counselling on financial management, prescription drug programmes, food stamps and energy assistance
Respite care	Home or institution 24-hour care for short periods of time
Spiritual, religious and cultural services	Meeting spiritual needs
Adult protective services	Assessment and services to prevent emotional and physical abuse

of meaningful and useful activities, leisure and self-care activities, and behavioural management approaches are more prominent in institutional settings as well. Historically institutional settings used the medical model and looked like hospital wards. The trend has shifted to a psychosocial, holistic model, with small home-like settings and person-centred care, which emphasises the person's well-being [88,89].

Hospital settings

'Hospital-at-home' services provide care at home for patients with certain acute illnesses occurring on top of more chronic conditions and were an extension of the earlier discharge models where care was initiated in the home after a patient's brief hospital stay [90]. An interdisciplinary 'Hospital-at-Home' team for dementia care should at least include a physician, nursing staff, technicians, and rehabilitative therapists. Assessments, tests and treatments are provided in the home until the frail person with dementia recovers from the acute condition [91]. These targeted services can improve the patient's quality of life and reduce the duration of a stressful hospital stay and the ensuing healthcare costs [90].

Comprehensive hospital care models recommend a geriatric multidisciplinary approach to care. Inpatient geriatric consultation teams can help to preserve cognitive functions so that patients can return home, instead of being discharged too soon to institutional settings [92]. 'Acute Care for Elders' (ACE) units have been developed in the hospital setting and provide a specifically designed environment (e.g. safe flooring, safe wandering space, orientation cues and aids to mobility and self-care), patient-centred care, planning for discharge, and appropriate medical care for patients with dementia. These ACE units have been shown to improve the older person's ability to perform ADLs on discharge and reduce admissions to residential care facilities [93]. They also improve the process of care and increase patient and provider satisfaction without increasing hospital length of stay or cost [94,95]. A hospital model for managing delirium using the ACE unit has also been initiated: the 'delirium room' is a specialised four-bed unit that provides 24-hour intensive nursing care, free of physical restraints, comprehensive geriatric medical care and non-pharmacological interventions addressing problematic behaviours [96]. Nursing staff prepare hospitalised patients and family caregivers for discharge by facilitating smooth, safe and efficient transition from hospital to the next site of care, and these approaches can reduce hospital readmission rates and costs [90,97]. The literature discusses transitions from hospitals to home or other settings, but there is an important step missing: outpatient services need to be configured to respond to emergencies quickly, focus on pre-emptive approaches and anticipate the care needs of a person with dementia in order to enable a smooth discharge.

Summary

The middle stages of dementia are characterised by transition. Worsening cognition, decreasing functional ability and increasing behavioural disturbances require flexibility and adaptability in addressing needs. The interdependence of the caregiver–care recipient dyad becomes paramount, so that one cannot be assessed or assisted without the other.

Services vary based on country, culture and setting (see the various chapters in Section IV of this book), but they must accommodate disease progression, regardless of where they are being provided. Good service delivery will be multi-disciplinary, tailored to the individual needs and directed by the wishes of both the person with dementia and the caregiver, taking into account the relationship between the two. Even with optimal pro-active care emergencies will occur. Ideal crisis intervention adjusts the level and intensity of the response to what is appropriate in an individual case, and such approaches must therefore be informed by discussions with patients and caregivers on their views on matters related to quality of life, advanced care planning and end-of-life care.

References

1. Pickard S (1999) Co-ordinated care for older people with dementia. *Journal of Interprofessional Care* 13(4):345–354.
2. Mestheneos E (2005) *Supporting Family Carers of Older People in Europe – The Pan-European Background Report*. Münster: Lit Verlag.
3. Brodaty H, Thomson C, Thompson C, Fine M (2005) Why caregivers of people with dementia and memory loss don't use services. *International Journal of Geriatric Psychiatry* 20(6):537–546.
4. Cummings JL, Frank JC, Cherry D, Kohatsu ND, Kemp B, Hewett L, et al. (2002) Guidelines for managing Alzheimer's disease: part I. Assessment. *American Family Physician* 65(11):2263–2276.
5. Reisberg B, Ferris SH, de Leon MJ, Crook T (1982) The Global Deterioration Scale for assessment of primary degenerative dementia. *The American Journal of Psychiatry* 139(9):1136–1139.
6. Reisberg B (1988) Functional assessment staging (FAST). *Psychopharmacology Bulletin* 24(4):653.
7. Guerin O, Soto M, Brocker P, Robert P, Benoit M, Vellas B (2005) Nutritional status assessment during Alzheimer's disease: results after one year (the REAL French Study Group). *The Journal of Nutrition, Health & Aging* 9(2):81–84.
8. Alexander NB, Mollo J, Giordani B, Ashton-Miller J, Schultz A, Grunawalt J, et al. (1995) Maintenance of balance, gait patterns, and obstacle clearance in Alzheimer's disease. *Neurology* 45(5):908–914.
9. Feldman H, Woodward M (2005) The staging and assessment of moderate to severe Alzheimer disease. *Neurology* 65(6 Suppl 3):S10–S17.
10. Steffens DC, Maytan M, Helms MJ, Plassman BL (2005) Prevalence and clinical correlates of neuropsychiatric symptoms in dementia. *American Journal of Alzheimer's Disease and Other Dementias* 20(6):367–373.
11. Craig D, Mirakhur A, Hart DJ, McIlroy SP, Passmore AP (2005 Jun) A cross-sectional study of neuropsychiatric symptoms in 435 patients with Alzheimer's disease. *The American Journal of Geriatric Psychiatry* 13(6):460–468.
12. Fischer DC, Ladowsky-Brooks R, Millikin C, Norris M, Hansen K, Rourke S (2006) Neuropsychological functioning and delusions in dementia: a pilot study. *Aging & Mental Health* 10(1):27–32.

13. Mega MS, Cummings JL, Fiorello T, Gornbein J (1996) The spectrum of behavioral changes in Alzheimer's disease. *Neurology* 46(1):130–135.
14. Lovheim H, Sandman PO, Karlsson S, Gustafson Y (2008) Behavioral and psychological symptoms of dementia in relation to level of cognitive impairment. *International Psychogeriatrics* 20(4):777–789.
15. Chiu MJ, Chen TF, Yip PK, Hua MS, Tang LY (2006) Behavioral and psychologic symptoms in different types of dementia. *Journal of the Formosan Medical Association* 105(7):556–562.
16. Hughes CP, Berg L, Danziger WL, Coben LA, Martin RL (1982) A new clinical scale for the staging of dementia. *The British Journal of Psychiatry* 140(6):566–572.
17. Morris JC (1993) The Clinical Dementia Rating (CDR): current version and scoring rules. *Neurology* 43(11):2412–2414.
18. Gure TR, Kabeto MU, Plassman BL, Piette JD, Langa KM (2010) Differences in functional impairment across subtypes of dementia. *The Journals of Gerontology Series A: Biological Sciences and Medical Sciences* 65(4):434.
19. Waldemar G, Phung KTT, Burns A, Georges J, Hansen FR, Iliffe S, et al. (2007) Access to diagnostic evaluation and treatment for dementia in Europe. *International Journal of Geriatric Psychiatry* 22(1):47–54.
20. Fu C, Chute DJ, Farag ES, Garakian J, Cummings JL, Vinters HV (2004) Comorbidity in dementia. *Archives of Pathology & Laboratory Medicine* 128(1):32–38.
21. Waite A, Bebbington P, Skelton-Robinson M, Orrell M (2004) Life events, depression and social support in dementia. *The British Journal of Clinical Psychology* 43(3):313–324.
22. Gruffydd E, Randle J (2006) Alzheimer's disease and the psychosocial burden for caregivers. *Community Practitioner* 79(1):15–18.
23. Folstein MF, Folstein SE, McHugh PR (1975) *Mini-Mental State: A Practical Method for Grading the Cognitive State of Patients for the Clinician.* Oxford: Pergamon Press.
24. Sunderland T, Hill JL, Mellow AM, Lawlor BA (1989) Clock drawing in Alzheimer's disease: a novel measure of dementia severity. *Journal of the American Geriatrics Society* 37(8):725–729.
25. Shulman KI, Pushkar Gold D, Cohen CA, Zucchero CA (1993) Clock-drawing and dementia in the community: a longitudinal study. *International Journal of Geriatric Psychiatry* 8(6):487–496.
26. Katz S, Ford AB, Moskowitz RW, Jackson BA, Jaffe MW (1963) Studies of illness in the aged. *JAMA: The Journal of the American Medical Association* 185(12):914–919.
27. Lawton MP, Brody EM (1970) Assessment of older people: self-maintaining and instrumental activities of daily living. *Nursing Research* 19(3):278.
28. Galasko D, Bennett D, Sano M, Ernesto C, Thomas R, Grundman M, et al. (1997) An inventory to assess activities of daily living for clinical trials in Alzheimer's disease. The Alzheimer's Disease Cooperative Study. *Alzheimer Disease and Associated Disorders* 11:S33.
29. Galasko D, Edland S, Morris J, Clark C, Mohs R, Koss E (1995) The Consortium to Establish a Registry for Alzheimer's Disease (CERAD). Part XI. Clinical milestones in patients with Alzheimer's disease followed over 3 years. *Neurology* 45(8):1451–1455.
30. Andrieu S, Reynish W, Nourhashemi F, Ousset P, Grandjean H, Grand A, et al. (2001) Nutritional risk factors for institutional placement in Alzheimer's disease after one year follow-up. *Journal of Nutrition Health and Aging* 5(2):113–117.
31. Thomas P, Hazif-Thomas C, Clement J (2003) Influence of antidepressant therapies on weight and appetite in the elderly. *Journal of Nutrition Health and Aging* 7(3):166–171.
32. Guigoz Y, Lauque S, Vellas BJ (2002) Identifying the elderly at risk for malnutrition. The Mini Nutritional Assessment. *Clinics in Geriatric Medicine* 18(4):737.
33. Vellas B, Villars H, Abellan G, Soto M, Rolland Y, Guigoz Y, et al. (2006) Overview of the MNA®-Its history and challenges. *Journal of Nutrition Health and Aging* 10(6):456.
34. Kaiser M, Bauer J, Ramsch C, Uter W, Guigoz Y, Cederholm T, et al. (2009) Validation of the Mini Nutritional Assessment Short-Form (MNA®-SF): a practical tool for identification of nutritional status. *The Journal of Nutrition, Health & Aging* 13(9):782–788.
35. Ballard C, O'Brien J, James I, Mynt P, Lana M, Potkins D, et al. (2001) Quality of life for people with dementia living in residential and nursing home care: the impact of performance on activities of daily living, behavioral and psychological symptoms, language skills, and psychotropic drugs. *International Psychogeriatrics* 13(01):93–106.

36. Taylor DH, Schenkman M, Zhou J, Sloan FA (2001) The relative effect of Alzheimer's disease and related dementias, disability, and comorbidities on cost of care for elderly persons. *The Journals of Gerontology Series B: Psychological Sciences and Social Sciences* 56(5):S285–S293.

37. Blankevoort CG, van Heuvelen MJG, Boersma F, Luning H, de Jong J, Scherder EJA (2010) Review of effects of physical activity on strength, balance, mobility and ADL performance in elderly subjects with dementia. *Dementia and Geriatric Cognitive Disorders* 30(5):392–402.

38. Slaughter SE, Eliasziw M, Morgan D, Drummond N (2011) Incidence and predictors of excess disability in walking among nursing home residents with middle-stage dementia: a prospective cohort study. *International Psychogeriatrics* 23(1):54.

39. Mathias S, Nayak U, Isaacs B (1986) Balance in elderly patients: the 'get-up and go' test. *Archives of Physical Medicine and Rehabilitation* 67(6):387.

40. Podsiadlo D, Richardson S (1991) The timed 'Up & Go': a test of basic functional mobility for frail elderly persons. *Journal of the American Geriatrics Society* 39(2):142.

41. Finkel SI (2001) Behavioral and psychological symptoms of dementia: a current focus for clinicians, researchers, and caregivers. *The Journal of Clinical Psychiatry* 62(Suppl 21):3–6.

42. Bullock R, Hammond G (2003) Realistic expectations: the management of severe Alzheimer disease. *Alzheimer Disease & Associated Disorders* 17:S80–S85.

43. Sadik K, Wilcock G (2003) The increasing burden of Alzheimer disease. *Alzheimer Disease & Associated Disorders* 17:S75–S79.

44. Kilik LA, Hopkins RW, Day D, Prince CR, Prince PN, Rows C (2008) The progression of behavior in dementia: an in-office guide for clinicians. *American Journal of Alzheimer's Disease and Other Dementias* 23(3):242–249.

45. Cummings JL, Mega M, Gray K, Rosenberg-Thompson S, Carusi DA, Gornbein J (1994) The Neuropsychiatric Inventory comprehensive assessment of psychopathology in dementia. *Neurology* 44(12):2308.

46. Lee HB, Lyketsos CG (2003) Depression in Alzheimer's disease: heterogeneity and related issues. *Biological Psychiatry* 54(3):353.

47. Lyketsos CG, Steele C, Galik E, Rosenblatt A, Steinberg M, Warren A, et al. (1999) Physical aggression in dementia patients and its relationship to depression. *The American Journal of Psychiatry* 156(1):66–71.

48. Sheikh JI, Yesavage JA (1986) Geriatric Depression Scale (GDS): recent evidence and development of a shorter version. *Clinical Gerontologist: The Journal of Aging and Mental Health* 5:165–173.

49. Kodner DL (2006) Whole-system approaches to health and social care partnerships for the frail elderly: an exploration of North American models and lessons. *Health & Social Care in the Community* 14(5):384–390.

50. Onega LL (2006) Assessment of psychoemotional and behavioral status in patients with dementia. *The Nursing Clinics of North America* 41(1):23.

51. Zarit SH, Leitsch SA (2001) Developing and evaluating community based intervention programs for Alzheimer's patients and their caregivers. *Aging & Mental Health* 5(S1):84–98.

52. Georges J, Jansen S, Jackson J, Meyrieux A, Sadowska A, Selmes M (2008) Alzheimer's disease in real life–the dementia carer's survey. *International Journal of Geriatric Psychiatry* 23(5):546–551.

53. Zarit SH, Reever KE, Bach-Peterson J (1980) Relatives of the impaired elderly: correlates of feelings of burden. *The Gerontologist* 20(6):649–655.

54. Ankri J, Andrieu S, Beaufils B, Grand A, Henrard JC (2005) Beyond the global score of the Zarit Burden Interview: useful dimensions for clinicians. *International Journal of Geriatric Psychiatry* 20(3): 254–260.

55. Hébert R, Bravo G, Préville M (2000) Reliability, validity and reference values of the Zarit Burden Interview for assessing informal caregivers of community-dwelling older persons with dementia. *Canadian Journal on Aging/La Revue canadienne du vieillissement* 19(04):494–507.

56. Robinson BC (1983) Validation of a caregiver strain index. *Journal of Gerontology* 38(3):344–348.

57. Prince MJ, Acosta D, Castro-Costa E, Jackson J, Shaji K (2009) Packages of care for dementia in low-and middle-income countries. *PLoS Medicine* 6(11):e1000176.

58. Kitwood T (2004) Person and process in dementia. *International Journal of Geriatric Psychiatry* 8(7):541–545.

59. Younger D, Martin GW (2000) Dementia care mapping: an approach to quality audit of services for people with dementia in two health districts. *Journal of Advanced Nursing* 32(5):1206–1212.
60. Bamford C, Bruce E (2000) Defining the outcomes of community care: the perspectives of older people with dementia and their carers. *Ageing and Society* 20(5):543–570.
61. Scotland NHS (2004) Framework for mental health services in Scotland: section 3: service profiles, services for people with dementia. Available at: http://www.show.scot.nhs.uk/publications/mental_health_services/mhs/Framework%20Document.pdf (last accessed on 27 February 2012.
62. Aneshensel CS, Pearlin LI, Mullan JT, Zarit SH, Whitlatch CJ (1995) *Profiles in Caregiving: The Unexpected Career.* San Diego, CA: Academic Press.
63. Mittelman MS, Haley WE, Clay OJ, Roth DL (2006) Improving caregiver well-being delays nursing home placement of patients with Alzheimer disease. *Neurology* 67(9):1592–1599.
64. Brookmeyer R, Johnson E, Ziegler-Graham K, Arrighi HM (2007) Forecasting the global burden of Alzheimer's disease. *Alzheimer's and Dementia* 3(3):186–191.
65. Association AM (1999) *Diagnosis, Management and Treatment of Dementia: A Practical Guide for Primary Care Physicians.* Chicago, IL: AMA Press.
66. Farlow MR, Miller ML, Pejovic V (2008) Treatment options in Alzheimer's disease: maximizing benefit, managing expectations. *Dementia and Geriatric Cognitive Disorders* 25(5):408–422.
67. Callahan CM, Boustani MA, Unverzagt FW, Austrom MG, Damush TM, Perkins AJ, et al. (2006) Effectiveness of collaborative care for older adults with Alzheimer disease in primary care. *JAMA: The Journal of the American Medical Association* 295(18):2148–2157.
68. Teshuva K, Laurence B, Nelms L, Johnson V, Foreman P, Stanley J (2007) Outcomes for Older People with Chronic and Complex Needs: A Longitudinal Examination of the Use of Community Services Following an Aged Care Assessment in Victoria: Brotherhood of St Laurence.
69. Fortinsky RH, Unson CG, Garcia RI (2002) Helping family caregivers by linking primary care physicians with community-based dementia care services. *Dementia* 1(2):227–240.
70. Banerjee S, Willis R, Matthews D, Contell F, Chan J, Murray J (2007) Improving the quality of care for mild to moderate dementia: an evaluation of the Croydon Memory Service Model. *International Journal of Geriatric Psychiatry* 22(8):782–788.
71. Vernooij-Dassen M, Olde Rikkert MGM (2004) Personal disease management in dementia care. *International Journal of Geriatric Psychiatry* 19(8):715–717.
72. Williams I (2000) What help do GPs want from specialist services in managing patients with dementia? *International Journal of Geriatric Psychiatry* 15(8):758–761.
73. Dupuis SL, Gillies J, Carson J, Whyte C, Genoe R, Loiselle L, et al. (2012) Moving beyond patient and client approaches: mobilizing 'authentic partnerships' in dementia care, support and services. *Dementia* 11(4):427–452.
74. Gwyther LP (1997) The perspective of the person with Alzheimer disease: which outcomes matter in early to middle stages of dementia? *Alzheimer Disease and Associated Disorders* 11(6):18–24.
75. Nolan M, Ryan T, Enderby P, Reid D (2002) Towards a more inclusive vision of dementia care practice and research. *Dementia* 1(2):193–211.
76. Eng C, Pedulla J, Eleazer GP, McCann R, Fox N (1997) Program of All-inclusive Care for the Elderly (PACE): an innovative model of integrated geriatric care and financing. *Journal of the American Geriatrics Society* 45(2):223–232.
77. Bergman H, Béland F, Lebel P, Contandriopoulos AP, Tousignant P, Brunelle Y, et al. (1997) Care for Canada's frail elderly population: fragmentation or integration? *Canadian Medical Association Journal* 157(8):1116–1121.
78. Hébert R, Durand PJ, Dubuc N, Tourigny A (2003) PRISMA: a new model of integrated service delivery for the frail older people in Canada. *International Journal of Integrated Care* 3 Epub 18 March 2003.:e08.
79. Schols J, Crebolder H, Van Weel C (2004) Nursing home and nursing home physician: the Dutch experience. *Journal of the American Medical Directors Association* 5(3):207–212.
80. van der Eerden WJ, Jones GMM (2011) Dutch large-scale dementia-care environments: a village within the community. *Journal of Care Services Management* 5(3):137–146.
81. Hertogh C, Deerenberg-Kessler W, Ribbe M (1996) The problem-oriented multidisciplinary approach in Dutch nursing home care. *Clinical Rehabilitation* 10(2):135–142.

82. Pinquart M, Sorensen S (2006) Helping caregivers of persons with dementia: which interventions work and how large are their effects? *International Psychogeriatrics* 18(4):577–596.

83. Gaugler JE, Kane RL, Kane RA, Newcomer R (2005) Early community-based service utilization and its effects on institutionalization in dementia caregiving. *The Gerontologist* 45(2):177–185.

84. Teri L, McCurry SM, Logsdon R, Gibbons LE (2005) Training community consultants to help family members improve dementia care: a randomized controlled trial. *The Gerontologist* 45(6):802–811.

85. Teri L, Gibbons LE, McCurry SM, Logsdon RG, Buchner DM, Barlow WE, et al. (2003) Exercise plus behavioral management in patients with Alzheimer disease. *JAMA: The Journal of the American Medical Association* 290(15):2015–2022.

86. Graff MJL, Vernooij-Dassen MJM, Thijssen M, Dekker J, Hoefnagels WHL, Rikkert MGM (2006) Community based occupational therapy for patients with dementia and their care givers: randomised controlled trial. *British Medical Journal* 333(7580):1196.

87. Hébert R, Lévesque L, Vézina J, Lavoie JP, Ducharme F, Gendron C, et al. (2003) Efficacy of a psychoeducative group program for caregivers of demented persons living at home. *The Journals of Gerontology Series B: Psychological Sciences and Social Sciences* 58(1):S58–S67.

88. Briller S, Calkins MP (2000) Defining place-based models of care: conceptualizing care settings as home, resort, or hospital. *Alzheimer's Care Quarterly* 1(1):17–23.

89. Finnema E, Dröes RM, Ribbe M, van Tilburg W (2000) A review of psychosocial models in psychogeriatrics: implications for care and research. *Alzheimer Disease & Associated Disorders* 14(2):68.

90. Boult C, Green AF, Boult LB, Pacala JT, Snyder C, Leff B (2009) Successful models of comprehensive care for older adults with chronic conditions: evidence for the Institute of Medicine's 'Retooling for an Aging America' report. *Journal of the American Geriatrics Society* 57(12):2328–2337.

91. Tibaldi V, Aimonino N, Ponzetto M, Stasi M, Amati D, Raspo S, et al. (2004) A randomized controlled trial of a home hospital intervention for frail elderly demented patients: behavioral disturbances and caregiver's stress. *Archives of Gerontology and Geriatrics* 38:431–436.

92. Stuck AE, Siu AL, Wieland GD, Rubenstein L, Adams J (1993) Comprehensive geriatric assessment: a meta-analysis of controlled trials. *The Lancet* 342(8878):1032–1036.

93. Landefeld CS, Palmer RM, Kresevic DM, Fortinsky RH, Kowal J (1995) A randomized trial of care in a hospital medical unit especially designed to improve the functional outcomes of acutely ill older patients. *New England Journal of Medicine* 332(20):1338–1344.

94. Counsell SR, Holder CM, Liebenauer LL, Palmer RM, Fortinsky RH, Kresevic DM, et al. (2000) Effects of a multicomponent intervention on functional outcomes and process of care in hospitalized older patients: a randomized controlled trial of Acute Care for Elders (ACE) in a community hospital. *Journal of the American Geriatrics Society* 48(12):1572.

95. Hickman L, Newton P, Halcomb EJ, Chang E, Davidson P (2007) Best practice interventions to improve the management of older people in acute care settings: a literature review. *Journal of Advanced Nursing* 60(2):113–126.

96. Flaherty JH, Tariq SH, Raghavan S, Bakshi S, Moinuddin A, Morley JE (2003) A model for managing delirious older inpatients. *Journal of the American Geriatrics Society* 51(7):1031–1035.

97. Coleman EA, Parry C, Chalmers S, Min SJ (2006) The care transitions intervention: results of a randomized controlled trial. *Archives of Internal Medicine* 166(17):1822.

98. Gauthier S, Feldman H, Hecker J, Vellas B, Ames D, Subbiah P, et al. (2002) Efficacy of donepezil on behavioral symptoms in patients with moderate to severe Alzheimer's disease. *International Psychogeriatrics* 14(4):389–404.

Chapter 7

Services for people with severe dementia

Betty S. Black[a], and Peter V. Rabins[b]

[a]Department of Psychiatry and Behavioral Sciences, the Johns Hopkins University School of Medicine and the Johns Hopkins Berman Institute of Bioethics, Johns Hopkins Hospital, USA
[b]Department of Psychiatry and Behavioral Sciences, the Johns Hopkins University School of Medicine and the Johns Hopkins Berman Institute of Bioethics, Johns Hopkins Hospital, USA

A typical person with onset of Alzheimer's disease (AD) at age 70 will spend the last four of the next 10 years in the severe stage of dementia [1]. This individual will require an array of services to address the complexity of her needs and those of her family caregivers. Those needs relate to a complex array of cognitive and functional impairments, psychiatric and behavioural disturbances and medical co-morbidities. The severity of dementia-related symptoms influences decisions about what care setting is best suited for the individual, determines the level of assistance that is required for daily functioning, suggests the types of therapeutic interventions that may improve the person's quality of life and that of their caregiver, affects how treatment decisions are made, and is related to caregiver burdens and needs.

Characteristics of persons with severe dementia

Severe dementia is the late or advanced stage of primary or secondary dementia, regardless of its aetiology [2]. Since progression of dementia is on a continuum, there is variability in the characteristics of those who reach the severe stage of dementia, and there is no single validated definition of severe or advanced dementia. Instead, clinical rating scales are commonly used operationally to define the stages of dementia, but these nominal scales vary in the domains they include [3]. The most widely used dementia staging tools are the Clinical Dementia Rating (CDR) [4,5] and the Functional Assessment Staging (FAST) [6]. Table 7.1 illustrates the differences in how these two measures characterise individuals who meet scale criteria for severe dementia. While the extended CDR [7,8] includes stages 3–5 that define respectively severe dementia, profound dementia and terminal dementia, the FAST categories of 6a-7e define moderately severe and severe dementia.

An alternative approach to identifying individuals with severe dementia relies on global measures of cognitive function, such as the Mini-Mental State Examination (MMSE) [9]. Individuals with MMSE scores of 10 or below on this 30-point measure are often considered to have severe dementia. However, the MMSE has a floor effect when communication abilities are severely affected. While the Severe Impairment Battery (SIB) [10]) has been used in drug trials, the Test for Severe Impair-

Designing and Delivering Dementia Services, First Edition. Edited by Hugo de Waal, Constantine Lyketsos, David Ames, and John O'Brien.

Table 7.1 Clinical staging of severe dementia based on CDR and FAST criteria

Clinical Dementia Rating (CDR) scale extended version[a]	Functional Assessment Staging of Alzheimer's disease (FAST)[c]
0 – None	1 – Normal adult
0.5 – Questionable dementia	2 – Normal older adult
1 – Mild dementia	3 – Early dementia
2 – Moderate dementia	4 – Mild dementia
3 – Severe dementia	5 – Moderate dementia
Memory – severe memory loss; only fragments remain	6 – Moderately severe dementia
Orientation – oriented to person only	Difficulty putting clothing on properly without assistance
Judgment and problem-solving – unable to make judgments or solve problems	Unable to bathe properly (e.g. difficulty adjusting bath water temperature) occasionally or more frequently over the past week
Community affairs – no pretence of independent function outside home; appears too ill to be taken to functions outside a family home	Inability to handle mechanics of toileting (e.g. forgets to flush the toilet, does not wipe properly or properly dispose of toilet tissue) occasionally or more frequently over the past weeks
Home and hobbies – no significant function in home	
Personal care – requires much help with personal care; frequent incontinence	Urinary incontinence, occasional or more frequent
4 – Profoundly demented[b]	Faecal incontinence, occasional or more frequently over the past week
Speech unintelligible or irrelevant	7 – Severe dementia
Unable to follow simple instructions or comprehend commands	Ability to speak limited to approximately a half dozen different words or fewer, in the course of an average day or in the course of an intensive interview
Only occasionally recognise spouse or caregiver	Speech ability limited to the use of a single intelligible word in an average day or in the course of an interview (the person may repeat the word over and over)
Uses fingers more than utensils or requires much assistance to eat	
Frequently incontinent	Ambulatory ability lost (cannot walk without personal assistance)
Usually chair-bound	
Rarely out of their residence	Ability to sit up without assistance lost [e.g. the individual will fall over if there are no lateral rests (arms) on the chair]
Limb movements often purposeless	
5 – Terminal dementia[b]	
Shows no comprehension or recognition	Loss of the ability to smile
Needs to be fed or has tube feedings	
Totally incontinent	
Bedridden	

[a]Hughes et al. (1982) [4]; Morris (1993) [3].
[b]Criteria specified by Dooneief et al. (1996) [8].
[c]Reisberg (1988) [6].

ment (TSI) [11] and Severe Impairment Rating Scale (SIRS) [12] are more user friendly and have been developed specifically to assess individuals with advanced dementia. For individuals in long-term care (LTC) settings, the severity of dementia can be determined using the Cognitive Performance Scale (CPS), derived from the Minimum Data Set (MDS) [13]. The MDS is a standardised comprehensive assessment instrument used in all licensed LTC facilities in the USA. CPS groups individuals based on five MDS items into one of seven categories (0–6), with category 5 reflecting severe impairment and 6 indicating very severe impairment with eating problems [14].

While memory impairment is one of the first indicators of most causes of dementia (excluding fronto-temporal dementia), by the severe stage of dementia, all cognitive systems are affected to a significant extent [15]. In their review, Boller and colleagues note that memory of one's own past (episodic memory) and linguistic and general knowledge (semantic memory) are profoundly impaired in advanced dementia [15]. Short-term memory (e.g. recalling a very limited number of items in a very limited time period), some aspects of implicit memory that enable one to perform a task without conscious awareness and over learned skills or habits, may be relatively spared until the late stages of dementia.

Cognitive and functional impairments are primary indicators of disease severity. In advanced dementia, language disturbances (*aphasia*) are common. These include difficulties in understanding others and in making oneself understood, and manifest as severe loss of fluency, echolalia, palilalia (verbal perseverations) and non-verbal utterances (e.g. groaning or single nonsense syllables) [15]. These impairments can interfere with the person's ability to make even the most basic needs known and lead to misunderstanding or misinterpreting care interventions and the precipitation of catastrophic reactions [16]. Individuals may retain the rhythm, intonation and gestures of speech (prosody) after they lose the ability to communicate with words [17]. When individuals with advanced dementia can no longer understand words, they may still respond to and return non-verbal communication through facial expressions and gestures. *Agnosia* (failure to recognise or identify objects, people, sounds, shapes and smells) can interfere with daily activities and social interactions. For example, some individuals may be unable to recognise themselves in a mirror or recognise their caregivers and as a result become uncooperative [17]. Impaired ability to carry out motor function (*apraxia*) results in the need for support with basic activities of daily living (ADLs) (e.g. dressing, bathing and toileting), including assistance with eating. Even the basic abilities of chewing and swallowing can be impaired with extreme apraxia [16]. Persons with advanced dementia are frequently, and often totally, incontinent due to impaired cortical control mechanisms of bladder and bowel function [18].

Neuropsychiatric symptoms (NPS) that occur in severe dementia include psychomotor disorders (e.g. pacing and agitation), psychiatric symptoms (e.g. hallucinations, delusions, depression and anxiety) and psychobehavioural disorders (e.g. aggressiveness, inappropriate shouting/screaming and sleep disturbances) [15,19]. NPS are distressing to those with dementia and their caregivers, are associated with lower quality of life [20,21], and often contribute to decisions to place individuals in nursing homes [22].

Severe dementia is associated with motor disorders and neurological signs, such as Parkinsonism and myoclonus [15]. Gait impairment, poor balance and difficulty transferring (moving from one place to another) put individuals with severe dementia at high risk of falling [17]. Ultimately, many individuals with severe dementia lose the ability to maintain upright posture and are at risk of becoming bedridden. This further predisposes to developing contractures, decubitus ulcers and infections [15,16]. Pneumonia, often resulting from aspiration associated with swallowing difficulties, is the most common cause of death in dementia [23].

Settings of care

Individuals with severe dementia may reside and receive care in their own homes or those of family caregivers in the community, in residential care or assisted living (RC/AL) facilities or in nursing homes. Estimating the prevalence of severe dementia in these care settings is challenging because of differences across studies in demographics, subjects' length of survival, study location, sociocultural factors, whether both community-residing individuals and institutional residents are included in a sample, and how severe dementia is defined and identified. In addition, some studies do not distinguish between individuals with moderate and severe dementia.

While the majority of people who have dementia in all stages are cared for in the community [24], only a minority of individuals with severe dementia receive community-based care because of their extensive needs for support. For example, the Canadian Study of Health and Aging [25] found that 0.4% of individuals age 65 and older living in the community had severe dementia. Studies of community residents who have dementia have found that 25–32% of those with dementia were considered to be in the severe stage of illness [26,27]. In one community-based sample, 20% of all persons with any diagnosis of dementia progressed to having a MMSE $\leq$ 10 or a CDR = 3 [28]. This translates to more than one million individuals with severe dementia in the USA.

Most of the care given to community-residing people with dementia is provided by family members and other unpaid carers [24]. As dementia progresses, the likelihood of placement in a residential facility or skilled nursing home increases. For example, Knopman and colleagues found that community-residing persons with dementia who participated in the Alzheimer's Disease Cooperative Study and reached the stage of severe dementia were eight times more likely to be institutionalised than those who remained in the moderate stage [29]. However, the range of factors that influence institutional placement include caregiver variables (e.g. perception of burden, health status, symptoms of depression and relationship to patient), patient variables (e.g. behavioural problems, incontinence, aggressive behaviour and severity of dementia) and other variables (e.g. income, use of services and support network) [18].

Dementia is common in RC/AL facilities in the USA. For example, the Maryland Assisted Living study found that 68% of participating residents had dementia [30]. However, the prevalence of severe dementia in these settings is less clear. The Collaborative Studies of Long-Term Care, which included a random sample of RC/AL facilities and nursing homes in four US states, reported that 29% of RC/AL residents with dementia met criteria for moderate to severe dementia (i.e. required physical assistance with one or more ADLs) [31]. After 1 year, 25% of the RC/AL residents with moderate to severe dementia required a higher level of care and were discharged to nursing homes, settings that are better able to manage major medical care needs.

In US nursing homes, 60–80% of residents suffer from dementia [17], with an estimated 41% (ranging from 29% to 61%) having moderate to severe dementia [24]. The Canadian Study of Health and Aging found that 31% of persons 65 or older who lived in institutions had severe dementia [25]. Nursing homes are often the final setting of care. In fact, approximately 70% of people who die from dementia do so in nursing homes [32]. A small proportion (5%) of nursing home residents with dementia are cared for in dementia special care (DSC) units of nursing homes [24]. While DSC units may be better able to care for individuals who have serious behavioural impairments, there is no convincing evidence that these specialised settings of care are necessary for providing an appropriate level of care for those with advanced dementia [17].

Much of what is known about individuals with severe dementia comes from studies of nursing home (NH) residents, such as CASCADE [33] and CareAD [34]. NH residents with dementia suffer from a high prevalence of co-morbid illnesses, including skin problems (95%), nutrition and hydration problems (85%), gastrointestinal problems (81%), febrile episodes (51%), and pneumonia (41%) [33,34]. In addition, people with advanced dementia are likely to be suffering from other chronic health conditions prevalent in older adults (e.g. arthritis, coronary heart disease, diabetes, congestive heart failure, cancer or Parkinson's disease) [35]. Given these prevalent co-morbidities pain is common in severe dementia but the presence of severe aphasia increases the risk that it will be unrecognised. In CareAD, 63% of NH residents with advanced dementia had staff-identified pain [34], but because the identification of pain by the staff was significantly associated with higher resident cognitive function, those with more severe cognitive impairment may have been at greater risk of unrecognised pain. Distressing pain and dyspnea increase as death approaches [36].

Regardless of where individuals with severe dementia reside, they are at high risk of admission to an emergency department (ED) or general hospital ward [33,37,38]. For example, in a comparison of persons with advanced dementia receiving community-based care versus NH care 44% of NH residents and 32% of those receiving home care were admitted to the hospital prior to death [37].

In the CareAD study, 44% of NH residents with advanced dementia were transferred at least once to the ED or to hospital during the 6 months before death [38], with 12% transferred more than once. Transfers to hospital in advanced dementia are often due to pulmonary problems (e.g. pneumonia) or urinary tract infections [38,39]. While transfer to hospital may be needed in a minority of cases to reduce physical suffering (e.g. due to a fracture), transferring individuals with severe dementia to hospital can be burdensome and may be of limited benefit [33].

Care and management of symptoms and co-morbidities in severe dementia

As the earlier descriptions of people with severe dementia suggest, the care and management of their symptoms involve a complexity of social, environmental, neuropsychiatric and medical interventions that consider the setting of care and the individual's likely proximity to death. Despite the severity of illness, interventions are available that can have a positive effect on symptoms, functioning and quality of life. However, as Tariot suggests:

> 'A balance must be struck between aggressive intervention and palliative care, continued treatment and withdrawal of medication, patient benefit and caregiver burden'. [18, p. S305]

Cognitive symptoms

Memantine has been approved for the treatment of severe AD in many jurisdictions, and donepezil has been approved for the treatment of severe dementia in the USA. While memantine was associated with a lower decline in ADLs in moderate to severe AD patients [40] and donepezil had a beneficial effect on SIB and ADL scores [41], further study is needed to identify the optimum use of cholinesterase inhibitors and memantine in advanced dementia and to determine the effects on patient outcomes of withdrawing these medications [42]. The benefit of anti-Parkinson's medications on cognition likely extends to persons with severe dementia, but this is not well studied.

Function and engagement

Individuals with severe dementia are partially or fully dependent on others for all of the basic ADLs (ambulation, dressing, bathing, grooming, toileting, transferring and eating). In general, individuals with severe dementia who reside in nursing homes have greater functional impairment than those who receive home-based care [37]. However, it is as important to recognise and support an individual's preserved functions, as it is to provide needed assistance with impaired functions in order to preserve individual dignity [17].

Continued residence at home for people with severe dementia requires 24-hour, 7 days-per-week care and depends on the support of highly committed informal caregivers (e.g. family members and/or friends), usually with additional support from paid individuals (e.g. personal and home care aides and nursing assistants). To provide this level of care successfully, informal and formal home-based care providers need training in how to manage and assist with basic ADLs, provide structure and meaningful daily activities, use exercise and range-of-motion techniques, manage behavioural problems, and modify the home environment to maximise safety and quality of life for the person with dementia and the caregiver. Occupational and physical therapists can provide valuable consultation, advice and training. The COPE randomised trial found that a 4-month training programme for caregivers by an occupational therapist and advanced practice nurse significantly improved the caregivers' well-being and the engagement of the person with dementia [43]. Family caregivers may also benefit from the services of a geriatric case manager or dementia care coordinator in helping to identify unmet needs and in coordinating health care, psychological care and home care services, as well as financial and legal planning. Providing home-based care requires the support of healthcare providers, such as nurses and physicians trained in geriatric medicine or geriatric psychiatry, to manage the complex medical co-morbidities and neuropsychiatric symptoms associated with advanced dementia.

One of the most challenging transitions that many people with dementia and their families face is the move from home-based care to a residential care facility, particularly a nursing home [44]. While nursing homes have traditionally had more of the 'look and feel' of a hospital than of a home, this is changing, with greater emphasis on person-centred care [45] and recognition that the physical environment has a significant impact on the person with dementia, their visiting family and friends, as well as the care providers who work in these facilities [46]. The 'culture change' movement is an effort to transform nursing homes from healthcare institutions to person-centred homes that provide LTC services [47]. This movement emphasises choice for residents, a homelike atmosphere, close relationships between residents, family members and staff, staff empowerment, collaborative decision-making and a quality improvement process.

Margaret Calkins, with degrees in psychology and architecture, outlines a set of therapeutic goals or user needs that have been derived over the past two decades by environment-behaviour researchers in relation to the care of persons with dementia in LTC settings [48]. These needs include: support for ADLs, aesthetics, affective experience, increased personalisation, autonomy, privacy, stimulation, safety and security, orientation, and socialisation. For example, different aspects of the environment may have an impact on the psychological and emotional states of the residents. Large rooms with poor acoustics and potentially multiple groups of people moving about in the space may be overstimulating and cause anxiety or distress for a person with severe dementia. Likewise, the environment may facilitate or discourage social contact and interaction. For NH residents with severe dementia, human contact may be all that can be expected and interaction does not necessarily imply verbalisation [48]. Nursing homes are increasingly moving away from the concept of 'units' housing large numbers of residents, to those of 'households' or 'neighbourhoods' in which fewer people reside. The spaces and layout of rooms can be designed, furnished and lighted to better accommodate the needs and limitations of persons with dementia, and inviting outdoor spaces provide additional opportunities for sensory stimulation, socialisation and meaningful activity in a safe and secure environment.

Engagement has been defined as the act of being occupied or involved with an external stimulus, such as concrete objects, activities and other persons [49]. In a sample of nursing home residents with severe dementia, Cohen-Mansfield and colleagues found that a variety of different stimuli (e.g. live human social stimuli, simulated social stimuli, music, a reading stimulus and inanimate social stimuli) significantly increased engagement and that level of engagement was associated with personal attributes (e.g. cognitive function), environmental factors (e.g. sound and lighting) and characteristics of the stimulus (e.g. one-on-one interaction) [49]. Such stimuli, particularly in an environment with moderate noise levels, can have an observable impact on pleasure in persons with advanced dementia [50]. These findings suggest that being occupied and involved has a positive influence on the well-being of individuals even in advanced dementia.

Neuropsychiatric symptoms (NPS)

Few studies of treatment efficacy have analysed outcomes specifically in persons with NPS and severe dementia, but many studies of NPS include a number of persons with severe dementia. For example, Gitlin et al. found that the Advancing Caregiver Training (ACT) programme, which relies on occupational therapists to help families manage distressing behaviours, significantly improved behavioural symptoms and caregiver well-being [51]. Activities tailored to the capabilities of the individual can benefit both the person with dementia and the caregiver [52]. Studies of behaviour therapy-based treatments targeting common behaviours, such as calling out [53] and treatment trials of music therapy [54], suggest that many non-pharmacological therapies are likely to improve NPS, but further studies are needed to conclude this with confidence. A review of studies, which evaluated the effect of non-pharmacological interventions on neuropsychiatric symptoms in advanced dementia, found limited moderate to high-quality evidence for the use of sensory-focused strategies, including aromatherapy, preferred or live music, and multisensory stimulation [55]. While the evidence is still limited, non-pharmacological interventions should be the first-line approach for NPS in severe dementia.

Similarly, few studies of pharmacological interventions targeting NPS have been designed to study only persons with severe dementia. However, the modest efficacy of anti-psychotic neuroleptic drugs in treating agitation and delusions in persons with dementia, combined with the increased risk of mortality and falls in persons treated with these drugs, suggests that pharmacological treatment of NPS should be limited to situations in which the risk of adverse outcomes due to NPS is significant and non-pharmacological interventions have failed. Use of psychotropic medications should be limited to the lowest effective dose for the shortest time [18]. Some NPS (e.g. agitation) may be due to other pathologies (e.g. urinary retention, impaction, pneumonia and pain), which should be ruled out before pursuing other interventions [15]. For example, the systematic treatment of pain can significantly reduce agitation in persons with moderate to severe dementia [56]. There are no trials of antidepressant efficacy for major depression that include only individuals with severe dementia, but the lack of convincing evidence of their effectiveness in individuals with dementia of milder severity has led some to recommend against their use [57]. However, our clinical experience suggests efficacy in some patients.

Medical co-morbidities

Severe dementia increases the risk of malnutrition, dehydration, skin problems and infections [34]. Careful monitoring and early intervention would seem likely to lessen adverse outcomes, but there is little empirical evidence to support this widely held belief. Because dementia is a major risk factor for delirium, the treatment of coexisting medical illness requires careful selection of medication dosage and monitoring of side effects. The minimum effective dose of all medications and cautious monitoring of oral intake and electrolytes should lessen the risk of an adverse outcome. The high prevalence of impaired communication (aphasia) means that regular assessments of level of consciousness and pain are particularly important, since pain often goes undetected and undertreated [58]. While there is limited evidence of the psychometric quality and clinical utility of existing tools, current findings support the use of the PAINAD (Pain Assessment in Advanced Dementia) for daily assessment and the PACSLAC (Pain Assessment Checklist for Seniors with Limited Ability to Communicate) as a longer interval assessment tool [59].

Ethical issues in severe dementia

A range of ethical issues arises for families and care providers over the course of dementia including in the final stages of these illnesses. Ideally, the physician should disclose the diagnosis and need for long term planning while the patient has the capacity to engage. Early in the illness the individual is usually capable of expressing wishes regarding issues, such as involvement in dementia research and preferences for end-of-life care and can implement advance directives, unless illness denial is present. Physicians and healthcare professionals, such as social workers and advanced practice nurses, can present scenarios of common difficult issues that require thoughtful decision-making: this may assist persons with dementia and their families in identifying prior wishes and/ or values of the person with dementia. Such decisions should consider potential burdens and benefits that the alternatives would have on both the person with dementia and their caregivers. Addressing these issues at an early stage may help in resolving some ethical challenges that families face when the individual no longer has the capacity to participate.

Balancing the person's autonomy with her safety and best interests, as well as with the interests of caregivers, may become more difficult with the gradual loss of cognitive and functional capacity. In severe dementia, deprivation of liberty occurs whether the individual is living in the community, in a form of assisted living or in a nursing home. Nevertheless, the goal should be to allow the individual as much freedom of choice in daily activities as possible while ensuring the individual's safety and well-being regardless of the setting. For example, environmental modifications should be made so that individuals who still have the ability to ambulate are free to walk and wander in safe areas, since walking may be an important means of lessening stress or agitation. Restraints (physical or chemical) should not be used as substitutes for environmental, social and activity modifications [57]. Physical restraints can result in unnecessary immobility, are likely to cause functional decline, incontinence and pressure ulcers, are frequently hazardous when someone seeks freedom, and violate the dignity of the individual [60].

Administering medications to individuals with advanced dementia can pose challenges for care providers if an individual who lacks decisional capacity is refusing (i.e. dissenting) to take medication. Haw and Stubbs [61] suggest that covert administration of medication is only appropriate in patients who lack capacity to consent, following a discussion with the multidisciplinary team, relatives and caregivers regarding the individual's best interests and then only if medication is necessary. They note the importance of consulting a pharmacist if a proposed plan is to crush tablets or open capsules and of documenting the care plan.

The care of individuals with severe dementia often leads to decision points in which the alternatives are to provide aggressive medical interventions or comfort measures. Examples are whether to use surgery, artificial feeding, antibiotic treatment or to transfer to a higher level of care, such as an ED or hospital. It is important to acknowledge that progressive dementia is a terminal illness and that in advanced dementia the individual has a limited remaining lifespan, even though prognostication remains challenging in dementia. Decisions about initiating or withdrawing treatments should be based on the goals of care [36]. The CASCADE study showed that most healthcare proxies, advocating for nursing home residents with advanced dementia, believe that comfort is the primary goal of care [33]. The occurrence of eating problems, infections (e.g. pneumonia) and dyspnea suggest that the end of life is near [33]. Assisted oral feeding is advised for eating problems given that there is no evidence that tube feeding prolongs survival, prevents aspiration pneumonia or helps heal pressure ulcers, and its risks are substantial [62]. It remains unclear whether the use of antibiotics can meaningfully extend life or improve comfort in individuals with end-stage dementia, and hospitalisation near the end-of-life can be traumatic and may be of limited benefit [36]. Therefore, infections and co-morbidities of dementia should be treated in the LTC setting as much as possible to prevent the risks associated with transitions to acute care facilities [63].

A palliative approach to care management can help prevent unnecessary suffering for individuals with advanced dementia [64]. Palliative care, which focuses on relieving pain and suffering and maximising quality of life, is a broader concept than hospice-based care, is not dependent on prognosis and does not exclude all disease-modifying therapies if a treatment is the best method to reduce discomfort. The Center to Advance Palliative Care has identified four models of integration of palliative care into nursing homes [65]:

1. palliative care consultation service
2. nursing home services integrated palliative care

3. hospice-based consultation service
4. hospice care.

For individuals in the USA who are eligible for Medicare hospice benefits (i.e. certified by a physician to have six months or less to live), hospice providers can bring an interdisciplinary approach to end-of-life care for people with dementia and their families. Based on survey data from family members of persons who died with dementia, Teno and colleagues found that those who received hospice care reported fewer unmet needs, higher quality of care, and better quality of dying than those without hospice services [66]. They concluded that both access to hospice services and timely enrolment into a hospice are important to quality end-of-life care.

Support for caregivers of people with severe dementia

A fundamental principle of caring for people with dementia is that the patient and family are a unit [18]. By the time an individual reaches the severe stage of dementia, a family caregiver has usually spent years assisting the person with dementia, coordinating healthcare needs, coping with and managing behavioural problems, and serving as the person's advocate and proxy decision-maker. Given the substantial burden imposed on family caregivers, their need for supportive services exists over the entire course of the illness (regardless of the settings of care) and continues after the death of the person with dementia. A fundamental source of support for caregivers is a steadfast, knowledgeable physician who can provide guidance, education and emotional support, and is able to refer to specialty care providers and allied health professionals as needed, but knowledgeable non-physicians can play an equally important role.

For families who are caring for persons with severe dementia in the community, caregiver skills counselling may provide the necessary knowledge and skills. Respite care can provide temporary time away from the person with dementia and enable the caregiver to attend to his or her own needs. These periodic breaks may enable the caregiver to continue providing home-based care if that is desired and is in the best interests of the person with dementia and caregiver.

Regardless of where the person with dementia lives, family caregivers have an ongoing need for dementia-related education and emotional support. Organisations, such as Alzheimer's Disease International or local Alzheimer's Associations, are important resources for caregivers. In many countries, they provide a range of resources, which may include educational information, support groups, a 24-hour help line, and information on research and clinical trials. Over time, caring for a person with dementia can impose a heavy toll on the physical and mental health of family caregivers. All too often caregivers neglect their own needs until they reach their own healthcare crisis. It is important for caregivers to see their own personal physician on a regular basis to address their healthcare needs. Given the emotional strain, losses, risk of depression, and anticipatory grief associated with the experience of having a loved one who is suffering from dementia, some caregivers may need to obtain emotional support or mental health care from a mental health professional.

The death of the person with dementia may mark the end of a long journey for family caregivers. However, the pattern of grief for some caregivers is prolonged, beginning prior to and lasting for months or more after the loved one's death. The CASCADE study found that the most common symptoms of grief among family members of nursing home residents who died with dementia were feelings of separation and yearning [67]. Caregivers may benefit from bereavement services that are offered by hospice programmes, hospitals, self-help organisation and support groups. Factors associated with the use of bereavement services among dementia caregivers include symptoms of depression, anxiety and complicated grief [68]. Givens and colleagues [67] suggest that caregivers who experience greater pre-loss grief, particularly those who lived with the person with dementia prior to a NH admission, may benefit from bereavement services.

Conclusions

At the final stage of this prolonged illness, severe dementia represents a challenging time for those affected by it. A range of services, skilled healthcare professionals and effective interventions can enable people with severe dementia and their family caregivers not only to weather this period but help maximise quality of life even in the face of death. It is important to remember that people with severe dementia are aware, even in the most severe or end stage and the humanity of the person remains undiminished, even when the individual is completely dependent on others [69]. This emphasises the need to provide quality care, an environment that optimises the person's engagement and quality of life and compassionate interactions that respect and protect the individual's dignity.

Acknowledgements

Dr Black has received funding from the National Institute on Aging (Grant AG038440) and the National Institute on Neurological Disorders and Stroke (Grant NS39810). Dr Rabins has received funding from the National Institute on Neurological Disorders and Stroke (Grant NS39810), has provided legal testimony for Janssen Pharmaceutica and is on the board of SeniorBridge.

References

1. Arrighi HM, Neumann PJ, Lieberburg IM, Townsend RJ (2010) Lethality of Alzheimer disease and its impact on nursing home placement. *Alzheimer Dis Assoc Disord* 24:90–95.
2. Winblad B, Wimo A, Mobius H, et al. (1999) Severe dementia: a common condition entailing high costs at individual and societal levels. *Int J Geriatr Psychiatry* 14:911–914.
3. Rikkert M, Tona K, Janssen L, et al. (2011) Validity, reliability, and feasibility of clinical staging scales in dementia: a systematic review. *Am J Alzheimers Dis Other Demen* 26:357–365.
4. Hughes CP, Berg L, Danzinger WL, et al. (1982) A new clinical scale for staging of dementia. *Br J Psychiatry* 140:566–572.
5. Morris JC (1993) The Clinical Dementia Rating (CDR): current version and scoring rules. *Neurology* 43:2412–2414.
6. Reisberg B (1988) Functional Assessment Staging (FAST). *Psychopharmacol Bull* 24:653–659.
7. Heyman A, Wilkinson WE, Hurwitz BJ, et al. (1987) Early-onset Alzheimer's disease: clnical predictors of institutionalization and death. *Neurology* 37:980–984.
8. Dooneief G, Marder K, Tang M, et al. (1996) The Clinical Dementia Rating scale: community-based validation of 'profound' and 'terminal' stages. *Neurology* 46:1746–1749.
9. Folstein MF, Folstein SE, McHugh PR (1975) 'Mini-mental state'. A practical method for grading the cognitive state of patients for the clinician. *J Psychiatr Res* 12:189–198.
10. Panisset M, Roudier M, Saxton J, et al. (1994) Severe impairment battery: a neuropsychological test for severely demented patients. *Arch Neurol* 51:41–45.
11. Albert M, Cohen C (1992) The test for severe impairment: an instrument for the assessment of patients with severe cognitive dysfunction. *J Am Geriatr Soc* 40:449–453.
12. Rabins PV, Steele CD (1996) A scale to measure impairment in severe dementia and similar conditions. *Am J Geriatr Psychiatry* 4:247–251.
13. Miller SC, Lima JC, Looze J, et al. (2012) Dying in U.S. nursing homes with advanced dementia: how does healthcare use differe for residents with versus without end-of-life Medicare skilled nursing facility care? *J Palliat Med* 15:1–8.

14. Morris JN, Fries BE, Mehr DR, et al. (1994) MDS cognitive performance scale. *J Gerontol* 49: M174–M182.
15. Boller F, Verny M, Hugonot-Diener L, et al. (2002) Clinical features and assessment of severe dementia. A review. *Eur J Neurol* 9:125–136.
16. Förstl H (2000) What is Alzheimer's disease? In: Ames D, Burns A, O'Brien J (eds), *Dementia*, 4th edn. London: Hodder Education, pp. 359–368.
17. Rabins PV, Lyketsos C, Steele C (2006) *Practical Dementia Care*. New York: Oxford University Press.
18. Tariot PN (2003) Medical management of advanced dementia. *J Am Geriatr Soc* 51:S305–S313.
19. Kverno KS, Rabins PV, Blass DM, et al. (2008) Prevalence and treatment of neuropsychiatric symptoms in advanced dementia. *J Gerontol Nurs* 34:8–15.
20. Samus QM, Rosenblatt A, Steele C, et al. (2005) The association of neuropsychiatric symptoms and environment with quality of life in assisted living residents with dementia. *Gerontologist* 45:19–26.
21. Black BS, Johnston D, Morrison A, et al. (2012) Quality of life of community-residing persons with dementia based on self-rated and caregiver rated measures. *Qual Life Res* 21(8):1379–1389. Epub ahead of print.
22. Chan DC, Kasper JD, Black BS, et al. (2003) Presence of behavioral and psychological symptoms predicts nursing home placement in community-dwelling elders with cognitive impairment in univariate but not multivariate analysis. *J Gerontol A Biol Sci Med Sci* 58:548–554.
23. Hicks KL, Rabins PV, Black BS (2010) Predictors of mortality in nursing home residents with advanced dementia. *Am J Alzheimers Dis Other Demen* 25:439–445.
24. Alzheimer's Association (2011) Alzheimer's disease facts and figures. *Alzheimers Demen* 7:208–244.
25. Graham JE, Rockwood K, Beattie BL, et al. (1997) Prevalence and severity of cognitive impairment with and without dementia in an elderly population. *Lancet* 349:1793–1796.
26. Evans DA, Funkenstein HH, Albert MS, et al. (1989) Prevalence of Alzheimer's disease in a community population of older persons. *JAMA* 262:2551–2556.
27. Lyketsos C, Steinberg M, Tschanz JT, et al. (2000) Mental and behavioral disturbances in dementia: findings from the Cache County Study on Memory in Aging. *Am J Psychiatry* 157:708–714.
28. Rabins PV, Schwartz S, Black BS, et al. (2012 November 1) Predictors of progression to severe Alzheimer's disease in an incidence sample. *Alzheimers Demen* pii: S1552–5260(12)00019-2.
29. Knopman DS, Berg JD, Thomas R, et al. (1999) Nursing home placement is related to dementia progression: experience from a clinical trial: Alzheimer Disease Cooperative Study. *Neurology* 52:714–718.
30. Rosenblatt A, Samus QM, Steele CD, et al. (2004) The Maryland Assisted Living Study: prevalence, recognition, and treatment of dementia and other psychiatric disorders in the assisted living population of central Maryland. *J Am Geriatr Soc* 52:1618–1625.
31. Sloane PD, Zimmerman S, Gruber-Baldini AL, et al. (2005) Health and functional outcomes and health care utilization of persons with dementia in residential care and assisted living facilities: comparison with nursing homes. *Gerontologist* 45:124–132.
32. Mitchell SL, Teno JM, Miller SC, et al. (2005) A national study of the location of death for older persons with dementia. *J Am Geriatr Soc* 53:299–305.
33. Mitchell SL, Teno JM, Kiely DK, et al. (2009) The clinical course of advanced dementia. *NEJM* 361:1529–1538.
34. Black BS, Finucane T, Baker A, et al. (2006) Health problems and correlates of pain in nursing home residents with advanced dementia. *Alzheimer Dis Assoc Disord* 20:283–290.
35. Maslow K (2006) How many people with dementia are hospitalized? In: Silverstein N, Maslow K (eds), *Improving Hospital Care for People with Dementia*. New York: Springer Publishing Co., pp. 3–23.
36. Mitchell SL, Black BS, Ersek M, et al. (2012) Advanced dementia: state of the art and priorities for the next decade. *Ann Intern Med* 156:45–51.
37. Mitchell SL, Morris JN, Park PS, et al. (2004) Terminal care for persons with advanced dementia in nursing home and home care settings. *J Palliat Med* 7:803–816.
38. Black BS, Hicks KL, Finucane T, et al. (2010) Transfers to hospital near the end of life among nursing home residents with advanced dementia. At: Gerontological Society of America Annual Meeting, New Orleans, LA.
39. Thune-Boyle ICV, Sampson EL, Jones L, et al. (2010) Challenges to improving end of life care of people with advanced dementia in the UK. *Dementia* 9:259–284.

40. Winblad B, Gauthier S, Astrom D, et al. (2010) Memantine benefits functional abilities in moderate to severe Alzheimer's disease. *J Nutr Health Aging* 14:770–774.
41. Cummings J, Jones R, Wildinson D, et al. (2010) Effect of donepezil on cognition in severe Alzheimer's disease: a pooled data analysis. *J Alzheimers Dis* 21:843–851.
42. Parsons C, Briesacher BA, Givens JL, et al. (2011) Cholinesterase inhibitors and memantine use in newly admitted nursing home residents with dementia. *Am J Geriat Soc* 59:1253–1259.
43. Gitlin LN, Winter L, Dennis MP, et al. (2010) A biobehavioral home-based intervention and the well-being of patients with dementia and their caregivers: the COPE randomized trial. *JAMA* 304:983–991.
44. Schulz R, Belle SH, Czaja SJ, et al. (2004) Long-term care placement of dementia patients and caregiver health and well-being. *JAMA* 292:961–967.
45. Hill L, Roberts G, Woldgoose J, et al. (2010) Recovery and person-centered care in dementia: common purpose, common practice? *Adv Psychiatr Treat* 16:288–298.
46. Grant-Savela S (2012) Care setting configuration and size. *Dementia Design Info*. Available at: http://www4.uwm.edu/dementiadesigninfo (last accessed on 21 Ferbruary 2013).
47. Koren MJ (2010) Person-centered care for nursing home residents: the Culture-Change Movement. *Health Aff* 29:1–6.
48. Calkins MP (2012) History of creating settings for people with dementia. *Dementia Design Info*. Available at: http://www4.uwm.edu/dementiadesigninfo (last accessed on 21 February 2013).
49. Cohen-Mansfield J, Marx MS, Freedman LS, et al. (2011) The comprehensive process model of engagement. *Am J Geriatr Psychiatry* 19:859–870.
50. Cohen-Mansfield J, Marx MS, Freedman LS, et al. (2012) What affects pleasure in persons with advanced stage dementia? *J Psychiatr Res* 46(3):402–406. doi: 10.1016/j.jpsychires.2011.12.003
51. Gitlin LN, Winter L, Dennis MP, et al. (2010) Targeting and managing behavioral symptoms in individuals with dementia: a randomized trial of a nonpharmacological intervention. *JAGS* 58:1467–1474.
52. Gitlin LN, Winter L, Burke J, et al. (2008) Tailored activities to manage neuropsychiatric behaviors in persons with dementia and reduce caregiver burden: a randomized pilot study. *Am J Geriatr Psychiatry* 16:229–239.
53. Cohen-Mansfield J (2001) Nonpharmacologic interventions for inappropriate behaviors in dementia: a review, summary, and critique. *Am J Geriatr Psychiatry* 9:361–381.
54. Garland K, Beer E, Eppingstall B, et al. (2007) A comparison of two treatments of agitated behavior in nursing home residents with dementia: simulated family presence and preferred music. *Am J Geriatric Psychiatry* 15:514–521.
55. Kverno KS, Black BS, Nolan MT, et al. (2009) Research on treating neuropsychiatric symptoms of advanced dementia with non-pharmacological strategies, 1998–2008: a systematic review. *Int Psychogeriatr* 21:825–843.
56. Husebo BS, Ballard C, Sandvik R, Nilsen OB, Aarsland D (2011 July 15) Efficacy of treating pain to reduce behavioural disturbances in residents of nursing homes with dementia: Cluster randomized clinical trial. *BMJ* 343:d4065.
57. Brodaty H (2011) Antidepressant treatment in Alzheimer's disease. *Lancet* 378:375–376.
58. Morrison RS, Siu AL (2000) A comparison of pain and its treatment in advanced dementia and cognitively intact patients with hip fracture. *J Pain Symptom Manage* 19:240–248.
59. Herr K, Bursch H, Ersek M, et al. (2010) Use of pain-behavioral assessment tools in the nursing home: expert consensus recommendations for practice. *J Gerontol Nurs* 36:18–29.
60. Post S (2000) *The Moral Challenge of Alzheimer Disease: Ethical Issues from Diagnosis to Dying*, 2nd edn. Baltimore, MD: The Johns Hopkins University Press.
61. Haw C, Stubbs J (2010) Covert administration of medication to older adults: A review of the literature and published studies. *J Psychiatr Ment Health Nurs* 17:761–768.
62. Finucane TE, Christmas C, Travis K (1999) Tube feeding in patients with advanced dementia: a review of the evidence. *JAMA* 282:1365–1370.
63. Fulton AT, Rhodes-Kroft J, Corcoran AM, et al. (2011) Palliative care for patients with dementia in long-term care. *Clin Geriatr Med* 27:153–170.
64. Casey DA, Northcott C, Stowell K, Shihabuddin L, Radriguez-Suarez M (2012) Dementia and palliative care. *Clin Geriatr* 20(1):36–41.

65. Center to Advance Palliative Care (2007) Improving palliative care in nursing homes. Available at: http://www.capc.org/support-from-capc/capc_publications/nursing_home_report.pdf (last accessed on 7 February 2012).
66. Teno JM, Gozalo PL, Lee IC, et al. (2011) Does hospice improve quality of care for persons dying from dementia? *J Am Geriatr Soc* 59:1532–1536.
67. Givens JL, Prigerson HG, Kiely DK, et al. (2011) Grief among family members of nursing home residents with advanced dementia. *Am J Geriatr Psychiatry* 19:543–550.
68. Bergman EJ, Haley WE, Small BJ (2011) Who uses bereavement services? An examination of service use by bereaved dementia caregivers. *Aging Ment Health* 15:531–540.
69. Clare L (2010) Awareness of people with severe dementia: review and integration. *Aging Ment Health* 14:20–32.

Section 3

External drivers of service development

Chapter 8

How to get results in public policy for Alzheimer's and dementia services

Alzheimer's disease international

Marc Wortmann

Alzheimer's Disease International, UK

Introduction

Alzheimer's Disease International (ADI) is the worldwide federation of almost 80 Alzheimer associations. Each member is the leading organisation in its country and represents the people with Alzheimer's disease and other dementias as well as their families. In 2006, ADI decided on a key strategic objective: making dementia a global health priority. By that time, there was only one country in the world that made dementia a national health priority: Australia. We were in official relations with the World Health Organisation (WHO), the main global health agency, but hardly had any influence on their agenda. Just having conversations with WHO officers or writing a letter was not enough. ADI started a strategy to stronger influence the WHO, and in April 2012, the WHO launched a report with the title 'Dementia: A Public Health Priority'. How could this happen and what were the key factors contributing to this success?

Strategic objective and arguments

We believed that especially for developing countries, it would be crucial to come onto the list of priorities of WHO, as many health departments let them steer the public health agenda.

To make this happen it was first of all crucial to get the figures right. There is no policy without data, or, in the words of Dr Margaret Chan, Director General of the WHO: what gets measured, gets done. The fact that people suffer from a disease is not enough to convince policymakers, as this is the same for many other diseases as well. ADI was in a position to commission a report on the global data. At its annual conference in 1998 in India, the 10/66 Dementia Research group was established with the aim to carry out population based research in lower and middle income countries (where at that time it was thought 66% of people with dementia lived and less than 10% of the research was done). The first task of this global network of researchers was to develop a methodology for prevalence research that was appropriate for all countries in the world, despite cultural

Designing and Delivering Dementia Services, First Edition. Edited by Hugo de Waal, Constantine Lyketsos, David Ames, and John O'Brien.

differences and biases. When this was done, they started to do studies in 11 lower and middle-income countries, including China, India, Nigeria and a number of Latin American countries.

With the results of these studies, it was possible to do a comprehensive systematic review of all the prevalence data in the world of both higher and lower and middle-income countries and come up with a landmark report, the World Alzheimer Report 2009.[1] The report calculated the number of people with dementia worldwide at 35.6 million by 2010 and made a forecast based on UN population data that this number will rise up to 66 million by the year 2030 and 115 million by 2050, fully due to global ageing.

The economic argument

In most countries with successful dementia policy, having the numbers was not enough and cost of illness studies helped very much to convince politicians and policymakers to pay more attention. With the global prevalence data, a number of cost studies and a survey within the ADI network, it was possible to put together a second World Alzheimer Report in 2010 with the economic impact of the disease. The global cost of dementia was calculated at US$604 billion, based on direct medical costs, direct societal costs and indirect informal care costs. This amount accounts for 1% of global GDP.

Organisational infrastructure and mobilisation

Having the right arguments still does not guarantee any success if you do not have the organisational infrastructure to talk to the right people at all levels. It also does not work if you do not find policymakers who are receptive to the message. We were in a position to establish both a group of regional advocates that were able to visit regional WHO meetings, make statements and network with government and WHO officials, as well as finding policymakers that championed for the cause in their own organisations. This happened at the country level as well, in countries like Australia, the UK, South Korea, Switzerland, the Scandinavian countries, the Netherlands, Singapore and New Zealand. These countries not only developed their own policies, but also supported international initiatives. All these were responses to grassroots initiatives. The only exception is France were President Sarkozy himself initiated an Alzheimer policy for his country and the European Union. Very recently, the USA has been coming on board as well with its own Alzheimer plan, and this fact might give the global movement a strong push forward.

Another success factor is mobilisation. Most Alzheimer associations have a network that they can use to collect signatures of people signing a petition or contribute with input through meetings, hearings or online. In various countries this proved to be effective. ADI developed a Global Alzheimer's Disease Charter that was signed by 54,000 people worldwide and presented to the WHO in the year 2010. The main purpose of these actions is to show that Alzheimer's disease and dementia is a topic that affects a large part of the community and that people are willing to participate.

Implementation

The next and probably even more difficult step will be the implementation of these plans and policies into day to day health and social care, legislation, health insurance and cost reimbursement.

---

[1] http://www.alz.co.uk/research/files/WorldAlzheimerReport.pdf

This is an area were Alzheimer associations still need to learn how they can effectively influence public policy. The French plan was the third in a row, but the first Alzheimer plan with very detailed and measurable actions, for instance the number of new memory clinics that should be established. An overall objective like decreasing the prescription of antipsychotics is also measured now. The English plan did not have a firm implementation commitment from the beginning, so when little results could be shown after a year, a national director was appointed and implementation became more important.

Part of the implementation is of course the budget, and we see big differences between the commitments that governments are making to fund these plans or relocate money from existing budgets. Ideally, this should be secured from the beginning. But the reality is often different. If there is not enough money attached, advocates need to continue to campaign for it.

Finally . . .

In my view, there is an unsatisfactory element in lobbying on behalf of disease areas. There is a clear misbalance between attention paid to some diseases and others. Those disease areas that lack high-level spokespersons or strong advocacy organisations are hardly seen by policymakers or donors. In an ideal world, these things should not matter. The reality is that it does matter, and the reality is that Alzheimer's disease and dementia has gained more and more attention on the country level and in international settings like the WHO and the European Union. Research funding, however, is still far from the level of HIV or cancer. Over time, we will learn if funding will increase and how this affects finding the right solutions for people with dementia and their families.

Politics, dementia and ageing in Australia

Glenn Rees

Alzheimer's Australia, Australia

Aged care policy and within it, dementia, is largely the responsibility of the Commonwealth Government. It is a second-order political issue in Australia.

The lack of political attention to issues of ageing is evidenced by how ageing has been represented in Parliament. Only twice in over 25 years has aged care or ageing more broadly been represented in Cabinet by a Minister. Between 1984 and 1987, the then Minister for Community Services, the Hon Don Grimes, was a member of Cabinet and more recently, the Minister for Mental Health and Ageing, the Hon Mark Butler, was elevated to Cabinet in December 2011.

For the remainder of the period, aged care and dementia has been the responsibility of a junior Minister within the Health portfolio.

It is true that the financial impacts of population and ageing issues have received political and community attention in the form of Intergenerational Reports[1] that have documented the economic consequences of an ageing population. These reports have been somewhat controversial as they have focused largely on the potential economic impacts of an ageing population and have suggested that the only way to address the impact is to cut spending or increase taxes. It is partly because of

---

[1]Australian Government (2010). *Intergenerational Report 2010: Australia to 2050: Future Challenges*. Canberra: Commonwealth of Australia.

these reports that the ageing of the Australian population has come to be perceived as a problem and a burden in political and economic terms.

In contrast, there has been little focus in political discussions on what we can do to help older people stay healthy, to reduce chronic disease in old age and to maximise quality of life. Or how we can ensure that those who have major chronic diseases like dementia receive quality care and support they so desperately need. At the same time, from the consumer perspective, there has been increasing concern about the quality of services and supports available to people in old age. Until very recently, the obvious need for reform of aged care has not been given political priority by either side of politics. When it has received attention, it has been the financial and regulatory aspects rather than the needs of older people that have been the policy focus.

However, in 2011, the report of the Productivity Commission's inquiry into 'Caring for Older Australians'[2] put beyond doubt the urgency of aged care reforms in Australia and made recommendations from the perspective of the needs of older people rather than the needs of service providers or policymakers. The Productivity Commission is the Australian Government's independent research and advisory body, and the inquiry was commissioned by the Government as a first step in its commitment to aged care reform.

The Governments responded to the Productivity Commission with an aged care reform package, Living Longer Living Better, as part of the 2012–2013 Federal Budget.[3] It sets the scene for much needed generational change in aged care policy, funding and service delivery that will benefit people with dementia as well as others.

Where does responsibility for dementia rest?

Responsibility for dementia rests within the aged care portfolio in Australia. This arguably has had two unfortunate consequences. First, it has all too easily been assumed that aged care services will provide appropriate care for people with dementia. Furthermore, until the last decade, there has been little recognition of the additional financial costs of providing care for people with dementia, the special care needs of people with dementia or the training needs of the workforce.

The second consequence of aged care having responsibility for dementia is that dementia has been incorrectly assumed by policymakers to be simply a natural part of ageing. As a result, the health system has taken next to no interest. Key issues concerning early diagnosis, making hospitals safer places for people with cognitive impairment, dementia risk reduction and investment in dementia research have been hastily passed to those responsible for aged care. Unfortunately, as aged care has rarely had any priority or standing in political decision making, it has been next to impossible for those with an interest in improving care for people with dementia to gain any traction in the broader health system.

To illustrate the point, the high-profile political reforms of the health and hospital system, primary care and preventive health since 2008 have provided no recognition of the impact of dementia on the health and care system, nor responded directly in any way to dementia. The Living Longer Living Better package, which includes funding to address dementia across both the health and aged care system and the commitment to make dementia a National Health Priority Area alongside eight other chronic diseases, including cancer and vascular disease, holds the prospect of dramatic policy change.

[2]Productivity Commission 2011, *Caring for Older Australians*, Report No. 53, Final Inquiry Report, Canberra.
[3]Australian Government, *Living Longer Living Better* (2012).

Much has been achieved

There has been a remarkable change in the political and policy environment since 2000 that has laid the basis for tackling dementia within a public health framework.

There have been a number of drivers.

First, Alzheimer's Australia has been able to work in close partnership with successive governments to contribute to policy and programme development. As the national peak body advocating on behalf of people with dementia and their carers in Australia, Alzheimer's Australia has also been funded by Government to undertake a range of activities including awareness, advocacy and services.

Second, there has been the development of intellectual capital to provide the evidence base for action on dementia and making it a health priority. The seminal document, commissioned by Alzheimer's Australia, was *The Dementia Epidemic: Economic and Social Impact and Positive Solutions for Australia*[4] in 2003. This publication documented the prevalence and incidence of dementia and the direct and indirect cost of dementia and a plan for the future. It has served as a model for reports in other countries.

Third, the implementation of the Dementia Initiative by the Commonwealth in 2005 with additional funding of AU $320 million over 5 years provided a focus for action on dementia. The main elements of the Initiative were:

- high-care, dementia-specific community support packages (the *Extended Aged Care at Home – Dementia*)
- Dementia Care Essentials Training
- Dementia Behaviour Management Advisory Services (DBMAS) that provide advice to those working with people with dementia in the community and residential care facilities
- the National Dementia Support Program, which includes support and counselling, and a 24-hour helpline
- funding for dementia care research, including dementia research grants, and funding for the Dementia Collaborative Research Centres
- community support grants.

Fourth, advances in medical science, while still well short of identifying interventions to address the causes of dementia, have contributed to a more positive understanding of dementia and the importance of identifying those at risk and intervening before the brain is too badly damaged. In these ways, it has become possible to advocate for dementia as for cancer, heart disease or diabetes – namely within a public health framework based on risk reduction, timely diagnosis, good management and quality care, including at the end of life.

Lastly, and perhaps most importantly, in the political and social context, people with dementia have been empowered to self advocate. In the life of Alzheimer's Australia, it took two decades – from the early 1980's to 2000 – to change from a carer's organisation to one inclusive of people with dementia. To have people with dementia of all ages as well as family carers telling their stories, has helped to remove some of the negativity and stigma associated with dementia. Over the past year, we have also grown in our sophistication of utilising social media to enable these stories to reach a much wider audience.

[4]Access Economics 2003, Dementia Epidemic: Economic and Social Impact and Positive Solutions for Australia.

Recent developments

The 2005 Dementia Initiative gave those of us in Alzheimer's Australia some confidence that there was a political platform that could be used to address concerns of patients and carers and particularly those in health policy.

This confidence was misplaced.

Lack of action on dementia in the healthcare reforms in Australia and a bad outcome in the 2011 Budget that effectively terminated the Dementia Initiative led Alzheimer's Australia to radically rethink its political strategy.

The response was to mobilise a social movement to pressure the Government and the Opposition to commit to the action required. This was achieved through the Fight Dementia Campaign, with a view to telling the stories of people with dementia and their family carers with greater impact. We advocated:

- For dementia to be tackled within a public health framework like any other chronic disease.
- For investment in medical science to beat dementia as we have with cancer, heart disease and HIV Aids.
- Additional funding of AU$500m over 5 years in key priority areas including dementia awareness, diagnosis, care, research and risk reduction.

The evidence base of the Campaign had been developed over the last decade. What was new was a strategy which embraces a new marketing and branding strategy with a more sophisticated approach to communications strategy, including social media, and a high-profile president.

A window of opportunity?

The Living Longer Living Better policy and funding framework provides a window of opportunity for genuine reform of aged care and dementia care.

From a customer perspective, the principal aged care elements are:

- a commitment to consumer-directed models of care to empower consumers to take decisions on the services they need
- a priority for community services and especially flexible respite to better support the carer
- access to information for consumers and provision for link workers to guide consumers through the system
- access to end of life care, advance care planning and palliative care
- development of meaningful quality indicators in residential care
- user charges that balance the requirement for the system to be sustainable with equitable access.

From the perspective of the politics of dementia, the Living Longer Living Better package offers new hope in tackling the two great challenges in dementia care.

First, the challenge of getting recognition within aged care reform that improved access to quality dementia care will only come about if there is recognition of the special needs of those with dementia. This includes:

- a funding supplement to account for the extra costs of dementia care in community and residential settings

- extra funding for those with severe behavioural and psychological symptoms of dementia
- age-appropriate services for younger people with dementia.

The second major challenge has been the recognition for the first time in Australian health policy of the need to address dementia as a chronic disease. The Living Longer Living Better package contains action to:

- Make dementia a National Health Priority Area.
- Achieve timely diagnosis.
- Hospital care of people with dementia rate alongside concerns about the need for more community care and the quality of residential care.
- Improve the quality of dementia care in hospitals.
- Introduce a publicly funded education programme on risk reduction delivered through Alzheimer's Australia. Possibly a world first.

Conclusion

There is new hope for tackling dementia in Australia within a public health framework. The missing element is adequate funding of dementia research which continues to be grossly underfunded in relation to other chronic diseases. This is now the sole focus of the Fight Dementia Campaign for the 2013 Budget.

Making dementia a European priority

Jean Georges

Alzheimer Europe, Luxembourg

When the member organisations of Alzheimer Europe unanimously approved the Paris Declaration of the political priorities of the European Alzheimer movement at the organisation's annual meeting in Paris in 2006, no one could have foreseen the incredible progress that would be achieved in such a short time.

The Paris Declaration[1] was a call for action highlighting 19 priorities for policymakers on a European and national level. The declaration highlights the necessity for governments to declare dementia a public health priority and to develop national dementia strategies or Alzheimer's programmes. It based this argument on existing prevalence figures and on research predicting a continued rise in the number of people with dementia due to the ageing of the European population.

In addition to this public health appeal, the declaration contained research and medical priorities (early diagnosis, access to treatment, increased funding for research and greater EU collaboration on research), care and social support priorities (support of Alzheimer associations, development of care services and carer support, and exchange of best practices), as well as legal and ethical issues (right to a diagnosis, recognition of advance directives, and exchange of information on legal issues and guardianship systems) to be addressed.

Alzheimer Europe and its national member organisations used the Paris Declaration to raise awareness of its priorities among Members of the European Parliament, and in 2007 set up the

---

[1]The Paris Declaration of Alzheimer Europe is available on: http://www.alzheimer-europe.org/Policy-in-Practice2/Paris-Declaration.

European Alzheimer's Alliance. This was chaired by Françoise Grossetête (France) and consisted of MEPs supporting Alzheimer Europe's goal of making dementia a European priority. By the end of 2007, 30 MEPs had shown their commitment to the cause by becoming members of the Alliance.[2] The year 2008 proved to be a pivotal year for greater European collaboration in the field of dementia. France took over the rotating Presidency of the European Union during the second semester of 2008 and included, for the first time, Alzheimer's disease and other forms of dementia as a priority for its 6-month Presidency.

In October 2008, Roselyne Bachelot, the French Health Minister, organised a European conference entitled 'The fight against Alzheimer's disease and related disorders', with the aim of identifying areas for joint actions on a European level. At the end of the conference, French President Nicolas Sarkozy summed up his ambitions for Europe in this field: 'Europe can take action, in my view, by working along three avenues: understanding the disease and performing research, sharing experiences on care and management, and engaging in an ethical manner'.[3]

The European Parliament gave its backing to these plans and launched a Written Declaration that was formally adopted on 5 February 2009. Initiated by Members of the European Alzheimer's Alliance, the Declaration was signed by 465 Members of the European Parliament (59.24% of all Members) from all 27 Member States of the European Union. The signatories called 'on the Commission, the Council and the governments of the Member States to recognise Alzheimer's disease as a European public health priority and to develop a European action plan with a view to: promoting pan-European research on the causes, prevention and treatment of Alzheimer's disease, improving early diagnosis, simplifying procedures for patients and carers and improving their quality of life, promoting the role of Alzheimer's associations, and giving them regular support'.[4]

In July 2009, the European Commission responded to the Parliament Declaration and the call issued during the French presidency by issuing two Communications:

1. a proposal for a Council recommendation on measures to combat neurodegenerative diseases, in particular Alzheimer's disease, through joint programming of research activities
2. a communication on a European initiative on Alzheimer's disease and other dementias.

Joint programming is a new collaborative approach in which European countries come together to define a common vision, a strategic research agenda and a management structure, in order to address the 'grand challenges' facing EU society in the coming years. It is a clear sign of the emergence of Alzheimer's disease and other forms of dementia as research priorities that Europe decided that the pilot for this unprecedented type of approach should be dedicated to this field.

The 'EU Joint Programme – Neurodegenerative Disease Research (JPND)' currently brings together 25 full member countries and Canada, which has recently been granted third country status. The aims of the programme are to 'identify common research goals that would benefit from joint action between countries in order to accelerate progress on solutions that can alleviate the symptoms, and lessen the social and economic impact for patients, families and health care systems'.[5]

The initiative has already passed three important milestones, in that it has conducted a mapping exercise of national and European funding programmes, it has adopted its European Research

---

[2]In 2012, this number stands at 66.
[3]http://www.plan-alzheimer.gouv.fr/IMG/pdf/president_sarkozy_081031_uk.pdf.
[4]Written Declaration 80/2008 on the priorities in the fight against Alzheimer's disease: http://www.europarl.europa.eu/sides/getDoc.do?pubRef=-%2f%2fEP%2f%2fNONSGML%2bWDECL%2bP6-DCL-2008-0080%2b0%2bDOC%2bPDF%2bV0%2f%2fEN.
[5]http://www.neurodegenerationresearch.eu/about/.

Strategy to guide research activity in the field and it has launched funding calls for Centres of Excellence in Neurodegeneration (COEN) and the harmonisation of biomarkers.

In the Communication on a European Alzheimer's initiative, the Commission highlighted four areas, where it felt Community action could be beneficial:

1. acting early to diagnose dementia and to reduce the risk of dementia in the first place
2. improving research coordination between EU countries
3. sharing of best practice
4. providing a forum to reflect on the rights, autonomy and dignity of patients.

This Communication led to a different type of concrete collaboration between European countries. Joint Actions were identified as a new mechanism for funding from the EU public health programme and one of the first Joint Actions to be launched was dedicated to Alzheimer's disease. ALCOVE, the 'ALzheimer COoperative Valuation in Europe' is a Joint Action between 30 partners from 19 EU Member States and the European Commission that 'aims to both improve knowledge on dementia and its consequences and to promote the exchange of information to preserve health, quality of life, autonomy and dignity of people living with dementia and their carers in European Union Member States'.[6]

The 2-year collaboration aims to develop public policy recommendations for the following issues:

1. how to improve data for better knowledge about dementia prevalence
2. how to improve access to dementia diagnosis as early as possible
3. how to improve care for people living with dementia and particularly those with behavioural disorders
4. how to improve the rights of people with dementia, particularly in respect to advance declarations of will.

In parallel to these important European developments, the past years saw great advances with regard to the recognition of dementia as a national health priority. When Alzheimer Europe launched its Paris Declaration in 2006, France was the only country to have an Alzheimer's strategy, albeit one with relatively modest aims. By 2012, the number of countries with a dementia strategy has grown to eight (Belgium, Denmark, Finland, France, the Netherlands, Norway, Sweden and the UK). Separate regional strategies are in place in the four countries of the UK (England, Northern Ireland, Scotland and Wales), in Wallonia and Flanders, and in the Italian region of Emilia-Romagna. There are an additional six countries (Cyprus, Czech Republic, Ireland, Italy, Luxembourg and Malta) where a dementia strategy is currently in development at a governmental level.

In Europe, France was the first country to develop an Alzheimer's Plan on a national level,[7] and also spearheaded the idea of greater European collaboration in this field. The country continues to provide leadership to the two EU wide collaborations, with Professor Philippe Amouyel as the chair of the EU Joint Programme – Neurodegenerative Disease Research (JPND) and the 'Haute Autorité de Santé' coordinating the ALCOVE project.[8]

---

[6] http://www.alcove-project.eu/.
[7] The current Alzheimer's Plan covering the period of 2008–2013 is in fact the third French Alzheimer's Plan.
[8] ALCOVE differentiates between partners contractually involved in the management and funding of the Joint Action (Associates) and more loosely involved partners (Collaborator).

Table 8.1 European recognition of dementia as a national priority by national governments

Member state	Dementia strategy	Involved in JPND	Involved in ALCOVE
Austria	No	Yes	No
Belgium	Yes	Yes	Associate
Bulgaria	No	No	No
Cyprus	In development	No	Collaborator
Czech Republic	In development	Yes	Collaborator
Denmark	Yes	Yes	No
Estonia	No	No	No
Finland	Yes	Yes	Associate
France	Yes	Yes	Associate
Germany	No	Yes	No
Greece	No	Yes	Associate
Hungary	No	Yes	Collaborator
Ireland	In development	Yes	No
Italy	In development	Yes	Associate
Latvia	No	No	Associate
Lithuania	No	No	Associate
Luxembourg	In development	Yes	Collaborator
Malta	In development	No	Collaborator
Netherlands	Yes	Yes	Collaborator
Poland	No	Yes	No
Portugal	No	Yes	Collaborator
Romania	No	No	No
Slovakia	No	Yes	Associate
Slovenia	No	Yes	No
Spain	No	Yes	Associate
Sweden	Yes	Yes	Associate
United Kingdom	Yes	Yes	Associate
Countries outside European Union			
Albania	No	Yes	No
Croatia	No	Yes	No
Israel	No	Yes	No
Norway	Yes	Yes	Collaborator
Switzerland	No	Yes	No

As can be seen from Table 8.1, the recognition of dementia as a national priority by national governments varies hugely across Europe. Currently, dementia strategies are limited to countries in Western and Northern Europe, with fewer promising developments in this field in Southern and Eastern European countries.

With regard to the JPND and the ALCOVE Joint Action, the involvement of European countries also differs significantly. Most countries participate in both, while others prioritise one type of collaboration over the other. Bulgaria, Estonia and Romania do not participate in either programme.

The progress achieved since the adoption of Alzheimer Europe's Paris Declaration is truly impressive. Alzheimer's disease and other forms of dementia have been given a higher priority by the European Union than some other chronic conditions. However, as the European institutions are discussing the future of the European public health and research programmes in a climate of economic down turn, organisations need to remain vigilant to ensure that dementia continues to be considered as a key European priority.

Dementia and politics in England

Andrew Chidgey

Policy and Public Affairs, Alzheimer's Society, UK

Ten years ago, in 2002, dementia was not receiving public or political attention in England. Yet now in 2012, England is 3 years into a National Dementia Strategy, and the Prime Minister has just announced that there will be a specific series of policy initiatives related to dementia contained within the Prime Minister's Challenge on Dementia – the only such health challenge he has issued. How has dementia become such a political force? I will argue that this has happened because of growing evidence about the impact of dementia and also because of the growing political potency of dementia as an issue.

The journey to a National Dementia Strategy

By the end of the first Blair government (1997–2001), the demographic challenge of our ageing population was becoming firmly established as a cross-government issue worthy of attention. The Treasury had recognised ageing as one of the five greatest challenges facing us, along with issues such as climate change. However, dementia was not recognised strongly within the policy agenda. In 2001, the Department of Health published a National Service Framework (NSF) for Older People, setting out the major areas of action that were needed in relation to older people. In the initial discussions about the NSF, dementia did not feature at all, and this was also true in relatively late drafts of the policy. However, eventually dementia featured, albeit fleetingly, under Standard 7 – Mental Health in the NSF. This limited reference was symptomatic of the fact that dementia was not recognised as a policy priority.

The main public advocate for action on dementia 10 years ago was the Alzheimer's Society and some leading clinicians who specialised in the treatment and care of people with dementia and their carers. However, dementia was not featuring strongly in public discussion or the media, and political attention was very limited – certainly no party manifesto for a general election had commitments specifically on dementia in it in the way that cancer, for example featured so strongly.

The Alzheimer's Society had for some time been developing networks of influence to ensure that the voice of people with dementia and their carers was featuring in political debate. This focused initially on gathering evidence and stories from people affected by dementia, publishing reports and encouraging people to become campaigners for change. As the charity grew, the scale of this activity and the evidence amassed increased as well.

In 2004, the National Institute for Health and Clinical Excellence published a review of a technology appraisal (assessment of value for money of a health intervention) that said that the four drugs available for people with Alzheimer's disease were not cost-effective and should not be prescribed on the NHS. This led to the development of the most assertive and focused campaign the Alzheimer's Society had held to date to reverse the decision. An umbrella body 'Action on Alzheimer's Drugs' was launched with many Royal Colleges and charities as members. *The Daily Mail* agreed to support the campaign, and campaigners organised activity in MPs' constituency surgeries, through letter-writing and by going on protest marches. This established a profile for dementia which had not been seen before.

Through the NICE review process, the drug guidelines changed so that they advised doctors to prescribe only to people in the moderate stage of Alzheimer's disease. However, this decision was taken to judicial review (JR) by pharmaceutical companies, with the Alzheimer's Society registering as an interested party to the JR. The JR secured some changes to the NICE guidance that gave more flexibility to clinicians in interpreting the guidance while leaving the stated guidance largely unchanged. The effect of the campaign on Alzheimer's drugs was noticeable in the interactions that the Society had with politicians and in terms of the access that the organisation had to Ministers and officials.

At the same time as the NICE decision on access to drug treatments was being debated, NICE had been working to create a clinical guideline on dementia with the Social Care Institute for Excellence. This was published in 2006 and set out the evidence for treatment and care of people with dementia and their carers. This was an important step in securing agreement on what the approach and interventions should be on dementia on the basis of the evidence available.

In February 2007, the Alzheimer's Society published work it had commissioned from King's College London and the London School of Economics. This for the first time set out the estimated numbers of people with dementia in the UK (700,000 in 2007) and the estimated economic cost (£17 billion in 2007). This evidence was used by the National Audit Office when it published its report on dementia in July 2007 in which it stated that dementia was a condition requiring urgent attention from the government given the low rates of diagnosis and the poor use of resources on dementia delivering poor outcomes for people. In response the government committed to develop a National Dementia Strategy. A draft was developed, consulted upon, re-worked and then published in February 2009. The national dementia strategy established three key areas of priority:

- improving public and professional awareness about dementia
- early diagnosis and intervention
- improving quality of care.

Has having a National Dementia Strategy made a difference?

Proving cause of effect is difficult when trying to understand the specific impact of the National Strategy. So, for example one might ask whether having a National Strategy is simply an expression of a growing recognition that there needs to be action on dementia, or, whether, in fact having a National Strategy is in fact what has led to increased action. I would argue that as in many things, the truth lies somewhere between the two.

National leverage from a National Strategy

Having a National Strategy has provided the basis on which further national 'system levers' and requirements could be developed. For example, inclusion in the annual NHS Operating Framework, which sets out priorities for action by the NHS, NICE Quality Standards, demonstrator sites and a National Clinical Director for Dementia have sprung from the National Dementia Strategy and NICE-SCIE guideline.

The Department of Health has a National Dementia Strategy Programme Board with senior people looking at how to implement the Strategy. There have also been a number of nationally funded dementia awareness campaigns that spring from the Government's commitment to the Strategy.

One might go so far as to argue that having a National Dementia Strategy for England has encouraged other parts of the UK to develop their own plans, but this is difficult to prove.

In 2010, the Alzheimer's Society brought together 40 interested organisations to develop a National Dementia Declaration, setting out shared commitment to action on dementia, and in October 2010, the Dementia Action Alliance was launched. The membership of that alliance has now grown to over 100 organisations. This could not have happened without the growing interest in dementia and the commitment shown through the national strategy.

Local action in line with the strategy

The National Strategy has provided an evidenced framework (linked to the NICE-SCIE dementia guideline) on what action should be taken locally. It has been used in business cases across the country for the development of dementia services, such as memory services, dementia advisers and workforce development plans. The requirement in the NHS Operating Framework that local plans should be published in line with the Strategy has also helped to ensure action.

Are things getting better for people living with dementia and their carers?

The experience for many people living with dementia and their carers remains as difficult as it was in 2009, when the National Dementia Strategy was published. Less than half of people with dementia are identified as having been diagnosed on GP dementia registers, many carers and families report not having access to information and care. Numerous reports explain the poor experience and outcomes for people with dementia in hospitals and care homes.

However, there are reasons for optimism. The amount of activity underway to tackle the challenge of dementia and political commitment to action is very high:

- All three political parties had manifesto commitments on dementia in their election manifestos in 2010.
- There have been large awareness campaigns underway, which evaluation shows are changing public attitudes to dementia.
- The number of memory services and the number of people using them has grown.
- The Dementia Action Alliance is encouraging organisations to work together on shared dementia action.
- There is now far more public discussion and attention on dementia, whether one measures this in column inches or the number of people speaking publicly about their experience of dementia. In opinion surveys, people over 55 years old state that Alzheimer's is the medical condition they most fear – a YouGov survey for Cancer Research UK in August 2011 shows that for people over 55, Alzheimer's is the most feared medical condition for 39% of respondents, followed by cancer (25%), stroke (8%) and motor neurone disease (8%).
- Many MPs report that on the doorstep caring for older relatives with dementia now features prominently as an issue of public concern.[1]

In March 2012, the Prime Minister published his Challenge on Dementia which calls on people and organisations across society to act on dementia. In a speech to the Alzheimer's Society's Dementia 2012 conference, David Cameron said:

'This is simply a terrible disease. And it is a scandal that we as a country haven't kept pace with it. The level of diagnosis, understanding and awareness of dementia is shockingly low. It is as though we've been in collective denial. Already a quarter of hospital beds are occupied by someone with dementia. Already the total cost of the disease is around £19 billion in England . . . that is higher than the costs of cancer, heart disease or stroke. And in less than ten years, as we all live longer, the number of people

[1]Source: Alzheimer's Society parliamentary contact programme.

with dementia will reach a million. So my argument today is that we've got to treat this like the national crisis it is. We need an all-out fight-back against this disease; one that cuts across society. We did it with cancer in the 70s. With HIV in the 80s and 90s. We fought the stigma, stepped up to the challenge and made massive in-roads into fighting these killers. Now we've got to do the same with dementia. This is a personal priority of mine, and it's got an ambition to match. That ambition: nothing less than for Britain to be a world leader in dementia research and care'.

With the launch of the Prime Minister's Challenge on Dementia, he made 14 commitments to action, including raising the amount government spends on dementia research from £26 million a year to £66 million by 2015, sustained awareness campaigns and the inclusion of dementia in health checks by GPs.

Conclusion

There is no doubt that dementia has become a high public and political concern. This is being reflected in public conversation, the media and government policy. This concern is leading to significant action. However, the evidence as to whether this is leading to change yet in terms of quality of life for people with dementia and carers is limited. It is likely to be some time before we know the outcome.

Chapter 9

Developing policy that works for dementia: National and global lessons in what makes a difference

Sube Banerjee

Centre for Dementia Studies, Brighton and Sussex Medical School, University of Sussex, UK

Dementia as a health issue

As discussed by Glenn Rees, one problem that dementia can have in policy terms is a lack of clarity of ownership. In political terms, ownership is a paramount characteristic because the development of strategy always requires resource and the implementation of strategy even more. There are trade-offs that need to be made in all areas of politics and policy, and this means hard choices. If there are not clear lines of ownership then what is likely to happen is nothing, as those things that are clearly owned by protagonists (be they ministers, managerial healthcare officials or civil servants) are given priority for thought and action. Dementia can get lost between health and social care, between mental health and physical health, and when it gets lost nothing happens. For things to happen, political capital needs to be invested and spent. For political capital to be invested and spent means there needs to be the likelihood of a return (i.e. there needs to be value creation, where value is equal to outcomes [clinical or political] divided by cost). How then do we get dementia the executive bandwidth that it needs? Recognition that dementia is a legitimate health issue, one where intervention is of value, is of profound importance. A fundamental that the contributions in chapter 8 have in common is primary work to locate responsibility with health, be that at the World Health Organisation (WHO), in the European Union or in specific countries.

Health is the right place for dementia to be considered. Health is firmly on the economic and political radar. This is understandable given the size and importance of the sector across both developed and low- and middle-income countries. Health, whether provided by insurance in the USA, by direct state funding in the UK or by direct payment in much of the developing world, is big business. OECD data suggest that in 2009 the proportion of gross domestic product spent on health care varied between 6.4% in Mexico and 17.4% in the USA, with the UK at 9.8% and Germany, Switzerland and Canada around 11% [1]. These are considerable amounts of money and they are growing, and in many cases, exemplified by the USA, are growing fast. Demographic ageing fuels this growth.

Health care works. Because of this, the world population is getting older, people are living longer, and old age carries a set of risks for illness. Dementia can be presented as the primary exemplar of such an illness and challenge. Taking the USA, in 2000, 4.5% of the population was over 65, and there were 411,000 new cases of Alzheimer's disease; by 2010 the proportion had increased to

Designing and Delivering Dementia Services, First Edition. Edited by Hugo de Waal, Constantine Lyketsos, David Ames, and John O'Brien.
© 2013 John Wiley & Sons, Ltd. Published 2013 by John Wiley & Sons, Ltd.

5.1%, with an extra 50,000 cases a year (data from US Alzheimer Association website). In the UK and Europe the numbers with dementia are set to double in the next generation with no likelihood that the disability and costs inherent in dementia will do anything other than continue. This creates the start of a potentially engaging narrative for dementia as articulated in chapter 8.

The potential consequences of this are profound. In 2010 Standard and Poor identified that the cost of caring for older people is likely to be a major determinant of the viability of the developed world economies in the medium term, and will profoundly affect growth prospects across the world [2]. They advocated that immediate strategic action should be taken to prevent foreseeable age-related crises and that public finance policy debates should be focused on this worldwide. For them the response of countries to these health and care challenges was likely to be a major determinant of sovereign credit worthiness in the next decade, not the evils of bankers. In the 13th *Geneva Report on the World Economy*, the major barrier to growth in Japan was identified as the high level of health and social benefits paid to older people which were 'squeezing out many other forms of government spending as a result', while in the USA growth was seen as being retarded by gross inefficiencies in its health system [3]. The US economy is in peril from the cost of long-term diseases and the Medicare system.

Each of the contributors to the previous chapters has been successful in framing policy development for dementia in this context. They make clear just how much of that spend may be attributable to dementia, just how many ways there are for that money to be spent better and just how much more value can be generated by this investment.

A worldwide issue

The work of Alzheimer's Disease International (ADI) and Alzheimer Europe (AE) makes clear that we are all in this together, that no country or system escapes, that the blissful inaction of the past century with respect to dementia cannot hold. Importantly, ADI has caught the attention of the WHO by the work set out in its *World Alzheimer Reports* of 2009 and 2010 just as AE has in Europe [4,5]. In the first report, the data on the epidemiology of dementia are systematically reviewed to generate an estimate of the numbers with the illness and likely growth in the next decades. In the second report, the economic impacts of dementia are subject to similar review. Their best estimate is that dementia currently affects 35.6 million people, 0.5% of the global population, with the numbers set to double in the next 20 years.

At present, 50% of people with dementia live in high-income countries, 39% in middle-income countries and 14% in low-income countries. But these proportions will change profoundly in the next years. The demographic trend for increases in longevity, and with it the incidence of dementia, is most marked in rapidly developing countries such as China and India.The predictions are that the number of people with dementia will roughly double every 20 years, to 65.7 million in 2030 and 115.4 million in 2050, and that most of this increase will be in low- and middle income countries [4]. Quoted in an article in *Nature*, one of the report's authors, Anders Wimo, an epidemiologist with an interest in economics from the Karolinska Institute in Stockholm, stated: 'we are seeing a linear increase in prevalence in rich countries, but an exponential increase in low-income countries . . . the need for solutions is urgent' [6].

A shared language

There is a need for a shared language if the issues of dementia are to be communicated, and in 'numbers' and 'cost' the four contributors in chapter 8 have addressed two of the most widely understood concepts.

In their 2010 report, the ADI estimated the global economic impact of dementia to be $604 billion [5]. What is really striking about this is that these cost-of-illness figures dwarf those of the illnesses that are currently prioritised at a national and international level such as HIV, cancer, heart disease, stroke and diabetes [7]. Echoing the concerns of Standard and Poor, based on simple demographics, the costs of dementia are set to increase by 85% by 2030, with developing countries bearing an increasing share of the economic burden [2]. The ADI report used the best available data to determine the direct medical and social care costs, and the indirect opportunity costs of care (family care and reduced productivity). Currently, 90% of the global costs of dementia fall to the developed world, with 70% attributable to Western Europe and North America; at present less than 1% of costs are borne by low-income countries. However, this will change predictably and change quickly. There are interesting potential differences here between India and China. Both have high rates of growth of people with dementia, but India's demographics mean that there is likely to be a good supply of labour at a reasonable price with which to care for people with dementia when needed. However, in China, the one-child policy initiated in the 1970s is having its demographic effect. This is compounded by the massive migration of particularly younger people from rural to urbanised areas. The consequence is that parents who age and need home care in the next 20 years may not be able to rely on their families, and the costs of care may be prohibitive.

People in China are increasingly aware and fearful of this, and saving for health and long-term care is one of the motors behind the personal savings boom there. As Haldane stated in his paper on global imbalances and their causes:

'Much of the rise in saving propensities appears to be precautionary. Facing "three mountains" in the future – education, pensions and health care – Chinese consumers have taken the high (saving) road' [8].

The conclusion is clear: dementia has macroeconomic consequences.

This is a language and narrative that has been developed by each contributor in the previous chapter and increasingly by others across the globe. It is a language and narrative that can make the world change.

Intervention to manage the challenge: Development of public policy

At a political level, the nature of the problem must be clear at a national level for the need for policy and action to be recognised. We have clear descriptions of how this has been achieved at national and supra-national levels (and some are reported upon in Section IV of this book). Similar processes to the successes presented here have led to dementia being made a public health and social care priority in other developed countries, including France, Denmark, Australia, Japan, South Korea and Ireland. In the USA, the National Alzheimer Planning Act was passed into law with bipartisan support in 2010 in the midst of legislative meltdown. In the developing world, India is working towards policy in this area. Across the world, politicians and policymakers are waking to the need to do something, rather than nothing, about dementia.

How can things be changed?

In order to develop a good strategy you need to be able to understand how things have come to be the way they are, as well as what you are aiming for in the future. All the contributors have striven to understand why a disorder so serious, so complicated, so expensive and so common was at the bottom of a long list of clinical priorities, as it was in the Department of Health (DH) in England in 2005. Why was it acceptable for the very large majority of cases of dementia to go undiagnosed and untreated? How could things be changed? The answer to all these questions was to build the case. There were pieces of evidence that needed to be brought together. With some extra work to fill in gaps, a narrative could be generated that could establish dementia as a health and social care priority. It was like building a path of stepping stones across a broad river towards a formal National Dementia Strategy (NDS).

Building the narrative

Stories are powerful in policy and politics, and medicine is not all about the reductive empiricism of randomised controlled trials and test tubes. At the start of each of their processes, the problem with the information about dementia was that it was complicated, disorganised and equivocal. As formulated by Heath et al., there was a need to build a clear simple narrative, with unimpeachable logic, that made a compelling case for change [9]. One that others would remember, own and tell to others, spreading the word. This meant building a story and a constituency of allies. It is possible to derive a seven-point change plan, with the first five the big questions that needed simple answers leading to a sixth 'development phase' and then a seventh 'implementation phase'. Each needed to be operationalised and delivered internationally (see Box 9.1 for the outline change plan).

There are strengths and weaknesses to formulating an action plan in this way. It is simple, so tasks can be chunked into manageable bits, but it may miss sub-steps. Mapping the data from the reports and enquiries summarised by Andrew Chidgey for England onto this framework results in an outline with which to draft an effective narrative (see Box 9.2).

In this, in England, we had the bones of our clear story. The next step was to articulate it as a whole and ensure that everybody comes to be telling it the same way. In terms of the Heath brother's formulation of message types, this is one that moves from common sense ('dementia is bad') to uncommon sense ('we should spend to save') [9]. It has elements that correspond to the SUCCESs framework they suggest can help an idea or message to become 'sticky'. In this the narrative below (see Box 9.3) is

- Simple – finding the core of the idea – it's bad, it's big, we can do something
- Unexpected – grabbing attention by surprising them – more than stroke, heart disease and cancer put together
- Concrete – an idea that can be grasped and remembered later – 700,000 people, £17 billion
- Credible – believability – evidence based, referenced
- Emotional – so people see the importance – use of adjectives to describe impacts
- Stories – empower people to use an idea through narrative – a single through line

---

Box 9.1 Action plan to make and deliver an NDS

Step 1: What are the numbers? – how many people with dementia are there?
Step 2: What are the costs? – how much does dementia cost?
Step 3: What about the future? – what will happen to the numbers and the cost in the future?
Step 4: Is it broke? – if the system is not broke there will not be the necessary urgency to fix it.
Step 5: They would say that wouldn't they? – is there independent corroboration of the need for change?
Step 6: Develop the strategy – making sure it has all the right elements.
Step 7: Implement the strategy – then we can all go home.

Box 9.2 Action plan to make and deliver an NDS for England

Step 1: **What are the numbers?** – 700,000, a definitive estimate of people with dementia in the UK. There is no more powerful tool than locally derived and relevant data.

Step 2: **What are the costs?** – £17 billion per year, a sum equivalent to a fifth of the whole health budget and more than heart disease, stroke and cancer combined.

Step 3: **What about the future?** – In the UK in just 30 years (i.e. in 2027) there would be a doubling of the numbers of people with dementia to 1.4 million and a trebling of the costs to over £50 billion per year. These figures make clear the need for a strategic plan for dementia and strongly support the need for this to be at a national rather than a local level.

Step 4: **Is it broke?** – The Dementia UK report and the National Audit Office (NAO) report, along with external data, suggesting that the UK is in the bottom third of European performance, all make the case for the system being 'broke'.

Step 5: **They would say that wouldn't they?** – Independent corroboration is vital. To gain credibility, it is very useful if dispassionate external assessment can come to the same conclusions. The NAO report (2007)[1] and the subsequent enquiry by the UK House of Commons' Public Accounts Committee (PAC; 2008)[2] confirmed the findings of the Dementia UK report providing vital external validation.

[1]Improving Services and Support for People with Dementia. London, National Audit Office, 2007.
[2]Public Accounts Committee. Improving Services and Support for People with Dementia. London, TSO, 2008.

Box 9.3 The UK narrative

In the UK we have 700,000 people with dementia and 200,000 new cases a year. It is a devastating disorder for those affected causing irreversible decline in global intellectual, social and physical functioning. The cost of caring for people with dementia is immense, £17 billion per year, greater than stroke, heart disease, and cancer put together. There are major problems with the health and social care system for dementia. Only a third of people with dementia ever receive a diagnosis and then often late in the illness when it is too late to prevent harm. There are misconceptions that nothing can be done for dementia. This is not true. There is a vast amount that can be done to enable people to live well with dementia. Finally, better dementia care is cheaper than the poor quality care we now provide (including £8 billion pa on care home places). We need to change the system to improve diagnosis and care; this will improve the quality of life of people with dementia and their carers and save money by reducing unnecessary institutionalisation.

How are we doing?: Research

Research into dementia is vital and all of the contributors have attempted to address this with varying degrees of success. We would hope that we would be able to treat or prevent dementia in the future. That depends on research. There are three main sources of funds for this: governments, the pharmaceutical industry and charities. The charity sector in dementia is very young and so does not have the deep pocketed bequests of cancer and heart disease. The charity funds available are therefore very small.

If the prevalence and cost of dementia are considered from the viewpoint of the pharmaceutical industry, then it is no surprise that there is a very high degree of interest and investment in this area. The cholinesterase inhibitors have been blockbuster drugs for their makers and they only afford limited symptomatic support. Who could resist entering the market where there is a devastating disease which is perceived of as worse than death and cancer? A disease which is terminal but can last 7–12 years from diagnosis? A disease where there is no cure, so any advance is likely to be used? An illness which affects the developed world in particular, irrespective of income, ethnicity or region? A potential market of 36 million people guaranteed to double in the next generation? However, the complexity and cost of trials in dementia, along with some high-profile late-phase 3 trial failures, means that there is a withdrawal from the field in many countries, with a wait for new basic insights to emerge.

The allocation of public research funds does not seem to reflect the costs of illnesses. In *Dementia 2010* it was estimated that in 2010, the UK annual national cost of dementia was £23 billion, twice that of cancer (£12 billion) and much more than heart disease (£8 billion) and stroke (£5 billion) [7]. However, the UK public spend on cancer research was 12 times higher than on dementia. In the USA, the National Institutes of Health spend 13 times more on cancer than on dementia. In research terms, governments are still fighting the last century's wars. This needs to change.

How are we doing?: The NDS

It is important to look critically at what we have done for the sake of future developments and for other territories entering into this phase of policy formulation. So how did we do in England? Using Jick's [10] 'Ten Commandments' we can complete an appraisal of what we might have done to strengthen our work and what we did (generally entirely unmindfully) that was positive in our method of strategy formation (see Box 9.4).

Box 9.4 Ten commandment analysis of NDS development for England

1. **Analyse the organisation and its need for change** – the consultation and NDS formulation certainly did this on a whole system level and at a functional level. The system analysis has stood the test of time and the test of governmental change: indeed, having its status increased, most recently by the Prime Minister's Dementia Challenge [11] and previously in post-election positive revisions to the NHS Operating Framework.
2. **Create a shared vision and common direction** – the simple vision of enabling people to live well with dementia, the clear narrative on why this was needed and what we should do, and the subsequent emergent identification of three key themes are supportive of positive action in this domain.
3. **Separate from the past** – we took care to build on the past so as not to alienate past players, but we also acknowledged explicitly the failure of the past policy as set out in the National Service Framework for Older People (2001). This received external validation in the NAO and PAC reports.
4. **Create a sense of urgency** – this was provided by the NAO and PAC proceedings and report. This enabled the whole of the UK Department of Health (DH) to be mobilised to meet the challenge.
5. **Support a strong leader role** – the need for a National Clinical Director (NCD) for Dementia was identified, but there was high resistance to creating such a role within DH. This was in the end resolved and there is now an excellent NCD in place, but that took a further 2 years.
6. **Line up political sponsorship** – the PAC gave an understanding of the issues to the executives at DH. We also got the external bodies well aligned and kept them so during the consultation.
7. **Draft an implementation plan** – this was done but it was weaker than the strategy. This phase requires separate strategy formulation for execution, not just ad hoc activity.
8. **Develop enabling structures** – DH created a dementia team with a network of regional implementation leads and a national board.
9. **Communicate, involve people and be honest** – this really was a cooperative venture with the Alzheimer's Society. The strategy was fuller, stronger and more effective than it would have been otherwise because of the openness and honesty in its construction.
10. **Reinforce and institutionalise change** – the jury is still out on this!

Conclusion

The reports in Chapter 8 and in some of the contributions in Section IV of this book give good reason to hope that dementia will be addressed by the formulation and delivery of national and international strategies for quality improvement. We have a shared narrative that dementia is a clear and present economic challenge for the world, countries and individuals, from the macro level right down to the unique economic circumstances of individuals. Before the economic crisis, governmental structural primary deficits were generally improving, and this would have given time and resource to meet the challenges of ageing in general and dementia in particular. However, increasing government debt over the past 3 years has had the effect of our needing to implement reforms to contain the risks to sovereign budgets sooner rather than later. This is not an issue that can be ignored any longer. Inaction will only lead to further debt accumulation in the medium term and the death of systems of care in the long term. We can conclude that across the developed world, the main long-term fiscal challenges come from healthcare costs [3] and dementia is a major driver of those costs. There is a need for budgetary consolidation and pension reform more generally. But given that dementia is the highest ticket health and social care item that we have (making up 60% of long-term care spend by some estimates) investment into early intervention and into research (into causes, cure and care) is likely to be of major value in personal, societal, political and economic terms. If the world's economy is not to suffer from dementia, then it must 'get' Alzheimer's in terms of the need for explicit policy prioritisation, as David Cameron in the UK has done with his personal, prime-ministerial challenge that we should go further and faster with care and research in dementia [11]. Action is then needed to make that policy happen.

References

1. OECD (2011) OECD Health Data 2011 – Frequently Requested Data. Available at: http://www.oecd.org/document/60/0,3746,en_2649_33929_2085200_1_1_1_1,00.html (last accessed on 19 February 2013).
2. Standard and Poor (2011) *Global Ageing 2010: An Irreversible Truth*. New York: S&P.
3. Eichengreen B, Feldman R, Liebman J, von Hagen J, Wyplosz C (2011) *Public Debts: Nuts, Bolts and Worries*. Geneva: ICMB.
4. Alzheimer's Disease International (2009) *World Alzheimer Report 2009*. London: ADI.
5. Alzheimer's Disease International (2010) *World Alzheimer Report 2010*. London: ADI.
6. Abbott A (2010) Dementia: a problem for our age. *Nature* 475:S2–S4.
7. Alzheimer's Research Trust (2010) *Dementia 2010*. Cambridge: ART.
8. Haldane AG (2010) *Global Imbalances in Retrospect and Prospect*. London: Bank of England.
9. Heath C, Heath D (2007) *Made to Stick: Why Some Ideas Survive and Others Die*. New York: Random House.
10. Jick TD (1991) *Implementing Change: Note*. Harvard: Harvard Business Review.
11. Department of Health (2012) *Prime Minister's Challenge on Dementia. Delivering Major Improvements in Dementia Care and Research by 2015*. London: DH.

Chapter 10

Health economics, healthcare funding and service evaluation: International and Australian perspectives

Julie Ratcliffe[a], Lynne Pezzullo[b] and Colleen Doyle[c]

[a]School of Medicine, Flinders University, Repatriation General Hospital, Daw Park, Australia
[b]Health Economics and Social Policy, Deloitte Access Economics, Deloitte Touche Tohmatsu, Australia
[c]National Ageing Research Institute, Royal Melbourne Hospital, Australia

Introduction

Dementia was recently identified by the World Health Organisation (WHO) as a public health priority [1], and governments in a number of countries have begun to shape policy to account for the cost implications of this burgeoning population. A number of countries now have dementia strategies in place. In recognition of its importance as a health priority, dementia has been targeted for increases in health service funding twice in five-year national initiatives in Australia – in 1997 in a National Action Plan for Dementia Care and then again in 2005 in the Dementia National Health Priority Initiative. Both initiatives were evaluated to determine the effect of extra funding on population health, the second initiative more extensively than the first. In this chapter we will discuss a number of external drivers, encountered in the international arena and in Australia, as these influence dementia service delivery and development. This should enable the reader to form an overview of relevant aspects in the fields of health economics, healthcare funding and service evaluation (the latter particularly as being used to underpin decision-making processes, relative to economic and funding considerations). Examples will be provided from international literature and from Australian dementia care initiatives. The content of this chapter will set the scene for Section V, Chapter 15: 'Developing a Business Case, Negotiating, Securing Funding'.

The economic impact of dementia

Chronic diseases such as dementia have a substantial economic impact. Chronic disease costs are highest for heart disease, stroke, diabetes and lung disease, but costs for dementia follow closely in magnitude, are substantial and growing due to the age-related nature of the disease [2]. An

Designing and Delivering Dementia Services, First Edition. Edited by Hugo de Waal, Constantine Lyketsos, David Ames, and John O'Brien.
© 2013 John Wiley & Sons, Ltd. Published 2013 by John Wiley & Sons, Ltd.

influential report on the global economic impact of dementia published by Alzheimer's Disease International estimated the worldwide cost of dementia was US$604 billion in 2010. This cost highlighted the impact of dementia care on the world economy. According to the WHO, if dementia care were a country, it would rank as the world's 21st largest economy, between Poland and Saudi Arabia [1].

The costs associated with dementia include direct health and social care costs and informal family care costs. The costs of dementia care are due to a high proportion of people with dementia needing some form of care. At the mild stage of dementia, support may be in the form of education to the carer, activities of daily living aids, personal care and aids in the home. As dementia progresses, the cost of care also increases. At the moderate to severe stage of dementia, costs will be incurred for assistance with personal and instrumental activities of daily living. Once residential care is used in the later stages of dementia, the costs will continue to be higher than for people with mainly physical health conditions.

In a world of increasing resource constraints, the drive to promote efficiency in the delivery of dementia care treatment and service programmes is becoming ever more acute, and economic evaluation, with its focus upon the quantification of a systematic and transparent framework for evaluating the costs and benefits of competing healthcare interventions, is increasingly utilised to facilitate difficult decisions about the optimal allocation of scarce resources both within dementia care and across the healthcare sector more broadly.

Types of economic evaluation

Economic evaluation is defined as the comparative assessment of the costs and benefits of alternative healthcare interventions [3]. There are four main types of economic evaluation which can be used in the context of dementia care evaluation: cost-effectiveness analysis, cost-utility analysis, cost-benefit analysis and cost-consequence analysis [4]. The key feature that distinguishes the different types of economic evaluation is the unit for measuring the benefits of health care:

- Cost-effectiveness analysis determines what is the best method of achieving a given objective, usually measured in clinical or 'natural' units, and presents results in terms of cost per unit of effect (e.g. cost per symptom free day, cost per unit improvement in cognitive functioning).
- Cost-utility analysis compares the costs of alternative healthcare programmes with their utility, usually measured in terms of quality adjusted life years (QALYs).
- Cost-benefit analysis compares the benefits with costs of a healthcare programme, where all the benefits are valued in monetary terms, including health improvement.
- Cost-consequence analysis was developed as a response to concerns about the extent to which all the relevant considerations for the measurement of benefits could be incorporated within a single number in an economic evaluation [5]. The results of a cost-consequence analysis are therefore presented in the form of a table, where all the relevant factors are presented, but are not collapsed into a single number to enable a unique and complete ranking of different treatment options (as would be the case with e.g. results presented in terms of cost per QALY estimates).

The most widely applied technique of economic evaluation internationally within the healthcare sector is cost-utility analysis. Many regulatory authorities, including the National Institute of Health and Clinical Excellence [6] in England and Wales and the Pharmaceutical Benefits Advisory Committee in Australia [7], routinely require the presentation of a cost-utility analysis alongside information relating to the clinical safety and efficacy of a new health technology as part of their reimbursement decision-making process.

Economic evaluations in dementia

Historically, economic evaluations of treatments and service programmes for dementia are surprisingly rare in comparison with other clinical conditions. The National Institute for Health Research, Centre for Reviews and Dissemination NHS Economic Evaluation Database, which contains abstracts of published journal articles from around the world relating to the effectiveness and cost-effectiveness of healthcare interventions, records a total of only 22 abstracts (out of a possible total of 12,400 abstracts) relating to economic evaluations in dementia. However, as dementia is now increasingly being recognised as representing an accelerating projected expenditure burden for limited healthcare budgets internationally, it is reasonable to expect a greater focus upon economic evaluations of treatments and service programmes for dementia care in the future. Of the 22 studies currently identified by the NHS Economic Evaluation Database, 16 (73%) were defined as cost-effectiveness analyses, 2 (9%) were defined as cost-benefit analyses, and the remaining 4 studies (18%) were defined as cost-utility analyses.

An example of a recent cost-effectiveness study undertaken in dementia is a Canadian study by Wong and colleagues [8], which examined the cost-effectiveness of pharmacological treatments (cholinesterase inhibitors donepezil, galantamine, rivastigmine or memantine) for mild to moderate vascular dementia. This study developed a decision analytic model with costs and outcomes populated using data extracted from a systematic review to examine the costs associated with pharmacological treatments, adverse events, other medications and physician visits over a 28-week time horizon. Outcomes were assessed by the Alzheimer's Disease Assessment Scale cognitive (ADAS-cog) subscale which is commonly used to assess cognitive dysfunction in individuals with Alzheimer disease and other dementias [9]. The results indicated that the most cost-effective treatment option was Donepezil 10 mg daily with an incremental cost-effectiveness ratio of $401 per unit decline in the ADAS-cog subscale.

A further example is provided by a UK-based cost-effectiveness study of cognitive stimulation therapy for people with dementia [10]. This economic evaluation was undertaken alongside a clinical trial with a total of 91 people with dementia randomised to receive evidence-based cognitive stimulation therapy and a total of 70 people with dementia randomised to receive care as usual over an 8-week period. Cognitive function, as measured by the mini mental state examination score (MMSE) [11] was utilised as the primary measure of outcome for the cost-effectiveness analysis. The results indicated that cognitive stimulation therapy was associated with an incremental cost-effectiveness ratio of £75 per additional point improvement on the MMSE.

The main difficulty with studies of this nature is that it is very difficult to compare the findings across treatment options; for example, is it more cost-effective to devote limited healthcare resources to providing pharmacological treatments or psychological therapies to individuals with mild to moderate dementia? In order to address this type of question, two main conditions are required. Firstly, it is necessary for different treatment and service programmes to be evaluated using the same outcome measure. Secondly, information is required about the decision-makers' willingness to pay for a specified improvement in the main outcome measure of interest. Given that a healthcare decision-maker is often faced with the need to address 'allocative efficiency' issues, that is, the allocation of scarce healthcare resources across the healthcare system for the treatment of all diseases and conditions as opposed to 'technical efficiency' issues, that is, the allocation of scarce healthcare resources within one particular disease or condition, for example dementia, it is also preferable that the outcome measure is generic (applicable to all diseases and conditions) to facilitate meaningful comparisons of the cost-effectiveness of treatment and service programmes across the healthcare system. Cost-utility analysis, with its focus upon improvements in health status as defined by the QALY as the main measure of outcome (at least in principle), achieves these objectives.

Hence, it has become the preferred method of economic evaluation internationally for regulatory and other decision-making bodies in health care.

Examples of cost-utility studies in dementia include an economic evaluation conducted alongside a clinical trial to establish whether a structured befriending service improved the quality of life of carers of people with dementia and at what cost [12]. This study was conducted over a 15-month period and involved 236 carers of people with a primary progressive dementia who were randomised to receive a trained lay volunteer befriender versus no befriender contact. The results indicated that the befriender programme was associated with an additional mean total cost of £1813 per carer and an additional QALY gain of 0.017. The incremental cost-effectiveness ratio is calculated by dividing the additional mean total cost by the additional QALY gains (£1813/0.017). The befriender programme was therefore associated with a relatively high incremental cost-effectiveness ratio of £106,647 per QALY gained. The National Institute for Clinical Excellence (NICE) guidance for the NHS in England and Wales [6] recommends that interventions with an incremental cost-effectiveness ratio above £30,000 per QALY are generally not considered as cost-effective, and hence the authors concluded that befriending is unlikely to be considered a cost-effective intervention from the viewpoint of society.

A further example of a cost-utility analysis in dementia is a study to evaluate an integrated diagnostic approach for cognitively impaired older people in the Netherlands [13]. This economic evaluation was undertaken alongside a randomised controlled trial and compared costs and outcomes over a 1-year time horizon for 230 patients randomised to receive multidisciplinary assessment and advice through screening, psychogeriatric assessment and evaluation of required care levels for the patient and caregiver versus usual care provided by the patient's general practitioner. The results indicated that the integrated diagnostic approach for cognitively impaired older people was associated with an additional total cost of 65 euros per patient with an additional QALY gain of 0.05. The incremental cost effectiveness ratio was therefore 1300 euros (65/0.005). The authors concluded that this ratio was well within accepted cost per QALY thresholds for determining cost-effectiveness, and hence the use of an integrated multidisciplinary diagnostic facility is likely to be highly cost-effective for the diagnosis and management of dementia in ambulatory patients.

An example of a cost-benefit study in dementia is a Canadian study which aimed to measure the economic value of cholinesterase inhibitors in the treatment of Alzheimer's disease [14]. The willingness to pay approach was utilised with a relatively small study sample of 28 nonprofessional caregivers of outpatients diagnosed with mild to moderate dementia. The results indicated that caregivers were willing to pay $Can3686 to $Can4540 per year for the stabilisation of behavioural symptoms from cholinesterase inhibitors. The authors concluded that the caregivers were willing to pay more for cholinesterase inhibitors than the drugs' costs, even when the adverse effects of the drugs are taken into consideration, and this therefore indicates a net benefit for cholinesterase inhibitors in the treatment of mild to moderate dementia.

In practice, cost-benefit analysis is less widely applied than either cost-effectiveness or cost-utility analysis. One of the main reasons for this is the difficulty associated with valuing the benefits of health care in monetary terms. Economists have tended to favour stated preference or contingent valuation approaches in assessing how much individuals would be hypothetically willing to pay to receive a healthcare treatment or service programme. While the willingness-to-pay approach has been popular in other areas of economics, including environmental and transport economics, the approach has been less widely applied in health economics [4]. The approach raises concerns due to its distributional implications since willingness to pay is intrinsically linked with an individual's ability to pay. This effectively means that those individuals with higher income levels are able to express higher willingness to pay values and therefore their values may carry greater weight than those individuals with lower income levels who are unable to express high values due to their comparatively reduced income levels. In addition, another problem arises from the fact that many healthcare systems around the world are either largely or exclusively publically provided and financed from general taxation. As such, it is often difficult to elicit willingness to pay values from individuals who may be unwilling and/or unused to thinking about having to pay out of pocket expenditures for the consumption of health care.

Measuring and valuing quality of life in dementia

In order to conduct a cost-utility analysis, we need to collect and present data relating to the measurement and valuation of quality of life in addition to the presentation of data relating to the measurement and valuation of resource use (costs). Traditionally, QALYs have been used to value the benefits of healthcare services and programmes within cost-utility analysis [15]. To calculate QALYs, it is necessary to represent health-related quality of life on a scale where death and full health are assigned values of 0 and 1, respectively. Therefore, states rated as better than dead have values between 0 and 1, and states rated as worse than dead have negative scores which, in principle, are bounded by negative infinity [4]. Indirect valuation of quality of life through the usage of generic preference-based measures of physical and mental health such as the EQ-5D (EuroQol), AQoL (Assessment of Quality of Life) and the SF-6D have become the most popular mechanisms for the estimation of QALYs for cost-utility analyses [4]. Generic preference-based measures of health comprise two main elements: a descriptive system for completion by patients or members of the general population comprising a set of items with multiple response categories covering the different dimensions reflecting health-related quality of life and an off-the-shelf scoring algorithm which reflects society's strength of preference for the health states defined by the instrument. The scoring algorithms are typically generated from large general population surveys to elicit values for a selection of health states described by each descriptive system [4]. Statistical modelling techniques are then employed to infer health state values for all health states described by each descriptive system. The scoring algorithms are anchored on the numerical scale required to construct QALYs, where full health is 1 and 0 is equivalent to death. For some instruments, for example, EQ-5D, particularly severe health states are associated with negative values, reflecting the average general population view that these states are considered worse than death.

Both of the cost-utility studies highlighted in the previous section used a generic preference-based measure of health, the EQ-5D, to calculate QALY gains. In the befriending study by Wilson et al., the EQ-5D was administered at baseline, 6, 15 and 24 months by face-to-face and telephone interviews. The individual responses to the EQ-5D were then converted to health state values or utilities by applying the scoring algorithm attached to the instrument. The QALY gains for intervention and control groups were then estimated for the entire period using area under the curve methods. Similarly, the economic evaluation of an integrated diagnostic approach for older people by Wolfs et al. also administered the EQ-5D at baseline, 6 and 12 months and then estimated the QALY gains for intervention and control groups using area under the curve methods. However, generic instruments, such as the EQ-5D, have been criticised as lacking sensitivity and having questionable validity in people with dementia. For example, one study found that 48% of people diagnosed with dementia self-reported themselves as being in full health according to their individual responses to the EQ-5D, with no reported problems on any dimension, including anxiety and depression [16]. More recently, condition-specific preference-based single index measures for dementia have been developed using the DEMQoL and DEMQoL-Proxy instruments [17]. These instruments have been specifically developed and validated in a cognitively impaired population across the full range of dementia and are therefore likely to be more appropriate than generic instruments for assessing health-related quality of life in people with dementia. DEMQoL has been designed for self-report in people with mild to moderate dementia whereas DEMQoL-Proxy enables measurement (and longitudinal follow-up) via proxy (carer) report for people with severe dementia. These condition-specific preference-based single index measures are based upon the values of the general population and enable individuals' responses to the DEMQoL and DEMQoL-Proxy instruments to be converted into health state values or utilities. These utilities can then be applied to generate QALY gains to inform economic evaluations of treatment and service programmes in dementia using a system that is appropriate across the full range of the condition.

To calculate disability adjusted life years (DALYs), it is necessary to utilise the burden of disease approach originally developed by Harvard University and the World Bank [18], and subsequently adopted by the WHO, which now periodically develops global burden of disease estimates at regional levels for more than 135 disease and injury conditions [19] as well as DALYs attributable to particular health risk factors [20].

The DALY has two components – the years of life lost (YLL) from premature death and the years of life lived (YLD) in less than full health. YLLs are calculated from the number of deaths at each age multiplied by a global standard life expectancy for each age. YLDs are estimated as the number of cases of a condition in the period multiplied by the average duration of the condition and a 'disease weight'. The disease weights reflect the severity of the condition on a scale from 0 (perfect health) to 1 (death) and are listed online [19]. For dementia, the weights used are 0.270 for mild dementia, 0.630 for moderate dementia, and 0.940 for severe dementia, based on Dutch weights [21].

Advantages of using DALYs over QALYs in evaluating dementia interventions are that the premature mortality component is included, and health states are not rated worse than death by people with dementia who may have cognitive or psychological impairment, so associated policy dilemmas are precluded. The WHO also identifies cost-effectiveness thresholds in terms of dollars per DALY averted. Following the recommendations of the Organization's Commission on Macroeconomics and Health, WHO-CHOICE (CHOosing Interventions that are Cost Effective) uses gross domestic product (GDP) as a readily available indicator to derive the following three categories of cost-effectiveness per DALY averted: highly cost-effective (less than GDP per capita); cost-effective (between one and three times GDP per capita); and not cost-effective (more than three times GDP per capita). The WHO [22] has estimated threshold values of cost-effectiveness in international dollars for the year 2005 for each global region, and encourages use of these thresholds in considering funding for interventions.

Evaluation of Australia's dementia initiative

Australia has had two major federal strategies or initiatives that aimed to improve dementia care: in 1992–1996 and again in 2005–2009. Many of the programmes initiated in the latter strategy continue today. In the 2005 initiative, approximately AUD$320 million was provided over 5 years to support people with dementia and their carers through the 'Helping Australians with dementia and their carers – making dementia a National Health Priority Initiative'. The Initiative was evaluated extensively, and DEMQoL-Proxy was used in some of the evaluations to determine cost utility. The example is instructive as the economic evaluation was embedded in a broader evaluation of the impact of the initiative as measured through a series of key performance criteria or performance indicators.

The overarching aim of the Dementia Initiative was to support people with dementia and their carers, through the implementation of three 'measures': the first 'measure' provided for additional research, improved care initiatives, and early intervention programmes in a broad-ranging suite of projects.

The second 'measure' was a new programme of community care called Extended Aged Care at Home Dementia (EACHD). Fully two-thirds of the total Initiative's funding provided an extra 2000 dementia-specific community care packages. The key external driver in developing this part of the policy was strong community interest in maintaining care for people with dementia in their own homes, to the extent that individual packages of care were more expensive than providing the care in a residential aged care (RAC) facility. The third 'measure' of the initiative was an injection of funding to provide extra training to care for people with dementia. This part involved additional dementia-specific training for up to 9000 aged care workers, and up to 7000 carers and community workers.

The overall objective of the National Evaluation was to provide information to address two questions:

- What effect does the Dementia Initiative have on consumers, that is, people with dementia and their carers?
- What added value was given to current dementia care in Australia as a result of the activities funded by the Dementia Initiative?

The specific aims of the National Evaluation were to evaluate the extent to which the Dementia Initiative met eight key performance criteria. The eight key performance criteria as articulated in the evaluation framework were: appropriateness, effectiveness, efficiency, quality, accessibility, impact on collaboration, sustainability and outcomes. A summary of the performance criteria with definitions is provided in Table 10.1.

Table 10.1 Summary of key performance criteria used to frame an evaluation of the most recent Australian dementia strategy (*Source*: Reference [23]. Reproduced in part with permission of the Australian Government.)

Performance criterion	Definition
Appropriateness	Extent to which the projects, programmes and the overall Dementia Initiative were suitable or fitting for the group of clients targeted; for example, the extent to which an intervention to improve assessment is appropriate for people from culturally and linguistically diverse backgrounds if they are included in the target group.
Effectiveness	Extent to which the projects, programme and the overall Dementia Initiative are producing their desired effect as measured by standardised outcome measures
Efficiency	Level of effective or useful output given the total input or cost
Quality	Extent to which the projects, programme and the overall Dementia Initiative possess those attributes deemed to be desirable based on specified normative standards or criteria
Accessibility	Extent of the price, quantity or other barriers that result in unmet need in the target populations; an assessment of the reach of the intervention
Impact on collaboration	Extent to which the projects, programme and the overall Dementia Initiative encouraged stakeholders to operate jointly or in collaboration with other programmes
Sustainability	Extent to which the projects, programme and the overall Dementia Initiative are able to remain in existence beyond the period of special funding over the longer term, without the need for extraordinary funding injections
Outcomes	The end results or consequences, as measured by standardised outcome measurement tools, or qualitative information

The Dementia Initiative was implemented in the context of strong government and community advocacy for the development of aged care supports [23]. The economic evaluation of the Dementia Initiative set out to answer the question: was the Dementia Initiative value for money? In evaluating the performance of the Initiative as a whole and of each of the three measures, seven components of the initiative were subject to individual in-depth evaluations. Some of the results of these evaluations are presented here as illustrations. It was not possible to combine the separate in-depth evaluation programmes into one metric for the entire Initiative. Nor, in the case of measures 1 and 3, was it possible to create a single evaluation metric at the measure level. This was because the broad range of programmes included in the Initiative had necessitated the use of a variety of evaluation metrics, and many of the output or benefits measured were not comparable (e.g. outputs measured included QALYs/DALYs, publications, students trained, workload and work quality). It was possible, however, to make conclusions and recommendations based on the component parts, with a summary table to provide an overview by measure and across the whole Initiative [23].

Cost-effectiveness analysis – with benefits in natural units – was generally used as the economic evaluation method for measure 1 projects and sub-projects, although only Dementia Behavior Management Advisory Services (DBMASs) had sufficient data to support cost-benefit and cost-utility analysis. For each project, cost data were derived from the Department of Health and Ageing from financial reports, while outcome and output data were derived from progress reports together with

- for National Dementia Support Program (NDSP), satisfaction data from user surveys in 2006 and 2008;
- for DBMAS, a survey of RAC facilities where staff rated quality of life outcomes in relation to challenging behaviours of concern (using a scoring system which was converted to DALYs) for patients before and after the DBMAS service encounter (with gains tapered to zero 6 months after the intervention), as well as other success measures derived through a questionnaire;
- for Dementia Training Study Centres (DTSCs), a survey of the quality, usefulness and increase in knowledge, skills and work performance from the activities; and
- for Dementia Collaborative Research Centres (DCRCs), surveys similar to those for the DTSCs together with publication data (including reports, newsletters, literature reviews and other information in addition to formal peer-reviewed journal articles).

Key performance indicators (KPIs) relative to evaluation benchmarks are summarised in Table 10.2 (2009 dollars) [23].

Broadly, measure 1 projects were cost-effective and compared favourably with benchmarks. In the NDSP project, the Helpline cost less than the average of similar phone and other help services at AUD\$162–AUD\$191/hour. The Dementia and Memory Community Centres and early intervention/counselling elements were also less costly than alternatives provided through allied health, medical or specialist delivery models. There was no comparator for the information, awareness, education and training element of NDSP.

DBMAS showed a very favourable benefit/cost ratio of 7.25 to 1, costing an estimated AUD\$20,825 per DALY averted, ranked 'very cost-effective' by the WHO benchmarks. This was subject to the caveat of there being a study design and measurement of quality of life that was aimed at assessing primarily the response of the residential care facility to their experience with the DBMAS and only secondarily the response of the person with dementia.

The cost per student of DTSCs, at AUD\$1320 per student, although broadly aligned, is not strictly comparable with the cost/EFTSU in other Australian universities, since the DTSCs deliver a broad range of materials rather than standard tertiary education modules. It would be useful for future economic evaluations if DTSCs (or similar organisations) could measure and report their own outcomes in-terms of EFTSU.

Table 10.2 Summary of Economic Key Performance Indicators (KPI) relative to evaluation benchmarks, Measure 1 (*Source*: Reference [23]. Reproduced in part with permission of the Australian Government.)

Project/Sub-project	Economic KPIs	Comment on evaluation
National Dementia Support Programme		
1. National Dementia Helpline	AUD$67/call or AUD$162–AUD$191/hour AUD$71/satisfied caller	This cost was lower than the AUD$192–AUD$213/hour for average of comparable services.
2. Dementia and Memory Community Centres	AUD$3015/visitor AUD$1511/session AUD$170/satisfied participant	These costs per session were one-third of the cost of equivalent psychological group sessions, half of specialist group sessions costs and three-quarters of GP group sessions.
3. Early intervention/ counselling	AUD$1978/session = AUD$187/hour AUD$1101/satisfied participant	These costs were lower than the cost range for average of comparators.
4. Information, awareness, education and training	AUD$7625/session AUD$337/participant	Due to the diversity of the service mix, there was no appropriate comparator by which to benchmark this metric, but it was useful to provide for future reference.
Dementia Behaviour Management Advisory Service	Cost: AUD$980/PWD Benefit: AUD$7106/PWD	BCR: 7.25 (3.63–10.88) to 1 AUD$20,825/DALY averted (AUD$13,883–AUD$41,650), i.e. very cost-effective by WHO benchmark of less than GDP per capita/DALY.
Dementia Training Service Centres	AUD$1320 per student	This cost was not directly comparable with Effective Full-Time Student Units (EFTSU), but for comparison they were AUD$1326.
Dementia Collaborative Research Centres	AUD$52,677 per publication (AUD$43,897 to AUD$65,846)	These were very broad definitions, but were compared to the NHMRC benchmark of AUD$62,735 per publication.

PWD, person with dementia; BCR, benefit/cost ratio; DALY, disability adjusted life year; EFTSU, equivalent full-time student units.

For the DCRCs, the cost per publication was estimated as somewhat less than the NHMRC comparator, although the evaluation depended on a number of assumptions about outcomes that would occur in the future.

The second measure, the new community support programme EACHD (measure 2) was found to be cost-saving relative to RAC, the alternative model of care for people with high-level care needs, dementia and behavioural and psychological symptoms. The cost-effectiveness of EACHD was challenging to measure due to the intangible nature of many of the benefits of care, such as the provision of choice (see Table 10.3). Furthermore, due to the lack of availability of an appropriate control group, the benefits that were included in the analysis may have been underestimated (i.e. the person with dementia may have deteriorated relative to the measured outcomes were it not for the EACHD package).

Two final projects were evaluated under the third measure – the Dementia Caring Pilot (DCP) and the Dementia Care Essentials (DCE) programme, which provided dementia care education and skills training for family carers and aged care workers respectively. Both were evaluated through

Table 10.3 Summary of Economic Key Performance Indicators (KPI) relative to evaluation benchmarks, Measure 2 (*Source*: Reference [23]. Reproduced in part with permission of the Australian Government.)

Project/Sub-project	Economic KPIs	Evaluation
Extended Aged Care at Home Dementia (EACHD)	AUD$7199 per client saving relative to RAC (2007–2008) AUD$27.5 million total programme saving relative to RAC (to June 2008) AUD$0.39 in QoL benefits per AUD$ spent (2007–2008) AUD$0.44 in QoL benefits per AUD$ spent (to June 2008)	The overall conclusion was that the services provided in this programme were better value for money than RAC.

RAC, residential aged care; QoL, quality of life.

cost-effectiveness analysis using natural units, given data limitations – with extensions to cost-utility and cost-benefit analysis. Cost data comprised government funding information supplemented by data on co-contributions where applicable and numbers trained. The main benefits measured were workload reductions (i.e. productivity gains), work quality improvements and changes in quality of life for carers. Quality of life was measured using the Goal Attainment Scaling (GAS) tool.[1] Table 10.4 provides a summary of the results.

Two overarching issues affected the conclusions drawn from the economic evaluation of the Dementia Initiative[2]:

1. *The lack of control group data*: as with evaluations of many large government programmes where it is not possible to randomly allocate individuals to intervention and control services, a major difficulty with this economic evaluation was accurately to describe and estimate the null case, or what would have been the costs and outcomes (e.g. for health and quality of life) if the services provided by the programme did not exist. The degenerative nature of dementia means that in the absence of the Initiative, the person with dementia may have become more challenging to care for and had much reduced quality of life, but the extent of this deterioration was sometimes unable to be measured. Without the ability to measure a control group (for ethical and other reasons), some economic benefits may have been underestimated.
2. *Difficulties measuring the benefits of interventions*: a variety of issues arose in trying to capture the benefits of the health interventions included in the Initiative. There were some technical impediments, such as the inability to access participants in DCE in their workplaces in order to measure efficiency. In addition, the time horizon for the economic evaluation did not match the time horizon for the outputs of some projects (i.e. DCRCs). The intangible aspects of benefits were difficult to capture, since quality of life metrics tend to provide a single measure of well-being and may not pick up important changes caused by the intervention, such as the benefit of

---

[1]The GAS score is determined at a post-intervention interview whereby the interviewer assigns scores depending on the level achieved (+2 = much better than expected, +1 = better than expected, 0 = as expected, −1 = less than expected, −2 = much less than expected). The scores are then converted to a GAS t-score using a formula or Conversion Key Tables.
[2]Reproduced in part with permission of the Australian Government [23].

Table 10.4 Summary of Economic Key Performance Indicators (KPI) relative to evaluation benchmarks, Measure 3 (*Source*: Reference [23]. Reproduced in part with permission of the Australian Government.)

Project/ Sub-project	Economic KPIs	Evaluation
Dementia Caring Pilot (DCP)	AUD$2741 per session AUD$969 per participant AUD$1253–AUD$1407 per participant that received an improvement in wellbeing AUD$2092–AUD$2510 per GAS point	Based on the descriptors in the GAS scale, it appeared likely that the cost-effectiveness measured for this programme met the standard of ≤AUD$155,200/QALY and so was a cost-effective programme. It was noted though that there is no established conversion for the GAS into a QALY measure.
Dementia Care Essentials (DCE)	AUD$1437 per student trained AUD$0.22 per AUD$improvement in workload [BCR: 4.55 (1.54–7.45) to 1] AUD$4.72 per 1% improvement in work quality	We found that the DCE training was both cost-saving (netting AUD$3.55 in productivity gains for each dollar spent) and quality-enhancing (by around 4.5% per annum sustained for 3 years). When considered together, the same costs are producing an improvement in both workload and work quality.

BCR, benefit/cost ratio; QALY, quality adjusted life year; GAS, Goal Attainment Scale.

having your own choice in where you receive care. All efforts were made to overcome or account for these difficulties in fully measuring benefits. Nevertheless, costs are generally more explicit and evident in their nature and hence more likely to be fully captured in the analysis.

On the whole, in this large evaluation, the majority of projects in the Initiative were cost-effective or otherwise represented value for money compared to available comparators. In some cases the comparators were not ideal, or comparisons needed qualification. The results of the evaluations of measures 1 and 3 particularly underscored the effectiveness of interventions that up-skilled care-workers and supported informal carers. Measure 3 was found to be highly cost-effective, with the DCP outcome comparing favourably to the cost-effectiveness benchmark of AUD$155,200/QALY and the DCE project proving to be cost-saving.

Together the above economic evaluations, it has been demonstrated that it was possible to evaluate a broad range of dementia care programmes, from research to service provision to education and training.

Discussion and summary

While economic evaluation is not as advanced in the area of dementia care as in other health areas, there is a developing evidence base for the effectiveness of interventions that can improve the quality of life of people living with dementia. Cost-effectiveness studies of non-pharmacological treatments are able to borrow from methodologies used traditionally to identify drug treatments with the potential to improve the population's health and quality of life. In dementia care, we are increasingly interested in examining the impact of non-pharmacological treatments such as befriending and psychosocial interventions. These more complex interventions can still be effectively evaluated using standardised outcome measures and quality of life tools that are specifically designed for use with people with dementia and their carers.

The challenge in applying economic evaluations to a degenerative disease such as dementia is that any long-term benefit of any intervention may not be apparent because a deterioration in the individual's condition may be slowed rather than completely eliminated by the service provided. At a programme level, we have found that evaluation can provide meaningful interpretations of the effect of programme developments when key performance indicators or performance criteria are applied. Dementia care evaluation can also be well informed by the effect of services on care-workers and informal or family carers as well. Depending on the focus of the evaluation then, the outcome measures used can include direct observation of the effect of the service on the condition of the person living with dementia, the effect on their family or informal carer, or the effect on care-workers. Quality of life is likely to feature as an important outcome to be demonstrated in any economic evaluation. In the future we are likely to see not only more complex but also more meaningful economic evaluations that can reflect the subtlety of caring for individuals with a degenerative disease such as dementia.

Acknowledgements

Lynne Pezzullo and Colleen Doyle were part of the LAMA consortium that evaluated the Australian federal government's Dementia Initiative 2005–2009, funded by a tender from Australian Government Department of Health and Ageing. The LAMA consortium consisted of La Trobe University (Colleen Doyle and Vanessa White), Access Economics (Lynne Pezzullo and Katie Yates), University of Melbourne (David Dunt, Susan Day, Rosemary McKenzie, Pauline van Doort) and Applied Aged Care Solutions (Richard Rosewarne, Janet Opie). Sections of this chapter have been reproduced in part from LAMA consortium National Evaluation Dementia Initiative; Overview and Summary of Findings. Report to Australian Government Department of Health and Ageing. Sourced from Department of Health and Ageing website, available via: http://www.health.gov.au/internet/publications/publishing.nsf/Content/ageing-dementia-evaluation-htmlversion-toc. Last accessed 27/03/2013 with permission of the Australian Government.

References

1. World Health Organisation (2012) Dementia a public health priority. London, UK.
2. American Diabetes Association (2012) Direct and Indirect costs of diabetes in the United States. American Diabetes Association Website. Available at: http://www.diabetes.org/diabetes-basics (last accessed on 27 March, 2013).
3. Drummond M, Sculpher M, Torrance G, O'Brien B, Stoddart G (2005) *Methods for the Economic Evaluation of Health Care Programmes*, 3rd edn. Oxford: Oxford University Press.
4. Brazier J, Ratcliffe J, Salomon J, Tsuchiya A (2007) *Measuring and Valuing Health Benefits for Economic Evaluation*. Oxford: Oxford University Press.
5. Coast J (2004) Is economic evaluation in touch with society's health values? *British Medical Journal* 329:1233–1236.
6. National Institute for Clinical Excellence (NICE) (2008) *Up-Dated Guide to the Methods of Technology Appraisal*. London: NICE.
7. Commonwealth Department of Health, Housing and Community Service (2002) *Guidelines for the Pharmaceutical Industry on the Submission to the Pharmaceutical Benefits Advisory Committee*. Canberra: Australian Government Publishing Service.

8. Wong C, Bansback N, Lee P, Anis A (2009) Cost effectiveness: cholinesterase inhibitors and memantine in vascular dementia. *Canadian Journal of Neurological Science* 36:735–739.

9. Rosen WG, Mohs RC, Davis KL (1984) A new rating scale for Alzheimer's disease. *American Journal of Psychiatry* 141:1356–1364.

10. Knapp M, Thorgrmsen L, Patel A, Spector A, Hallam A, Woods B, et al. (2006) Cognitive stimulation therapy for people with dementia: cost-effectiveness analysis. *The British Journal of Psychiatry* 188: 574–580.

11. Folstein M, Folstein S, McHugh P (1975) 'Mini-mental state'. A practical method for grading the cognitive state of patients for the clinician. *Journal of Psychiatric Research* 12:189–198.

12. Wilson E, Thalanany M, Shepstone L, et al. (2009) Befriending carers of people with dementia: a cost utility study. *International Journal of Geriatric Psychiatry* 24:610–623.

13. Wolfs C, Dirksen C, Kessels A, et al. (2009) Economic evaluation of an integrated diagnostic approach for psychogeriatric patients. *Archives of General Psychiatry* 66:313–323.

14. Wu G, Lanctot K, Hermann N, Moosa S, Oh P (2003) The cost benefit of cholinesterase inhibitors in mild to moderate dementia: a willingness to pay approach. *CNS Drugs* 17:1045–1057.

15. Weinstein M, Torrance G, McGuire A (2009) QALYs: the basics. *Value in Health* 12:S5–S9.

16. Coucill W, Bryan S, Bentham P, Buckley A, Laight A (2001) EQ-5D in patients with dementia: an investigation of inter-rater agreement. *Medical Care* 39:760–771.

17. Rowen D, Mulhern B, Banerjee S (2012) Estimating preference-based single index measures for dementia using DEMQOL and DEMQOL-Proxy. *Value in Health* 15:346–356.

18. Murray CJL, Lopez AD (1996) *The Global Burden of Disease*. Geneva: World Health Organization, Harvard School of Public Health, World Bank.

19. World Health Organization (2008) *The Global Burden of Disease: 2004 Update*. Geneva: World Health Organization.

20. World Health Organization (2009) *Global Health Risks: Mortality and Burden of Disease Attributable to Selected Major Risks*. Geneva: World Health Organization.

21. Mathers C, Vos T, Stevenson C (1999) *The Burden of Disease and Injury in Australia*. Canberra: Australian Institute of Health and Welfare. AIHW cat. No. PHE 17.

22. World Health Organization (2012) *CHOosing Interventions That Are Cost Effective (WHO-CHOICE)*. Geneva: World Health Organization. Available at: http://www.who.int/choice/en/ (last accessed on 27 March 2013).

23. LAMA consortium National Evaluation Dementia Initiative (2009, October) Overview and Summary of Findings. Report to Australian Government Department of Health and Ageing. Sourced from Department of Health and Ageing website, available via: http://www/health.gov.au/internet/publications/publishing.nsf/Content/ageing-dementia-evaluation-htmlversion-toc (last accessed 27 March 2013).

Section 4

Services and developments around the world

In this section succinct descriptions are presented of how dementia services are configured and are developing in various countries, with a particular emphasis on aspects that are unique to those countries, given the varying demographic, political and cultural backdrops and the way their health care in general and dementia care in particular is organised.

The section is divided in four chapters:

- Chapter 11.   The Americas
- Chapter 12.   Australasia
- Chapter 13.   Eastern Europe
- Chapter 14.   Western Europe

For each area we collated contributions from some countries in which we felt relevant service issues are identifiable. Limited space meant we had to decide which countries were likely to add most to the overall picture. The result is that readers may not find countries of their interest and we add that any selection, regardless of the rationale behind it, inevitably leads to such gaps. Certain countries, which would potentially have yielded interesting insights, were left off the list in order to decrease repetition if they were deemed to have similar services, solutions or issues to others. We also decided that for the purposes of this book, Turkey should be regarded as lying within Eastern Europe on the grounds that Turkey seems to orientate itself more to Europe than to Asia.

Readers will also note that there are no contributions from the African continent: on exploring possible candidates to contribute it became clear that the vast majority of African nations to a considerable degree have different priorities with regard to dementia care than elsewhere, in part as a result of demographic profiles leading to dementia currently presenting a less pressing concern (whether one agrees with that lower prioritising or not), in part as a result of various forms of political instability in many areas, which appears to have deprived health care in general from the attention it deserves.

Chapter 11

The Americas

In this chapter we present an overview of dementia services and the general state of affairs regarding dementia in four countries, representing North and South America:

- Argentina
- Brazil
- Chile
- the USA

All expect increases in incidence and prevalence of dementias.

Argentina reports not only inequitable access to healthcare funding as well as a concentrated provision of specialists mainly in large cities, but also improved resources for carers. There are various partnerships and initiatives to progress research into, for example, biomarkers.

Brazil describes a particular diverging pattern of morbidity due to high levels of socio-economic inequality and a relatively younger age of onset in Latin America in general. It reports inadequate provision of dementia care, and this is equally true with regard to postgraduate training in dementia. However, the picture overall is slowly improving, particularly through 'dementia reference centres' and other initiatives.

In Chile there is a comparable lack of attention to dementia care, in spite of a number of governmental health programmes. A number of professional organisations collaborate to counter this tendency, and there is an expectation that current low levels of training in dementia will reverse.

The USA reports a complex, fragmented patchwork of services, providers and financing mechanisms. However, it is hoped that recent legislation will address these issues, and specific national initiatives are observed to lead to improvements in practices and policy developments.

Designing and Delivering Dementia Services, First Edition. Edited by Hugo de Waal, Constantine Lyketsos, David Ames, and John O'Brien.
© 2013 John Wiley & Sons, Ltd. Published 2013 by John Wiley & Sons, Ltd.

Argentina

Pablo M. Bagnati[a], Janus L. Kremer[b], Fernando E. Taragano[c] and Ricardo F. Allegri[d]

[a]*Memory and Aging Center, Instituto de Investigaciones Neurológicas Raúl Carrea (FLENI), Argentina*
[b]*Instituto de Neuropsiquiatría Kremer, Argentina*
[c]*Department of Neurosciences, Centro de Estudios Médicos e Investigaciones Clínicas (CEMIC), Argentina*
[d]*Memory and Aging Center, Instituto de Investigaciones Neurológicas Raúl Carrea (FLENI), Argentina*

In the last decades, the Argentinian population has aged faster than anticipated, resulting in an exponential growth of age-dependent illnesses such as dementia. The increase in dementia in the next 20 years will be much faster in low- to medium-income countries than in richer nations.

In 2010, Argentina recorded just over 40 million inhabitants, with 4.7 million being over 60, proving that our country is not free from the problem [1]. The population pyramid is likely to change into a somewhat inverted pyramid, similar to that of developed countries, due to this increase. In this context the prevalence of dementia is estimated as 12.18% of people over 65 [2]. An epidemiological study in Cañuelas (a city in Buenos Aires province) found that 23% of those over 60 had cognitive impairment [3]. According to these numbers, we can infer that there are approximately 1 million people with cognitive impairment and 480,000 with dementia in the country [4] (see Figure 11.1).

However, there is a lack of epidemiological data needed properly to plan health strategies in dementia care. A recent initiative of the National Health Department to address this is the Registry of Cognitive Pathologies in Argentina (ReDeCAr, Registro de Deterioro Cognitivo en Argentina), which – so it is hoped – will in the short term lead to a national plan to tackle dementia [5]. ReDeCAr is a prospective case register in hospitals and health centres throughout the country, using standardised software, enabling epidemiological observations, centrally recorded by the National Health Department.

This allows us over time to build a centralised database of patients, which will produce a national and regional epidemiological picture, in turn enabling us to generate progressive policies in cognitive impairment and dementia, adapted to real needs [6].

Dementia creates an important economic, social and personal burden. Local studies were therefore conducted to establish the costs of dementia. A study carried out by Allegri et al. showed that the annual costs were US$3420.40 in mild Alzheimer's dementia and up to US$9657.60 in severe

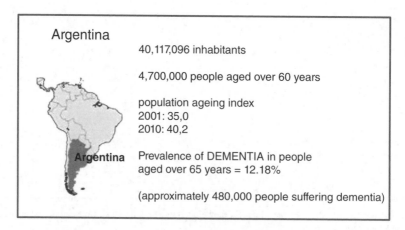

Argentina

40,117,096 inhabitants

4,700,000 people aged over 60 years

population ageing index
2001: 35,0
2010: 40,2

Prevalence of DEMENTIA in people
aged over 65 years = 12.18%

(approximately 480,000 people suffering dementia)

Figure 11.1 Epidemiological data showing ageing and dementia in Argentina

forms, increasing to US$14.447.68 if it included care paid for by the patient's family [7]. Another recent study showed that different types of dementia (Alzheimer's, vascular and frontotemporal dementia) have different costs. Vascular dementia is slightly more expensive, probably because of the presence of behavioural symptoms and impairment in functioning [8].

Dementia care in Argentina is shared between the public and private sectors. The public sector provides care to low- and middle-income populations, mainly in hospitals, whereas the private sector tends to provide care to middle- and high-income populations, including home assistance [9]. Unfortunately, this distribution is not equitable: more than 17 million people (43% of the population) have access which is limited to the Public Health System: this segment of healthcare receives only 28% of total health resources [10]. On the other hand, most elderly people (91% of people over 65) receive medical care from Social Security Support in a model which combines health with social care needs, but the economic instability over the years leads to variable efficacy in addressing the demands posed by the illness. Despite this, in the last 5 years, the system has shown a slight improvement [11].

With regard to assessment, diagnosis and treatment of dementia, Argentina has an unequal distribution of specialists (neurologists, psychiatrists and geriatricians): most are located in large cities, while there is a shortage in small towns and rural areas. The facilities needed for accurate diagnosis are scarce, except in Buenos Aires and a few other large provincial cities. There are few specialists trained in geriatric neuropsychiatry, and more education for lay people is needed as well [12].

In the last 10 years, the role of memory or dementia clinics has become more important. Most of these memory clinics are based on private initiatives. Recently, the directors of the 20 most important memory clinics were interviewed [13]. Among its main findings this survey showed that 70% of these memory clinics only cater to private patients. Sixty percent are run by neurologists. However, every clinic had at least one psychiatrist on their staff. Only 35% of the centres perform clinical trials, and only 20% of the groups present original papers or studies at meetings. Sixty percent of the centres have day-care services, 35% of the clinics provide training, and 80% offer counselling for spouses and caregivers [13].

Previous reviews have identified that in most countries, more than two-thirds of people with dementia live at home, and the majority is cared for by family members [14]. Argentina has a similar profile: most senior citizens live at home with their families, but approximately 15% live in nursing homes [15–17]. Family and non-family caregivers need information and counselling about dementia care. In our country, these resources are improving: ALMA ('Asociación de Lucha contra el Mal de Alzheimer' – Association against Alzheimer's Disease, a member organisation of Alzheimer's Disease International) is the main organisation fighting the disease: it works locally, to promote and offer care and support for people with dementia and their carers. It has more than 20 associations around the country [18]. Our group wrote the first book in the country about dementia family care in 2003, re-edited in 2010 [19]. More books and publications are being published, aimed to help families with early detection and treatment of dementia [20,21].

Early diagnosis of dementia is another challenge. It may be possible to increase the predictive validity of prodromal risk indicators based upon cognitive decline and subjective impairment. One widely advocated approach is the incorporation of disease biomarkers that may indirectly represent the extent of underlying neuropathology: structural neuro-imaging (medial temporal lobe or hippocampal volume), functional neuroimaging (Aβ ligands to visualise amyloid plaques *in vivo*) and cerebrospinal fluid [22]). In February 2011, FLENI ('Fundación para la Lucha contra las Enfermedades Neurológicas de la Infancia' – based in Buenos Aires [23]) joined ADNI ('Alzheimer Disease Neuro Imaging', a public sector-industry partnership founded in 2004 [24]) to develop biomarkers to predict the progression from normal ageing or mild cognitive impairment to the dementia phase of Alzheimer disease. This research involves volumetric magnetic resonance imaging and positron emission tomography with fluorine-18-labeled deoxyglucose and Aβ ligands (PiB and AV45), cog-

Table 11.1 Argentina: state of affairs regarding dementia

Weaknesses	Current reality	Future challenges
• Absence of complete rational epidemiological studies in dementia • Unequal distribution of and access to resources between private and public sectors • Absence of national prevention and care plans of dementia • Few trained in gerontoneuropsychiatry • Few trained caregivers	• Prime centralised registry of cognitive pathologies (ReDeCAR) • Memory clinics and dementia specialists working jointly • ALMA • ADNI/FLENI • Brain bank • Caregivers' training programmes • Books written by Argentine specialists about dementia family care	• National and regional epidemiological studies • Progressive state policies focusing on dementia • Psychogeriatrics' medical educational programmes • More education on dementia for the population and caregiver training; more equal distribution of resources between the private and public sectors

nitive and neurological evaluations, and analyses of cerebrospinal fluid biomarkers ($A\beta42$, tau and f-tau) [24,25]. In addition, FLENI houses the only brain bank in South America [23]. Another institution in Argentina ('CEMIC') studies the diagnosis of early Alzheimer's with PET and $A\beta$ ligands [26].

In summary, despite having weaknesses, Argentina is currently fighting strongly to improve the quality of life of people with cognitive impairment and dementia and their carers around the country (see Table 11.1). If our governments act urgently to develop research and care strategies, the impact of this disease can be reduced.

Conflict of interest: none.

References

1. INDEC (2010) Instituto Nacional de Estadísticas y Censos. Censo Nacional de Población y Viviendas 2001 y 2010. Available at: http://www.indec.gov.ar (last accessed on 20 February 2013).
2. Pages Larraya F, Grasso L, Mari G (2004) Prevalencia de las demencias de tipo Alzheimer, demencias vasculares y otras demencias en la República Argentina. *Revista Neurológica Argentina* 29:148–153.
3. Arizaga RL, Gogorza RE, Allegri RF, Barman D, Morales MC, Harris P, et al. (2005) Deterioro cognitivo en mayores de 60 años en Cañuelas (Argentina). Resultados del Piloto del Estudio Ceibo (Estudio Epidemiológico Poblacional de Demencia. *Revista Neurológica Argentina* 30(2):83–90.
4. Allegri RF (2011) Primer Registro Centralizado de Patologías Cognitivas en Argentina (ReDeCAr). Resultados del Estudio Piloto. *Publicación del Ministerio de Salud* 5:7–9.
5. Melcon CM, Bartoloni L, Katz M, Del Mónaco R, Mangone C, Melcon MO, et al. (2010) Propuesta de un Registro centralizado de casos con Deterioro Cognitivo en Argentina (ReDeCAr) basado en el Sistema Nacional de Vigilancia Epidemiológica. *Neurología Argentina* 2(3):161–166.
6. Katz M, Bartoloni LC, Melcon CM, Del Mónaco R, Mangone CA, Allegri RF, et al. (2011) Presentación del Primer Registro Centralizado de Patologías Cognitivas en Argentina (ReDeCAr). In: Sistema de Vigilancia Epidemiológica en Salud Mental y Adicciones, Boletín 5. Ministerio de Salud. 11–14.
7. Allegri RF, Butman J, Arizaga RL, Machnick G, Serrano C, Taragano FE, et al. (2006) Economic impact of dementia in developing countries: an evaluation of costs of Alzheimer-type dementia in Argentina. *International Psychogeriatrics* 18:1–14.
8. Galeno R, Bartoloni L, Dillon C, Serrano C, Iturry M, Allegri RF (2011) Clinical and economic characteristics associated with direct costs of Alzheimer's, frontotemporal and vascular dementia in Argentina. *International Psychogeriatrics* 23(4):554–561.

9. Ritchie CW, Ames D, Burke J, Bustin J, Connely P, Laczo J, et al. (2011) An international perspective on advanced neuroimaging: cometh the hour or ivory tower? *International Psychogeriatrics.* 23(Suppl): 558–564.

10. World Health Organization (2008) Countries: Argentina. Available at: http://www.who.int/countries/arg/ en (last accessed on 21 February 2013).

11. PAMI (2011) National Institute of Social Services for Retired People and Pensioners (INSSJP/PAMI). Available at: http://www.pami.org.ar (last accessed on 20 February 2013).

12. Sarasola D, Taragano F, Allegri R, Arizaga R, Bagnati P, Serrano C, et al. (2006) Geriatric Neuropsychiatry in Argentina. IPA Bulletin p 10 and 19.

13. Kremer J (2011) Memory Clinics in Argentina. Questionnaire. Available at: http://www.institutokremer.com.ar (last accessed on 20 February 2013). Data on file.

14. Rabins P, Lyketsos CG, Steele CD (1999) Practical Dementia Care. 7, p. 111.

15. Taragano TE (2011) Síntomas neuropsiquiátricos en la Enfermedad de Alzheimer. Revista de ALMA (Asoc. Lucha Mal de Alzheimer). pp. 10–11.

16. Pollero A, Gimenez M, Allegri RF, Taragano FE (2004) Síntomas Neuropsiquiátricos en pacientes con enfermedad de Alzheimer. *Vertex* 15(55):5–9.

17. Taragano F, Mangone C, Comesaña Diaz E (1995) Prevalence of neuropsychiatric disorders in nursing homes. Revista de la Asociación Argentina de Establecimientos Geriátricos.

18. ALMA – Asociación de Lucha contra el Mal de Alzheimer (2011) Misión de ALMA. Revista de ALMA. p. 7. Available at: http://www.alma-alzheimer.org.ar (last accessed on 20 February 2013).

19. Bagnati PM, Allegri RF, Kremer JL, Taragano FE (2010) Enfermedad de Alzheimer y otras demencias. Manual para la familia. Editorial Polemos, Buenos Aires, Argentina.

20. Manes F (2005) Convivir con personas con EA u otras demencias. D. Palais Ediciones, Buenos Aires, Argentina.

21. Gonzalez Salvia M (2006) Manual para familiares y cuidadores de personas con Enfermedad de Alzheimer. Editorial del Hospital Italiano, Buenos Aires, Argentina.

22. Alzheimer Disease International (ADI) (2011) World Alzheimer Report. p. 12.

23. Memory and Aging Center, Institute of Neurology, FLENI, Buenos Aires, Argentina Available at: http:// www.fleni.org.ar (last accessed on 21 February 2013).

24. ADNI (Alzheimer Disease Neuroimaging Initiative) (2011) FLENI partnership. Available at: http:// www.alz.org/research/funding/partnerships (last accessed on 20 February 2013).

25. Burton A (2011) Big science for a big problem: ADNI enters its second phase. *Lancet* 10:206–207.

26. Neurosciences Department, CEMIC (Centro de Estudios Médicos e Investigaciones Clínicas) Available at: http://www.cemic.edu.ar (last accessed on 20 February 2013).

Brazil

Cassio M. C. Bottino

Old Age Research Group (PROTER), Institute and Department of Psychiatry, University of São Paulo, Brazil

Ageing in Brazil

Traditionally considered a 'young' country, Brazil has in recent decades seen its population age significantly. This is set to continue: whereas the elderly population will increase by 2–4% per year, the young population will decline. According to United Nations projections, the elderly population in Brazil will increase from 3.1% of the total population in 1970 to 19% in 2050. In particular, the 'oldest old' will more than triple between 1990 and 2020, from 1.9 to 7.1 million [1].

Brazil has a heterogeneous ethnic and racial origin population with different socio-economic and cultural profiles. The majority of the population (84%) lives in urban areas. Thirteen cities have more than 1 million inhabitants, including Rio de Janeiro and São Paulo, which are among the 30 largest cities in the world.

According to the General Household Survey of 2009, the population over 60 is estimated at 21 million, the majority of whom are female (55.8%). The education level among the elderly is very low: 50.2% with less than 4 years of schooling. Less than 12% live in households with up to half minimum wage per capita, 77.4% receive retirement benefits and/or survival pensions from Social Security, and 37.5% of males and 14.4% of females still work after age 60 [2]. At the same time, traditional versions of family support are declining.

The ageing process has led to an increase in chronic and degenerative diseases and disabilities. Two patterns of morbidity currently coexist: one typical of poor living conditions (infectious and parasitic communicable diseases) and the other of more developed societies (chronic and degenerative non communicable diseases). The resulting 'epidemiologic polarisation' increases significant health gaps between different social groups and geographical areas within the country [3].

Prevalence of dementia

A review of population-based cohorts in Latin America showed the prevalence of dementia (7.1%) to be similar to that in developed countries, although a higher prevalence of dementia in relatively young subjects was evidenced: this may be associated with low educational levels and lower cognitive reserve, causing earlier emergence of clinical signs of dementia in Latin America [4].

In Brazil, the prevalence of dementia was similar to various regions of the world [5]. Prevalence ranged from 5.1% to 8.6% in subjects older than 65. Alzheimer's disease (AD) is the leading cause (55.1–59.8%), followed by mixed dementia or AD with cerebrovascular disease and vascular dementia. Moreover, older age and low educational level were in all studies significantly associated with a higher prevalence of dementia [6–8].

The incidence of dementia was also comparable to those reported in Western and Asian studies. According to the Catanduva Study, the incidence of dementia and AD was 13.8 and 7.7 per 1000 people per year, respectively, in those who are over 65 years old. The incidence of dementia almost doubled with every 5 years of age [9].

Organisation of services

In recent years, Health and Social Services have acknowledged the need for improvements in dementia care, with some progress being made.

After the publication of the National Policy Act for the Health of the Aged by the Ministry of Health in 1999, 48 reference centres were launched for the care of patients with dementia and their families. These centres offer free distribution of cholinesterase inhibitors under rigid medical control. Additionally, the Elderly Act was approved by the National Parliament in 2003 to ensure social, health, citizenship and human rights to the Brazilian elderly population.

The healthcare system in Brazil is a mix of public and private systems, with most elderly persons being served by the public system. The national programme of the health of the family (PSF) was initiated in 1994 with the provision of multidisciplinary teams in primary care settings in geographically defined areas, covering >95% of municipalities by 2009. However, at least 32.5% of elderly households were neither registered in PSF nor were covered by private health insurance, a figure that was even worse in the state of Rio de Janeiro at 49.1% [2].

Moreover, in most primary care settings, professionals work in inadequate conditions and are overstretched. Most general practitioners are lacking in diagnostic and management skills of dementia. Patients are not adequately investigated and often not or belatedly referred to the reference centres.

Dementia care services are fairly scarce across the country and not always readily accessible. Most are based in big cities at large teaching hospitals with the availability of structural and functional neuro-imaging and genetic and neuropsychological testing. Psychogeriatric units, dementia reference centres and memory clinics usually have insufficient numbers of properly trained professionals. Specialists (geriatricians, neurologists or psychiatrists) are mainly devoted to private practice, and multidisciplinary teams are rarely available [10].

Support groups for patients and their carers have sprung up over the past 20 years since the foundation of The Brazilian Association of Alzheimer's disease (ABRAz), which is organised in sub-regional branches in the five regions of the country. At present there are 19 support groups serving about 2000 families.

Education, training and research

Despite growing interest, a national framework for postgraduate education in dementia is lacking. Geriatric psychiatry is not recognised as a medical subspecialty by the Brazilian Medical Council other than as a special interest.

The Brazilian Society of Geriatrics and Gerontology, The Brazilian Association of Psychiatry and The Brazilian Academy of Neurology have special interest groups in dementia and cognitive disorders. The Brazilian Association of Geriatric Neuropsychiatry (ABNPG) was founded in 1997, acknowledging the importance of interdisciplinary approaches to dementia and other neuropsychiatric disorders and acting as a source of expertise. The Annual Meeting of Researchers on Alzheimer's Disease and Related Disorders (RPDA) has been convened since 1997 by the Scientific Department of Cognitive Neurology and Aging (DCNCE) of the Brazilian Academy of Neurology and is considered the most important national meeting for researchers in the field. Abstracts are published in the journal *Dementia & Neuropsychologia*.

Conclusions

Dementia care has undergone considerable and steady improvement in Brazil. In spite of this, governmental funds are currently insufficient, public awareness is low, socio-economic problems are significant, and there is a considerable shortage of specialists in the public and private sectors.

There are enormous opportunities to develop systems that differ from those in more developed countries by capitalising on the lack of a pre-existent infrastructure and configure more home-based rather than institution-based long-term care systems. Dementia care is dynamic and ideally should be approached through programmes that range from health promotion to the establishment of support networks for long-term care in the community. These programmes should form part of a public policy that involves all sectors of society and aims to provide adequate care for patients, with or without family support. Involvement of older people in the planning of their own future is equally of paramount importance.

References

1. Carvalho JA, Rodríguez-Wong LL (2008) The changing age distribution of the Brazilian population in the first half of the 21st century. *Cad Saude Publica* 24(3):597–605.
2. Instituto Brasileiro de Geografia e Estatística – IBGE (2010) Síntese de Indicadores Sociais. Uma Análise das Condições de Vida da População Brasileira 2010. Estudos e Pesquisas. Informação Demográfica e Socioeconômica número 27, Rio de Janeiro.
3. Pan American Health Organization (2002) Health in the Americas, Pan American Health. Washington, DC.
4. Nitrini R, Bottino CMC, Albala C, Capuñay NSC, Ketzoian C, Llibre Rodriguez JJ, et al. (2009) Prevalence of dementia in Latin America: a collaborative study of population-based cohorts. *International Psychogeriatrics* 21(4):622–630.
5. Lopes MA, Hototian SR, Reis GC, Elkis H, Bottino CMC, et al. (2007) Systematic review of dementia prevalence – 1994 to 2000. *Dementia & Neuropsychologia* 1(3):230–240.
6. Herrera E Jr, Caramelli P, Silveira ASB, Nitrini R (2002) Epidemiologic survey of dementia in a community-dwelling Brazilian population. *Alzheimer Disease and Associated Disorders* 16(2):103–108.
7. Scazufca M, Menezes PR, Vallada HP, Crepaldi AL, et al. (2008) High prevalence of dementia among older adults from poor socioeconomic backgrounds in São Paulo, Brazil. *International Psychogeriatrics* 20(2):394–405.
8. Bottino CM, Azevedo D Jr, Tatsch M, Hototian SR, Moscoso MA, Folquitto J, et al. (2008) Estimate of dementia prevalence in a community sample from São Paulo, Brazil. *Dementia and Geriatric Cognitive Disorders* 26(4):291–299.
9. Nitrini R, Caramelli P, Herrera E Jr, Bahia VS, et al. (2004) Incidence of dementia in a community-dwelling Brazilian population. *Alzheimer Disease and Associated Disorders* 18(4):241–246.
10. Machado JCB (2003) Evolving strategies for the integration of the related specialties devoted to the field of clinical neurosciences and aging: a view from geriatric medicine. *International Psychogeriatrics* 15(Suppl 2):66.

Chile

Patricio Fuentes

Cognitive Neurology and Dementia Unit, Neurology Service, Hospital of Salvador and Geriatrics Section, Clinical Hospital University of Chile, Chile

Demographic and health facts

Chile has a total population of about 17 million, with 13% being over 60. Life expectancy is estimated at 81.5 years for women and 75.5 years for men, meaning Chile is an ageing nation. Chile has the highest 'human development index' in Latin America, is considered an upper-middle income country and has a GDP per capita of $ 15,300 with an estimated $ 20,000 for 2015 [1].

The health system is mixed, with around 80% of the population accessing public sector services. For older adults, the majority of whom use public sector services and for whom there is evidence of socio-economic inequality, a law was passed in 2011 which decreased the cost of mandatory health contributions for all pensioners by around 7%. According to the latest National Health Survey, conducted in 2009, 10.4% of adults over 60 have cognitive impairment, reaching 20.9% in those over 80. If one considers the combination with functional impairment, 4.5% of older adults may meet criteria for dementia [2].

Clinical practice

There is no national strategy for dementia and any existing governmental health programmes, such as the National Program for the Elderly or the Mental Health Program, have paid only marginal attention to initiatives aimed at the care of people with dementia. Recent governments have not shown any greater sensitivity to the problem and have given it only secondary priority. In 2002, the government established 'El Senama' (Servicio Nacional del Adulto Mayor): its main task is the improvement of quality of life for older people, taking a gerontological perspective.

Only a few private clinics or large hospitals, concentrated in major cities, have integral units for the diagnosis and treatment of dementia with multidisciplinary professional teams. At the primary care level, there are basic standards and clinical guidelines for cognitive impairment and dementia: a screening instrument, called EFAM (Functional Assessment of the Elderly) is in regular use, validated in our setting, which allows the detection of older adults in the community who are at risk of losing functionality in the short and medium term and enables categorisation by level of independence [3]. Furthermore, since 2008, there is the Preventive Medical Examination for the Elderly (EMPAM), as part of the so-called GES guarantee or AUGE: this provides a comprehensive benefits package, free and guaranteed to be delivered both in the public and private health system. It prioritises certain diseases, but has not yet incorporated dementia despite its recognised disease burden.

There are memory clinics in public hospitals, where patients with cognitive disorders can be examined adequately and a probable diagnosis reached within reasonable time. However, therapeutic options are limited since it is not possible to prescribe approved anti-dementia medication as a result of lack of central funding. Neither are cognitive stimulation programmes readily available. Appropriate psychotropic drugs for the management of neuropsychiatric symptoms are equally difficult to prescribe. In general, people with dementia experiencing significant behavioural change have poor access to inpatient care in public hospitals. There are virtually no health structures that can be called acute psychogeriatric units, and the only public hospital in the country specialising in older adults, the National Institute on Aging, has important limitations in physical and human resources. It is noteworthy that the diagnosis and treatment of patients with dementia is mainly carried out by neurologists and geriatricians and in only a very small proportion by psychiatrists. Additionally, in recent years there has been little interest in the study and management of mental disorders in the elderly within specialist training, despite the obvious increase in prevalence of these diseases.

There are about 1700 long-term care homes, half of them concentrated in the capital and a third informal. Most are private and others, run by religious or philanthropic organisations, receive some help from the state. It is clear that the majority of patients with advanced dementia are being cared for by relatives. Day hospitals and day centres for patients with cognitive disorders are rare.

Complementary activities

Chile has only three or four research centres in neuroscience applied to neurodegenerative diseases (University of Chile, Catholic and Concepcion), which are able to compete internationally. Moreover, in the last decade, the country has become an important platform in Latin America to conduct clinical trials with new anti-dementia drugs at various stages of development. A significant contribution around training in and management and care of dementia is provided by the relevant scientific societies and the local association of family volunteers. The Society of Neurology, Psychiatry and Neurosurgery of Chile as well as the Society of Geriatrics and Gerontology of Chile collaborate in various workgroups and provide training and information to professionals and community representatives through courses, publications and media campaigns highlighting the enormous challenges Chilean society is facing in the near future. For 20 years or so the Corporation Alzheimer-Chile, affiliated with Alzheimer's Disease International, has provided education, medical care and psychological support to families and caregivers, mainly those on low income.

There is growing interest to include psychogeriatric training of cognitive impairment and dementia into under- and postgraduate curricula of health professions in most academic institutions, both public and private. This is expected soon to reverse the current low level of training of both professionals and non-professionals providing mental health care for older people.

Conclusion

Chile is faced with an ageing population and consequently a steep increase in the incidence and prevalence of dementia, a problem typical of developed countries. However, the dementia challenge is faced by a system applying standards more typically encountered in developing countries. Socioeconomic inequality and the structure and dynamics of the country's healthcare system prevent delivery of quality care to the majority of those affected by dementia. Hence, even small improvements in the various agencies and systems will lead to important redress in the medium term.

References

1. INE (Mayo 2010) Evolución de la población chilena en los últimos 200 años. Available at: http://www.ine.cl (last accessed on 20 February 2013).
2. Encuesta Nacional de Salud ENS Chile 2009–2010. Available at: http://www.minsal.gob.cl (last accessed on 20 February 2013).
3. Albala C, Icaza G, Vío F, Garcia C, Marin PP, Quiroga P, et al. (2001) A short test to evaluate cognitive impairment based on Folstein's MMSE. *Gerontology* 47(S1):S183.

The United States of America

Quincy M. Samus

Department of Psychiatry and Behavioral Sciences, Johns Hopkins Bayview, The Johns Hopkins School of Medicine, USA

In the USA – as elsewhere – dramatic demographic shifts and an absence of curative treatments means that the number of older Americans with dementia is expected to rise precipitously from 5.4 million in 2012 to 10.2–13.2 million by 2050 [1,2]. The long-term care (LTC) needs for persons with dementia (PWD) are substantial and increase over the course of the illness. This chapter provides a concise overview of the organisation of LTC for dementia in the USA and summarises key practice and policy issues. LTC refers to the provision of health, social and personal care services, necessary to manage chronic conditions across the span of care environments (e.g. private community homes, assisted living and nursing homes).

Best practice recommendations for dementia care focus on several key principles:

- timely and accurate clinical diagnosis
- provision of clinical care for memory symptoms, related neuropsychiatric symptoms and comorbid medical conditions
- long-term follow-up and reassessment
- assessment of non-medical care needs and provision of appropriate supportive care to patients and their families (e.g. safe living environments, assistance with Activities of Daily Living, homemaker services, senior centres, adult day care, nutritional services, transportation, meaningful activities, psychosocial services, caregiver respite, disease support groups) [3].

Thus, the ideal LTC system for dementia would be comprehensive, proactive, and coordinated; one that attends to a broad range of health and social service needs and that is adaptive to the changing needs of PWD and their carers over the course of the illness. The organisation of LTC in the USA falls short of this ideal and is often described as a complex, fragmented patchwork of different services, providers and financing mechanisms [4]. Medicare, a tax-based federal health insurance programme, is the primary provider of outpatient and inpatient medical care for the majority of older PWD. Medicaid, a federal/state health programme, serves as the nation's safety net for low-income Americans requiring long-term nursing home care [5]. However, the quality and effectiveness of these programmes for PWD continues to be plagued by factors such as

- mismatches between patient and carer needs and preferences and covered services (e.g. home-based care, social service and care coordination, preventive services)
- provider reimbursement policies
- lack of continuity and integrated service networks
- lack of provider education and specialisation in dementia care
- eligibility requirements for covered services [6].

Recent reforms as part of the Patient Protection and Affordable Care Act (PPACA) include provisions for dementia care, for example, programmes targeted at identification, prescription drug coverage, care coordination, transitional care, quality care and research [7]; it will take time to implement and evaluate the effects of these reforms.

The bulk of needed LTC support typically falls outside the purview of Medicare and Medicaid and is largely coordinated and provided by carers in the community [5], with 50–70% of dementia care costs shouldered by individuals and families [8,9]. US carers for PWD provide substantial, often unpaid, care for their loved ones and struggle to navigate loose networks of community-based supports and services to meet wide-ranging LTC needs. This is often a confusing and daunting task. Public awareness and education, stigma, misconceptions about dementia and a lack of culturally sensitive outreach programmes and services all present significant challenges to accessing and utilising needed services [1]. The availability, capacity and financing structure of supportive services and programmes also vary widely from community to community, or state to state, adding further complexity to achieving care quality and continuity. Also, many ageing service providers lack knowledge and dementia-specific training.

Several promising shifts in LTC practices and policies are underway in the USA. Promising practices include

- culture change movement towards consumer-directed, individualised care
- interdisciplinary service integration incorporating a wide range of disciplines in care management
- shifts to community-based care rather than more expensive and restrictive institutionalised care [4].

Several high-profile policy initiatives are also gaining momentum. In addition to the PPACA, the Obama administration signed into law a historic political act in January 2011 that explicitly recognised the need for further care reform, with dementia identified as a public health crisis. The National Alzheimer's Project Act (NAPA) aims to

- create and maintain an integrated national plan to overcome Alzheimer's disease
- coordinate Alzheimer's disease research and services across all federal agencies
- accelerate the development of treatments that would prevent, halt or reverse the course of Alzheimer's disease
- improve early diagnosis, coordination of care and treatment of Alzheimer's disease
- improve outcomes for ethnic and racial minority populations at higher risk
- coordinate with international bodies to fight Alzheimer's globally [10].

Table 11.2 summarises key practice and policy issues for dementia care in the USA. These issues reflect the nation's unique demographic, political and cultural attributes, such as

- generational differences in care expectations and preferences ('baby-boomers' vs prior generations)
- cultural emphasis on independence, dignity and personal rights
- preference of most older people to receive care in their own homes
- a rapidly increasing number of older Americans who belong to minority groups, many of whom are disproportionately affected by dementia
- a system that currently relies on primary care as the gateway and hub of dementia care
- the substantial care burdens placed on informal caregivers, including the *sandwich generation* phenomenon, that results in significant medical, financial and psychosocial needs
- presence of societal stigma related to memory loss and ageing.

Clearly, the organisation of the US LTC system as it exists today is inadequate to meet the chronic and wide-ranging needs of older people with dementia and their families. Promising shifts in practices and political developments are emerging, such as the passage of the NAPA. However, time is of the essence as in the coming years millions more will join the ranks of American families currently devastated by this disease. Significant health system improvements will necessarily encompass willingness to reorganise the system, long-term vision, collaboration and changes in how dementia and dementia care are viewed in the American culture.

Table 11.2 Key issues and considerations for dementia care in the USA (*Sources*: References 4–7, 10–12.)

Practice/Policy issue	Considerations
Mismatch between patient and carer needs/preferences and services	• Focus on models of person-centred care • Routinely assess and respond to carer needs • Evaluate services on patient-centred outcomes (e.g. ageing in place, quality of life and care satisfaction) • Configure care settings to maximise efficiency and convenience (e.g. availability of social work, mental health, nursing, lab testing/diagnostics, pharmacy at or near primary care practices) • Provide more care in homes and community-based settings by shifting public and private health insurance policies to cover community-based care • Expand state and national data collection systems for programme evaluation
Coordination/ integration of health, social and personal care services	• Increase primary care provider dementia knowledge • Encourage primary care practices to use multidisciplinary teams • Increase number of providers in geriatric specialties to support PCPs • Establish interagency networks to support PCP referrals to local specialist care, social or personal care services • Restructure health systems and reimbursement policies to support multidisciplinary care and care coordination/management services • Create standard health information systems to support timely exchange of information between providers
Financing dementia care	• Explore ways to reduce healthcare cost while improving quality and efficiency (e.g. fee-for-service vs fee capitation; community-based care vs institutional care) • Review policies that create disincentives for older adults planning for future needs (e.g. Medicaid eligibility policies requiring *spending down* life savings) • Establish systems that spread financial risk equitably between individuals and publicly financed insurance so impoverishment is not a common outcome in cases of high long-term care needs • Encourage, educate and incentivise individuals to plan for LTC needs • Expand availability and affordability of long-term care insurance programmes
Increasing racial and ethnic diversity	• Racial disparities in access and receipt of appropriate care abound • Efforts to increase availability and accessibility of culturally sensitive public education, outreach and services is critical
Cultural stigma-related to memory loss	• Increase public education campaigns underscoring the value of early detection to improve dementia treatment and outcomes • Increase available support for self-management and decision-making
Prioritise dementia research (all levels)	• Expand dementia-related research funding using a balanced approach (e.g. biomedical and pharmaceutical development vs intervention and service delivery; prevention vs treatment) • Accelerate translation of effective programmes to practice • Mechanisms to cultivate early career researchers • Explore public–private partnerships to accelerate and coordinate research initiatives

(Continued)

Table 11.2 (*Continued*)

Practice/Policy issue	Considerations
Workforce training and retention in dementia care	• Increase health care and community ageing service worker knowledge (e.g. social workers, pharmacists, senior building managers, home care workers) • Incentivise long-term employment in workforce possibly through access to specialised certification programmes, loan repayment programmes, creating incentives for continuing education for low- and mid-level direct care workers (e.g. certified nursing assistants, case managers) to reframe 'jobs' into 'careers', increasing pay and benefits and raising social position of workers by making dementia care a high public health priority

References

1. Alzheimer's Association (2012) Alzheimer's disease facts and figures. *Alzheimer's & Dementia* 8(2). Available at: http://www.alz.org/downloads/facts_figures_2012.pdf (last accessed on 21 February 2013).
2. Brookmeyer R, Evan DA, Hebert LE, Langa KM, Heeringa SG, Plassman BL, et al. (2011) National estimates of the prevalence of Alzheimer's disease in the United States. *Alzheimer's & Dementia* 7(1):61–73.
3. Lyketsos C, Colenda C, Beck C, Blank K, Doraiswamy M, Kalunian D, et al. (2006) Task Force of American Association for Geriatric Psychiatry Position statement of the American Association for Geriatric Psychiatry regarding principles of care for patients with dementia resulting from Alzheimer disease. *The American Journal of Geriatric Psychiatry* 14(7):561–572.
4. Lehning AJ, Austin MJ (2009) Long-term care in the United States: policy themes and promising practices. *Journal of Gerontological Social Work* 53(1):43–63.
5. Feder J, Komoisar H, Niefeld M (2000) Long-term care in the United States: an overview. *Health Affairs* 19(3):40–56.
6. Bartels S, Dums A, Oxman T, Schneider L, Areán P, Alexopoulos G, et al. (2003) Evidence-based practices in geriatric mental health care: an overview of systematic reviews and meta-analyses. *Psychiatry Clinics of North America* 26(4):971–990.
7. Alzheimer's Association (2012) Health Care Reform and Alzheimer's Disease. Available at: http://www.alz.org/living_with_alzheimers_healthcare_reform.asp (last accessed on 21 February 2013).
8. Stommel M, Collins CE, Given BA (1994) The costs of family contributions to the care of persons with dementia. *The Gerontologist* 34(2):199–205.
9. Wanless D, Forder J, Fernández J-L, Poole T, Beesley L, Henwood M, et al. (2006) *Wanless Social Care Review: Securing Good Care for Older People, Taking a Long-Term View*. London, UK.: King's Fund.
10. US Department of Health and Human Services (2012) National Plan to Address Alzheimer's Disease. Available at: http://aspe.hhs.gov/daltcp/napa/NatlPlan.pdf (last accessed on 21 February 2013).
11. Knapp M, Comas-Herrara A, Somani A, Banerjee S (2007) *Dementia: International Comparisons*. London, England: Institute of Psychiatry at the Maudsley. Unit PSSR.
12. Callahan CM, Boustani M, Sachs GA, Hendrie HC (2009) Integrating care for older adults with cognitive impairment. *Current Alzheimer Research* 6(4):368–374.

Chapter 12

Australasia

In this chapter we present an overview of dementia services and the general state of affairs regarding dementia in five countries, representing Australasia:

- Australia
- China
- India
- Japan
- South Korea

All expect increases in incidence and prevalence of dementias.

Australia describes a complex health system with three levels of government involvement plus private providers. There are a variety of multidisciplinary teams with varying service specifications. It has seen overall improvement of services and education and training over the past 20 years.

China adopts a number of centralised approaches in policy-setting, including in health insurance systems. There are doubts regarding proper implementation of centralised guidelines and suitable training of staff. The Peking University Institute of Mental Health plays a leading role in service development and research.

In India there is hardly any community service, although dementia services, including approximately 100 memory clinics exist, linked to general hospitals. The District Mental Health Programme (DMHP) is a public healthcare service which aims to decentralise mental health care and is expected to be rolled out across India.

In Japan there is a huge gap between the estimated number of persons with dementia and the numbers actually receiving a diagnosis. 'Medical Centres for Dementia' improved dementia care and this is being rolled out across the country. An Adult Guardianship Scheme was introduced to protect and support persons with limited mental capacity, including people with dementia.

South Korea reports a streamlined assessment process and 50% of people with dementia receiving anti-dementia medication. Professional care workers pass a national qualification exam, and there are minimum staff/user ratios prescribed by law.

Designing and Delivering Dementia Services, First Edition. Edited by Hugo de Waal, Constantine Lyketsos, David Ames, and John O'Brien.
© 2013 John Wiley & Sons, Ltd. Published 2013 by John Wiley & Sons, Ltd.

Australia

Eleanor Flynn[a], Dina Lo Giudice[b] and David Ames[c]

[a]University of Melbourne, Australia
[b]Royal Melbourne Hospital, Australia
[c]National Ageing Research Institute, National Ageing Research Institute, Royal Melbourne Hospital, Australia

Australia has three distinct groups of older people: the Anglo-Celtic majority, indigenous Australians and post-war migrants. Patterns of dementia and ageing and expectations of service provision differ between these groups. In June 2010, 35.7% of the 3 million Australians aged over 65 had been born overseas [1]. The majority (60%) of Australia's population lives in five large cities.

The number of people with dementia in 2011 is estimated to be 266,574 (total population = 22.5 million, 13.5% aged over 65), and that number will undergo a 254% increase by 2050 to 942,624, while the overall population will rise by only one-third [1].

The Australian health and welfare system is complex with three levels of government (federal, state and local) plus private organisations providing services. Medicare (the national universal health insurance system) reimburses part or all of the costs incurred by patients for primary medical care, specialist medical and diagnostic care and pharmaceuticals for ambulatory patients. Residential aged care for eligible people is heavily subsidised by the federal government. Six state and two territory governments provide free hospital care, primarily inpatient, but also some outpatient visits associated with inpatient stays. Funding for public hospitals comes from the federal government by way of grants to the states from funds raised by taxes. About one-third of the population has private health insurance which covers private hospital inpatient care and some inpatient specialist costs. War veterans, predominantly elderly, receive extra health and welfare services. Indigenous Australians are able to access services for those aged at 50 years. Community services (home care and delivered meals) are funded by state and federal governments and tendered out to private and not-for-profit organisations.

In Australia patients see a general practitioner (GP) for initial consultations, who bill their older and pensioner patients only the amount they are reimbursed by Medicare. Patients' visits to specialists are reimbursed if the patient has been referred by a GP.

The GP is often the first point of contact for a patient or carer seeking help, but many GPs have difficulties with both the diagnosis and management of dementia [2]. Although extra payment is provided to GPs for time spent meeting families or contacting specialised services, this remuneration does not cover the costs.

The state governments provide psychiatric services. The services in the state of Victoria consist of multidisciplinary community Aged Psychiatry Assessment and Treatment Teams (APATTs), which are linked to hospitals and cover all the state's regions. Patients are assessed at home at the request of the GP, another health worker, family member or other carer. Unlike the Aged Care Assessment Teams (ACATs), the APATTs provide a continuing care and support service to patients to enable them to remain in the community, with beds available for acute aged psychiatry. Old age psychiatry services in other states are variable, but improving.

The ACATs were set up in 1984 and cover all of Australia [3]. Most are co-located with regional bed-based geriatric services. The ACATs are funded by the federal government to ensure that all people referred to residential care actually need it and to assist people to remain at home with support. Referrals are taken from patients, carers and health workers, and assessments are carried out at home or in hospital by multidisciplinary teams. The majority of people assessed by an ACAT have evidence of dementia or other cognitive impairment [4].

In Victoria there are 15 regional Cognitive, Dementia and Memory Services (CDAMS) which provide multidisciplinary assessment of dementia patients and their carers. The aim is to provide integrated services at all levels of the healthcare system. Specialised memory clinics exist in the other capital cities, but none is state-funded and some are privately operated. Attendance at a memory clinic which provides education, counselling and referral to appropriate services improves the quality of life of carers of those with dementia [5].

Each state and territory has a Dementia Behaviour Management Service (DBMAS). These are funded by the national government and provide predominantly telephone advice as well as some rural outreach services.

Many patients with dementia see psychiatrists, neurologists or general physicians for diagnostic workup. Younger and wealthier persons with dementia are more likely initially to be referred to a private specialist. Depending on the specialist's or the carer's knowledge of the system, patients may later be referred to publicly funded assessment services.

Cholinesterase inhibitors have been subsidised for people with mild to moderate Alzheimer's disease since 2001 and are widely used, though the criterion that recipients must show a 2-point rise in Mini Mental State Examination score in the first 6 months of thereapy limits their availability. Memantine is subsidised for a few patients with moderate dementia. As in many other countries, antipsychotics, antidepressants and benzodiazepines are widely and probably overprescribed to people with dementia.

Family and other informal carers provide the bulk of care to persons with dementia. A range of community options is available for patients with dementia to continue living in the community, especially after discharge from hospital or specialist units. Many of these services are part of broader schemes to replace residential care with community care.

Alzheimer's Australia was set up in 1985 to provide advocacy for those with dementia and their carers. Branches operate in each state and territory, providing counselling, carer groups, educational material and a Dementia Helpline. Its goals include dementia policy development at a federal level, sharing of resources and expertise across Australia and liaison with Alzheimer's Disease International.

Residential care is provided by a variety of organisations, including state governments, private operators and charitable organisations, which are subsidised and regulated by the federal government. Care is classified as low level (providing meals and assistance with activities of daily living) or high level (providing 24-hour nursing care). Residents requiring an increased level of care can sometimes remain in their current residence with extra services.

Medical education has undergone expansion and change in the last two decades with both graduate and undergraduate entry courses available. Nursing and allied health education is university based. All clinicians are expected to undertake continuing professional education, which gives opportunities for academics to provide education on dementia assessment and management.

There is an expectation by both professionals and carers that there will be a continuation of the improvements in services for dementia patients seen in the last 20 years. All levels of government have acknowledged the demographic realities of a large increase in the older population and therefore of increasing numbers of dementia patients. The costs of providing world-class services to a rapidly growing elderly population may constrain further improvements and even the maintenance of services, but to date this has not been the case. The future of dementia care may depend as much on continued trade and business success as on the expertise of our professionals.

References

1. Deloitte Access Economics (2011) *Dementia Across Australia: 2011–2050*. Canberra: Alzheimer's Australia.

2. Brodaty H, Howarth GC, Mant A, Kurrle S (1994) General practice and dementia: a national survey of Australian GPs. *Medical Journal of Australia* 160:10–14.
3. Howe A (1997) From states of confusion to a National Action Plan for Dementia Care: the development of policies for dementia care in Australia. *International Journal of Geriatric Psychiatry* 12:165–171.
4. LoGiudice D, Waltrowicz W, McKenzie S, Ames D, Flicker L (1995) Dementia in patients and carers referred to an Aged Care Assessment Team, and stress in their carers. *Australian Journal of Public Health* 19:275–280.
5. LooGiudice D, Waltrowicz W, Brown K, Burrows C, Ames D, Flicker L (1999) Do memory clinics improve the quality of life of carers? A randomised trial. *International Journal of Geriatric Psychiatry* 14: 626–632.

China

Xin Yu and Huali Wang

Institute of Mental Health, Peking University, China

Epidemiology and burden of dementia in China

A population census conducted in 2010 showed the proportion of people over 65 growing from 4.9% in 1982 and 7.0% in 2000 to 8.9% in 2010, so in 2010 the population aged over 65 amounted to 118.8 million [1]. The prevalence of dementia is approximately 5% [2,3]. Therefore, it is estimated that there are approximately 6 million persons living with dementia in China, with Alzheimer's disease (AD) being the most common subtype [2]. The 10/66 Dementia Research Group reported the incidence of dementia in China as 24.0 per 1000 person-years. Although it is difficult to assess the contribution of dementia to mortality, the hazard ratio (HR) calculated was 3.02 (95% CI 2.13–4.28) in urban China and 3.59 (95% CI 2.47–5.21) in rural China [4].

In an observational cross-sectional study in a memory clinic, Wang et al. reported that caregiver time varied dramatically across different stages of dementia. For example, the caregiver time on personal activities of daily living (PADL) recorded using the Resource Utilization in Dementia (RUD) scale was 25 hours per month in mild cases and 172 hours per month in severe cases [5].

Ageing service policies

At the WHO/China Mental Health Awareness Event held in 1999 in Beijing, Dr Brundtland, former Director-General of the World Health Organisation, stated that mental health should be listed as a health priority in China. Dementia would be a great challenge to China as a simple consequence of demography and increase in life expectancy due to better physical health [6]. In 2001, Jiang Zemin, former President of the Peoples' Republic of China, in his response to Dr. Brundtland, reassured that promoting mental health care and reducing stigma against mental disorders are extremely important for the socioeconomic development of the country [7].

Following this response, national mental health action plans have been implemented in the past decade [8]. In the latest national mental health plan increasing public awareness, knowledge of mental health problems and improving early detection and intervention of dementia and depression are still listed as priorities [9]. In addition to these national mental health policies, a series of national ageing development plans have been released by the National Ageing Committee since the early 1990s [10]. The latest 12th five-year (2011–2015) National Plan for Ageing Development explicitly urges the whole society to promote mental health and psychological well-being of the elderly [11]. These social policies and documents have provided new guidance for social and other services for the elderly, closely related to mental health care. Notably, in 2006, in the White Paper on China Ageing Development, the State Council recognised the significant increase of the ageing population and its implications for long-term care [12].

By 2011 universal health insurance coverage was achieved through the implementation of a social medical insurance system, including the urban employee basic medical insurance (UEBMI), the new rural cooperative medical system (NRCMS) and the urban resident basic medical insurance system (URBMI). The universal health insurance coverage is particularly beneficial for rural dwelling elderly and those who have never been employed. These policies provide a great opportunity to develop a culturally appropriate mental healthcare delivery system in China, which integrates with the social and medical service system.

Guidelines on dementia care

There are two major sets of guidelines on the management of dementia. One was developed by the Chinese Society for Psychiatry (CSP) and the other by a professional group on cognitive impairment under the auspices of the Chinese Society for Neurology (CSN) [13,14]. Usually in China, one randomised controlled trial (RCT) with positive results is sufficient for drug registration and approval by our State Food and Drug Administration (SFDA): there are few RCTs designed to test the effectiveness of anti-dementia agents further, once these are approved for the treatment of AD. Therefore, the evidence described in both sets of guidelines is mostly adapted from trials conducted in other countries. Guidelines released by the European Federation of Neurological Societies, the American Psychiatric Association and the American College of Physicians (ACP) were the main sources of guidelines on dementia and cognitive impairment by CSN. Due to limited local evidence on dementia care in China, the CSP working group aimed to introduce certain standards for dementia care, including reducing risk factors, early detection of clinical features, introducing timely pharmacological and non-pharmacological interventions and care for people with dementia. The CSP guidelines place a strong focus on home care and long-term residential care for people with dementia and set an optimal framework for dementia care. However, more local evidence on dementia care is needed to develop evidence-based guidelines appropriate for China.

Another concern is the lack of efficient or effective ways to monitor physicians' performance, making it difficult to estimate how either dementia guideline is being applied in routine clinical practice. The inadequate implementation of dementia guidelines may result in extra barriers to access dementia care services.

Service resources for dementia care

People with cognitive impairment usually seek medical help from neurologists, psychiatrists or geriatricians. In the past decade, widespread public health education has contributed to an increased awareness of cognitive impairment among the general population. Now more and more people living with cognitive impairment and early dementia are seen in memory clinics. However, there is no specific certification requirement for subspecialty training in dementia and cognitive impairment, and the quality of care may vary across different areas. A national psychogeriatric service resource survey conducted in 2004 found there were only 93 hospitals providing a 'mental health service for the elderly'. The number of psychiatrists and psychiatric nurses providing elderly mental health care were too few. There were no social workers at all in the field of dementia care. These findings suggest that there is a great paucity of service resources for people with mental disorders, including dementia [15]. This is contrasted with the great demand for quality mental health care for the elderly. In addition to the implementation of continuous medical education programmes (CME), which have educated hundreds of physicians, the Peking University Institute of Mental Health initiated a subspecialty training programme in geriatric psychiatry. It is expected that this initiative will increase the availability of subspecialty training and will ultimately be scaled up in the whole country, so that there will be more well-trained psychogeriatricians delivering elderly mental health programmes.

Despite limited resources Chinese experts have provided and continue to provide valuable diagnostic services and care for people with dementia, as well as carrying out significant research. Memory clinics have been set up in major cities, providing diagnosis, treatment and management for people with dementia. In cities, such as Beijing, Guangzhou, Shanghai and Hangzhou, medical professionals also try to ensure dementia caregiver support groups are available. The caregiver support group at the Peking University Institute of Mental Health provides group intervention for caregivers of people with dementia. AD centres and collaborative networks are formed by well-established institutions, such as the national collaborative network for early diagnosis and research of dementia directed by the Peking University Institute of Mental Health. Meanwhile, institutions with a high scientific reputation have been and are involved in collaborative AD projects with international academic and scientific institutions. For example, in collaboration with Harvard Medical School, the development of the AD Care and Research Centre at the Peking University Institute of Mental Health was funded by the National Institute of Health in the USA. More than 10 hospitals have been enrolled as participating sites for several global AD trials. Investigators may also receive funding from the Ministry of Science and Technology, the Natural Science Foundation of China and some other research funding agencies. Investigators at universities, academic and research institutions carry out basic research on the neurobiological mechanism of AD and mild cognitive impairment (MCI).

Currently, care for the elderly primarily depends on family care and community-based social services, while private care may not be affordable to the majority of the elderly population. Therefore, in addition to hospital services, family and neighbourhood communities are still considered as the optimal setting for care and one of the key components of mental healthcare delivery. As is the Chinese tradition: a feeling of duty as the exemplary attitude for children and filial obligation and reciprocity are the two major philosophical underpinnings of caring for the elderly in China [16]. The newer entity of a National Ageing Committee has declared the importance and urgency of building elderly friendly communities and home-care service systems [17].

These strategies may to some extent urge our society to be engaged in the community-based services for the elderly. However, it will take a long time to reach a high-level readiness in the community. Community understanding and responsiveness at the very earliest stage and public awareness of mental health problems in general have been quite low [18]. With collaborations between academic institutions and several organisations, for example, Alzheimer's Disease Chinese (ADC, an ADI member), the Beijing Cuncaochunhui Mental Health Service Center (NGO) and the Chinese Alzheimer Project (NGO), efforts on raising awareness of mental health problems, such as dementia and depression, have met with considerable public acceptance, including among community-dwelling elderly, nursing home residents, college students, social welfare staff and the media.

In recent years, the issue of long-term care has been identified as one of the major concerns in dementia care. In addition to nursing homes established by the government, several privately owned nursing homes have been set up in cities such as Beijing and Shanghai. However, staff seldom receive training in professional caregiving skills for people with dementia. Therefore, improving the quality of dementia nursing care is critically important. The China Alzheimer Project (CAP) and ADC are collaborating in an online training programme for good quality dementia care which was launched in the autumn of 2012.

Future perspectives

Great strides in promoting quality dementia care have been made in the last two decades in China. However, there remain many challenges to establish quality care of dementia nationally. First, more work is needed to improve early detection and to explore an effective model of care for older persons with dementia or cognitive impairment, who live at home. Second, the competence of physicians in providing dementia care should be increased with more targeted CME programmes. Finally, social and medical care should be integrated in multidisciplinary teams to provide comprehensive and holistic care for persons with dementia.

References

1. Nation Bureau of Statistics, P. R. C. (2011) China's main demographic indicators from the 6th National Population Census. Available at: http://www.stats.gov.cn/tjgb/rkpcgb/qgrkpcgb/t20110428_402722232.htm (last accessed on 20 February 2013).
2. Zhang ZX, Zahner GE, Roman GC, Liu J, Hong Z, Qu QM, et al. (2005) Dementia subtypes in China: prevalence in Beijing, Xian, Shanghai, and Chengdu. *Archives of Neurology* 62(3):447–453.
3. World Health Organisation (2012) *Dementia: A Public Health Priority.* Geneva: World Health Organisation.
4. Prince M, Acosta D, Ferri CP, Guerra M, Huang Y, Libre Rodriguez JL, et al. (2012) Dementia incidence and mortality in middle-income countries, and associations with indicators of cognitive reserve: a 10/66 Dementia Research Group population-based cohort study. *The Lancet* 380(9836):50–58.
5. Wang H, Gao T, Wimo A, Yu Xin (2010) Caregiver time and cost of home care for Alzheimer's disease: a clinic-based observational study in Beijing, China. *Ageing International* 35(2):153–165.
6. Available at: http://www.who.int/director-general/speeches/1999/english/19991111_beijing.html (last accessed on 20 February 2013).
7. Available at: http://www.people.com.cn/GB/shizheng/16/20010407/435637.html (last accessed on 20 February 2013).
8. Ministry of Health, Ministry of Civil Affairs (2003) China Mental Health Work Plan. *Shanghai Archive of Psychiatry* 15(2):125–128.
9. Ministry of Health (2011) China Mental Health Work Plan (2011–2020).
10. Available at: http://wenku.baidu.com/view/1ef65545be1e650e52ea99fc.html (last accessed on 20 February 2013).
11. The State Council (2011) The 12th Five-Year Plan for China Aging Development. Availabale at: http://www.gov.cn/zwgk/2011-09/23/content_1954782.htm (last accessed on 20 February 2013).
12. Available at: http://news.sohu.com/20061212/n246981747.shtml (last accessed on 20 February 2013).
13. Zhang M (2007) *Management Guideline of Dementia in China.* Beijing: Peking University Medical Press.
14. Jia J (2010) *Diagnostic and Treatment Guideline of Dementia and Cognitive Impairment in China.* Beijing: People's Health Press.
15. Xue H, Yu X, Xiao, S (2006) Evaluation of present status of psychiatric services in elderly in China. *Journal of Clinical Psychological Medicine* 16(1):11–13.
16. Xiong Q, Wang H, Wang H, et al. (2011) Sociocultural beliefs on caregiver for the elderly in Chinese rural area. *Chinese Journal of Gerontology* 31(4):669–671.
17. Available at: http://www.cncaprc.gov.cn/info/17342.html (last accessed on 20 February 2013).
18. Li X, Fang W, Su N, Liu Y, Xiao S, Xiao Z (2011) Survey in Shanghai communities: the public awareness of and attitude towards dementia. *Psychogeriatrics* 11:83–89.

India

K. S. Shaji and T. P. Sumesh

Govt. Medical College, India

Introduction

There are about 3.7 million people with dementia in India, as per the estimates of the Dementia India Report released in 2010. This figure is expected to double by 2030 [1]. The prevailing low public awareness about dementia prevents early detection and causes delay in getting help. The formation of the Alzheimer's and Related Disorders Society of India (ARDSI) and later the formation of the 10/66 Dementia Research Group in 1998 have helped raise awareness to some extent.

Need for services

Though the estimated social and economic costs associated with dementia are high, dementia care remains unsupported by health services [2,3]. The current care provision is one of home-based care without any medical or social input. Facilities for institutional care are almost non-existent except in a few places. Home-based care by a co-resident family member, most often the spouse, children or their spouses, seems to be the norm. But families are becoming smaller, and more women are seeking employment. This will further limit the human resource available for home-based care. The medical input for home-based care is limited to occasional consultations, often with private providers. Home visits by doctors or nurses for evaluation or management are not common.

Health services in India

India has a large national network of government-run primary care health centres and hospitals. These work alongside private and not-for-profit healthcare providers. Public healthcare facilities are managed by the state governments. Resource limitations, especially manpower shortages and poor infrastructure are widespread. Though the services are free, many people choose to seek help from the costly private system [3]. The availability of services varies from state to state and access is generally poor, especially in rural and remote areas. Primary care doctors do not encounter many cases of dementia in their practices whereas health workers are aware of cases in the community [4]. Possibly the public primary care system is not responsive to the needs of people with dementia, and cases of dementia remain largely unattended. At present, public healthcare services do not offer any special services for older people. Outpatient services remain crowded and consultations are brief. The usual focus here is on 'treatable' acute pathologies and not on long-term care. Older people are reluctant to access these services as often services are not local, necessitating travel and long waits. Clinic-based services are thus of limited value for older people needing long-term support and care.

Dementia care services: The current situation

The availability of dementia care services in India is very limited [1]. There are only a few residential care facilities, which are exclusively for people with dementia. There are about 10 day-care centres offering professional care for people with dementia. Most of these services are situated in southern India. Residential care facilities, exclusively for persons with dementia, are even fewer.

Most of these services are run by registered non-profit organisations and are financed by public contributions and user fees. These centres usually cater for about 5 to 20 residents and employ trained carers. Some day-care facilities take older people with dementia, but most old-age homes refuse to care for older people with dementia. Local branches of the ARDSI and other organisations, such as the Dignity Foundation [5] and the Nightingales Trust (Bangalore) run day-care services for persons with dementia.

There are a few centres which provide support for people with dementia who live at home. These send out part time staff, social workers or volunteers to visit the homes of people with dementia and provide assistance or guidance in dementia care. Home-care services are available in major cities. Many support groups exist, and many of them liaise with local branches of the ARDSI or memory clinics. There are only about 10 helplines, and most of them are run by the ARDSI.

Clinic-based services

Dementia care services are available in many general hospitals through the departments of psychiatry and neurology. They focus on caregiver education and support. Special services like dementia clinics or memory clinics are available in general hospitals. It is estimated that there are nearly 100 such clinics in India. They usually offer the services of a clinician and will have a facility for neuropsychological assessments. Families find such services useful [6]. Development of clinic-based services help clinicians to acquire knowledge and skills necessary for providing specialised dementia care services.

The District Mental Health Programme (DMHP) is a public healthcare service which aims to decentralise mental health care and is currently operational in 125 out of 629 districts in India. Monthly psychiatric clinics are organised in various parts of the districts. Medicines are provided free. Older people with dementia and other mental health problems seek help in these clinics. Mental health professionals in the DMHP team can act as a resource to provide personalised guidance and to monitor dementia care. Community-based dementia care can get continued support if the DMHP is effectively linked to primary care and outreach services. The government wants to extend the DMHP programme to cover all districts in India.

People's participation in dementia care

People's participation is the key in sustaining community-based services. The Department of Psychiatry of the Medical College Thrissur assisted the local government in planning and implementing a dementia care service at Talikulam Block Panchayath in the Thrissur District of Kerala. A qualitative study of patients with Alzheimer's disease from the region highlighted the problems faced by the caregivers [2]. The findings were brought to the attention of the local government. This led to a project to provide mental health services for older people in the area. After a preliminary survey, a monthly geriatric psychiatry clinic was established in the local community health centre in 1999. The local government continues to fund this project. A caregiver guide in the local language was prepared and is available to health workers and caregivers. The ongoing programme serves a population of about 10,000 older people. Inputs from this initiative led to the development of a caregiver training module by the 10/66 Dementia Research Group to guide home-based interventions for people with dementia. Simple home-based interventions were found to be useful on evaluation in Goa [7]. In this study, the interventions were delivered by Home Care Advisors (HCA) trained to plan and provide interventions to suit the needs of the person with dementia. Dementia care ideally could be made part of broad-based community outreach programmes to support older people with disabling health conditions. This would ensure wider application in the community and cut costs.

Future directions

Development of dementia care services in India is likely to be driven by the increasing demand and gradual rise in awareness. The involvement of families and the local community is key to its success. Outreach services will have a pivotal role in supporting home-based care. Specialists need to support and guide the outreach services. The government is keen to develop geriatrics as a specialty. The Medical Council of India has recently approved Geriatric Mental Health as a sub-specialty of Psychiatry. Growth and development of specialties like Geriatrics and Geriatric Mental Health will help to generate manpower with expertise in dementia care. These experts can train and guide non-specialist healthcare providers working in primary and secondary care settings to deliver dementia care.

References

1. Shaji KS, Joteeshwaran AT, Girish N, Bharath S, Dias A, Pattabiraman M, et al. (2010) Dementia India Report: Prevalence, impact, costs and services for Dementia. Alzheimer's and Related Disorders Society of India.
2. Shaji KS, Smitha K, Praveen Lal K, Prince M (2002) Caregivers of patients with Alzheimer's disease: a qualitative study from the Indian 10/66 dementia research network. *International Journal of Geriatric Psychiatry* 18:1–6.
3. Prince M (2004) Care arrangements for people with dementia in developing countries. *International Journal of Geriatric Psychiatry* 19(2):170–177.
4. Patel V, Prince M (2001) Ageing and mental health in a developing country: who cares? Qualitative studies from Goa, India. *Psychological Medicine* 31(1):29–38.
5. Pednekar MS, Gupta PC, Hebert JR, Hakama M (2008) Joint effects of tobacco use and body mass on all-cause mortality in Mumbai, India: results from a population-based cohort study. *American Journal of Epidemiology* 167(3):330–340.
6. Shaji KS, Iype T, Praveenlal K (2009) Dementia clinic in general hospital settings. *Indian Journal of Psychiatry* 51(1):42–44.
7. Dias A, Dewey ME, D'Souza J, Dhume R, Motghare DD, Shaji KS, et al. (2008) The effectiveness of a home care program for supporting caregivers of persons with dementia in developing countries: a randomised controlled trial from Goa, India. *PLoS ONE [Electronic Resource]* 3(6):e2333.

Japan

Atsuhiro Yamada[a] and Miharu Nakanishi[b]

[a]*Research & Consulting Division, the Japan Research Institute Ltd, Japan*
[b]*Research Division, Institute for Health Economics and Policy, Japan*

Background

The elderly population (>65 years) in Japan was 29.6 million in 2010, being 23.1% of the total population [1]. In 2003, the National Ministry of Health, Labour and Welfare (MHLW) published a report 'Long-Term Care for the Elderly in 2015'. It estimated that the total number of people with dementia was 1.49 million in 2002 and would reach 2.50 million in 2015, 3.53 million in 2030, and 3.78 million in 2045.

Overview of dementia care

Dementia care services are mostly covered by Health Insurance (HI) or Long-Term Care Insurance (LTCI) with co-payments. Both are public. In April 2000, the National Long-Term Care Insurance programme for the elderly was implemented. Although municipal governments manage the programme as insurers, the provision of service is open to the private sector, including for-profit companies, voluntary groups, and non-profit organisations [2]. A care manager is assigned to a client to coordinate home-care services under the LTCI programme, but this is terminated when the client is admitted to residential care facilities or healthcare institutions. Japanese health insurance is mandatory and covers all citizens. Under the health insurance scheme, beneficiaries have guaranteed access to any healthcare provider (called 'free access') (Figure 12.1).

Features of dementia care

Memory clinic under the HI

There is no system of general practitioner registration such as in Western countries. In theory, any physician in any specialty can diagnose dementia. However, in practice, this is likely to occur at departments of psychiatry, neurology or geriatrics in hospitals. Some hospitals have outpatient memory clinics that can provide the diagnosis of dementia.

Home-care services under LTCI

Home-care services under LTCI cover personal care at home (home help), outreach nursing, day care, and short stay services for the aged. Clients of outreach nursing under LTCI included 79.6% of persons with dementia [3].

Community care services under LTCI

Community-based services were introduced under the LTCI programme in 2006 to establish one-stop home-care services for small groups of clients and small-scale residential care facilities.

Community-based care services provide some types of specialised care such as day care and group homes (group living). Group homes are small-scale homelike facilities that accommodate older adults with mild to moderate dementia.

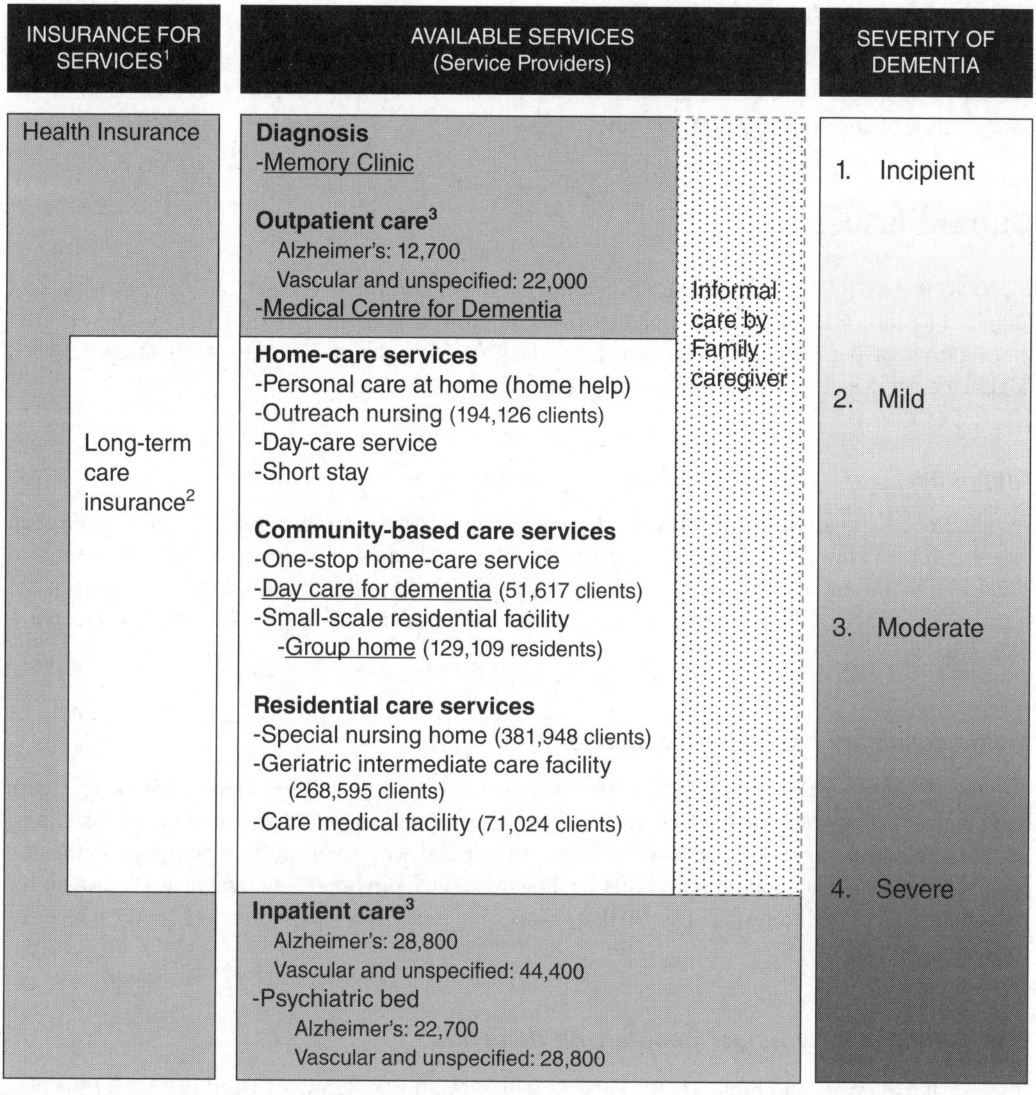

INSURANCE FOR SERVICES[1]	AVAILABLE SERVICES (Service Providers)	SEVERITY OF DEMENTIA

Health Insurance

Diagnosis
-Memory Clinic

1. Incipient

Outpatient care[3]
  Alzheimer's: 12,700
  Vascular and unspecified: 22,000
-Medical Centre for Dementia

Informal care by Family caregiver

Long-term care insurance[2]

Home-care services
-Personal care at home (home help)
-Outreach nursing (194,126 clients)
-Day-care service
-Short stay

2. Mild

Community-based care services
-One-stop home-care service
-Day care for dementia (51,617 clients)
-Small-scale residential facility
  -Group home (129,109 residents)

Residential care services
-Special nursing home (381,948 clients)
-Geriatric intermediate care facility
  (268,595 clients)
-Care medical facility (71,024 clients)

3. Moderate

Inpatient care[3]
  Alzheimer's: 28,800
  Vascular and unspecified: 44,400
-Psychiatric bed
  Alzheimer's: 22,700
  Vascular and unspecified: 28,800

4. Severe

Figure 12.1 Overview of dementia care services in Japan
Underline: specialised dementia care
[1]Most of dementia care services (except family care) are covered by insurances with co-payments
[2]The LTCI programme requires elderly people to undergo a standardised assessment by care managers to determine their eligibility for services covered under LTCI. Numbers of clients and residents under the Long-Term Care Insurance are at September 2010
[3]Numbers of inpatients and outpatients under the Health Insurance are at October 2008

Residential care services under the LTCI

Residential care services under the LTCI programme consist of special nursing homes, geriatric intermediate care facilities and medical care facilities. Special nursing homes are facilities for residents who require high intensity care. Geriatric intermediate care facilities are for residents who require rehabilitation. Care medical facilities are for high intensity care residents who require medical care [4]. More than 90% of residents in these care facilities are suspected of having dementia [2].

Psychiatric hospital under the HI

Most inpatients with dementia are treated in psychiatric facilities [5]. In October 2008, about a quarter of inpatients with dementia were deemed to have been admitted for non-medical reasons, such as lack of social care service or other support.

Current issues

In 2008, the MHLW launched the 'Emergency Project for Improvement of Medical Care and Quality of Life for People with Dementia' [6]. The project reported that the LTCI system covered the majority of persons with dementia, but a lack of early diagnosis and coordination between healthcare services and social care services caused some problems.

Diagnosis

As mentioned above, the total number of people with dementia has been estimated at more than one 1 million. However, the MHLW estimated the total number of patients with dementia at 112,100: 34,700 outpatients and 77,400 inpatients [5]. There is therefore a large gap between the estimated number of persons with dementia and the numbers of those who actually receive a diagnosis.

Multidisciplinary healthcare team/agency

Previously there was no multidisciplinary healthcare service providing support for people with dementia and behavioural and psychological symptoms of dementia (BPSD) in home-care settings. In 2008, Medical Centres for Dementia were established to provide the diagnosis of dementia, special healthcare consultation with other healthcare service providers and healthcare treatment for BPSD and other conditions [7]. The MHLW plans to increase the total number of Medical Centres for Dementia to 150.

Care services for younger people with dementia

In 2005, the Services and Supports for Persons with Disabilities Act was passed [8]. Under the new system, municipal governments manage social care services for the disabled, and the provision of services is open to the private sector as well as providers under the LTCI programme. The programme covers home-care services, residential care services and rehabilitation services for children and adult persons with physical, intellectual or mental disabilities.

Guardianship

In 2000, the Adult Guardianship Scheme was introduced to protect and support persons with limited mental capacity, mainly with regard to the management of their property. Guardians for persons with dementia, however, will also be involved when someone needs social care services under the LTCI programme and in cases of elder abuse. Since many providers under LTCI are private sector providers, advocacy services for persons with dementia are of importance. However, the annual number of guardianship stands at about 30,000, and therefore, this scheme appears to provide protection for only a small proportion of people with dementia [9].

End-of-life care

In Japan, there are no systematic approaches to advance directives, living wills or similar constructs regarding end-of-life care. National statistics indicate that around half of people with dementia die in healthcare institutions (hospitals and clinics) [10].

References

1. Japanese Cabinet Office (2011) Aged Society White Paper, 2011 (in Japanese).
2. Campbell JC, Ikegami N (2000) Long-term care insurance comes to Japan. *Health Affairs* 19:26–39.
3. Ministry of Health, Labour and Welfare (2012) Survey of Institutions and Establishments for Long-term Care, 2010 (in Japanese).
4. Ikegami N, Yamauchi K, Yamada Y (2003) The long term care insurance law in Japan: impact on institutional care facilities. *International Journal of Geriatric Psychiatry* 18:217–221.
5. Ministry of Health, Labour and Welfare (2009) Patient Survey, 2008 (in Japanese).
6. Takeda A, Tanaka N, Chiba T (2010) Prospects of future measures for persons with dementia in Japan. *Psychogeriatrics* 10:95–101.
7. Awata S (2010) New national health program against dementia in Japan: the medical center for dementia. *Psychogeriatrics* 10:102–106.
8. Takei T, Takahashi H, Nakatani H (2008) Developing a uniformed assessment tool to evaluate care service needs for disabled persons in Japan. *Health Policy* 86:373–380.
9. Supreme Court of Japan (2011) Summary of Adult Guardianship, 2010 (in Japanese).
10. Ministry of Health, Labour and Welfare (2011) Vital Statistics, 2010 (in Japanese).

South Korea

Guk-Hee Suh

Hallym University Hangang Sacred Heart Hospital, Korea

Chronic illnesses like dementia place a heavy psychological, physical and economic burden on those living with the illness. Family-based long-term care is reaching its limits as a result of diminishing supportive social networks, which in South Korea went hand in hand with rapid economic growth. Responding to the ensuing need of a more formal care system, South Korea adopted a long-term care insurance scheme in 2008. Since its inception, the number of people receiving support through this system has vastly increased from 76,000 in 2008 to around 312,128 in 2010 [1].

Long-term care insurance

By providing systematised nationwide services, Long-Term Care Insurance aims to improve the health and quality of life of senior citizens, to reduce the burden of long-term care on families, to resolve problems arising from family carers not being able to work and to vitalise the economy by creating new employment opportunities for care workers, nurses and social workers.

The National Health Insurance Corporation is the only social health insurer covering the entire Korean population of over 50 million people. The National Health Insurance Corporation administers Long-Term Care Insurance, which is financed through a combination of contributions from the insured, the government and co-payments of those receiving support. Its premiums have increased dramatically from 4.05% in 2008 to 6.55% in 2010. Co-payments from beneficiaries are means-tested and further depend on the services needed.

Who is entitled to receive long-term care services?

In 2010, about 50% of people with dementia (around 230,000) received anti-dementia drugs according to National Health Insurance Corporation data [2]. The Long-Term Care Needs Certification Committee at city, county and municipal level decides on entitlement of long-term care services. It examines the applicant's case files, carries out home visits and assesses needs, partially based on medical advice, and includes assessment of functional abilities, mental capacity and the need for rehabilitation. There are no strict age limits for people with dementia.

Care category decision

The Long-Term Care Needs Certification Committee decides the care category of applicants after collecting all information and data (Table 12.1).

Services provided

Long-term care services include home care, institutional care and financial benefits.

1. Home carers provide assistance with bathing, toileting, dressing, cooking, shopping, cleaning, and so on. Sometimes a vehicle equipped with a portable bath provides a bathing service at

Table 12.1 Three categories of dependence requiring long-term care

Category	Criteria	Services provided
1	Cannot get in and out of bed unaided; impaired memory and judgement; behavioural problems; needs full assistance with ADLs	All
2	Cannot feed or dress themselves; need full assistance with ADL; impaired memory and judgement	All
3	Needs partial assistance with feeding, dressing and self-care; needs assistance with household activities or activities outside	Only in-home services

home. Nurses provide home care under medical supervision. Day care or night care centres provide nursing care, functional therapy, medical treatment and assistance with Activities of Daily Living, again under medical supervision. Long-term welfare facilities also provide respite care when needed. Various aids, such as wheelchairs, portable bathtubs and sore-preventing mattresses can be rented for use at home.

2. Institutional services are provided by long-term care facilities, licensed nursing homes, homes for the aged and licensed residential care facilities.
3. Financial benefits are available to support family carers in case there are logistical or geographic difficulties hampering a necessary admission to institutional care. If someone is admitted to a geriatric hospital or a non-registered long-term care institution over a long period of time, the cost is partially reimbursed.

In July 2010, the total number of people receiving support through Long-Term Care Insurance was 246,726. More than twice as many people received home care than institutional care (170,181 and 78,203, respectively) [3].

Who can provide services?

Professional care workers must complete 240 hours of training and pass a national qualification exam. Provider organisations are required to hire carers according to minimum staff/user ratios which are defined officially by law. In 2010, this ratio stood at 3.3 care workers per 1000 over 65s. (OECD average 6.1 workers) [4].

Present condition and future prospect

The needs of people with dementia and their caregivers are diverse. Even those at the same stage of dementia differ considerably in their requirements for assistance and support. Thus, a wide range of service alternatives is necessary. Furthermore, needs change over time and therefore services must be responsive to those changes. Given this and the need for flexibility, a variety of services should be available. These services should provide medical treatment, stimulating activities, respite and relief from caregiving for the caregivers, and support and counselling to families as they build and maintain their resources for the long haul.

Home care is a common goal in almost all countries to preserve autonomy for as long as possible, but demand often outstrips resources. This is even more likely to be the case, given the sharp increases in the numbers of 'oldest old' people, whose illnesses are likely to be severe and whose needs are more complex. Current economic circumstances are likely to impede necessary investment into dementia care services, so governments must be even more focused on addressing the inevitable increase we all will have to face.

References

1. Choi ID (2010) Long-term financial perspective and health policies for the Long-term Care Insurance. National Health Insurance Corporation.
2. National Health Insurance Corporation (2011) 2010 Annual report of Elderly Long-term Care Insurance.
3. National Health Insurance Corporation (July 2010) Monthly report of Elderly Long-term Care Insurance.
4. OECD (2010) Health Data 2010, Paris.

Chapter 13

Eastern Europe

In the Czech Republic there are over 10 sites specialising in Alzheimer's disease and the country is involved in many international research projects, some into service delivery and quality of services. A National Alzheimer or Dementia plan is being finalised.

Hungary reports high alcohol consumption as a possible causative factor for relatively high prevalence rates of dementia, as well as higher than usual prevalence of vascular dementia. There is a network of specialised services called 'Dementia Centres', but these have limited efficiency. There are many non-governmental and some patient organisations active in dementia care.

Poland is seeing a gradual move from an institutional model of mental health care towards a model based in the person's environment. There is a plethora of services for people with dementia, but structure is lacking and the vast majority of people with dementia are looked after by their families. However, there is a government endorsed 'National Alzheimer's Program'.

In Turkey, most assessments are still carried out in specialist centres (neurology, geriatric medicine and psychiatry). There are high levels of traditional family support and since 2003, the Turkish Alzheimer Foundation operates a care centre for people with dementia in Istanbul, this being the first specialist care centre for people with dementia in Turkey. It recently expanded and now provides extensive home-based care, actively supporting caregivers.

Designing and Delivering Dementia Services, First Edition. Edited by Hugo de Waal, Constantine Lyketsos, David Ames, and John O'Brien.
© 2013 John Wiley & Sons, Ltd. Published 2013 by John Wiley & Sons, Ltd.

The Czech Republic

Katerina Sheardova[a], Iva Holmerova[b] and Jakub Hort[c,d]

[a]*International Clinical Research Center, Department of Neurology, St. Anne's University Hospital Brno, Czech Republic*
[b]*Centre of Gerontology and CELLO-ILC-CZ, Faculty of Humanities, Charles University in Prague, Czech Republic*
[c]*Memory Disorders Clinic, Department of Neurology, 2nd Faculty of Medicine, Charles University in Prague and University Hospital Motol V Úvalu 84, Czech Republic*
[d]*International Clinical Research Center, St. Anne's University Hospital Brno, Czech Republic*

The Czech Republic has a long history of dementia research. It is the homeland of Oskar Fischer (1876–1942) who first described the presence of plaques and tangles in 12 cases of presenile dementia, compared to one case described by Alois Alzheimer (1864–1915) [1]. Arnold Pick (1854–1924), working in Prague, found swollen brain cells known as Pick cells, together with abnormal staining within cells (Pick bodies) in a patient with fronto-temporal atrophy.

The Czech Republic has approximately 10.5 million inhabitants. According to the latest prevalence rates we estimate that there are about 125,000 people with dementia. The diagnosis is mostly established by neurologists in the earlier stages, while psychiatrists and geriatricians deal mainly with people in the moderate and severe stages [2]. There are approximately 11,400 people per 1 neurologist, 10,800 people per 1 psychiatrist and 51,500 people per 1 geriatrician. These numbers are comparable to other central and eastern European countries [3].

Prescribing of cholinesterase inhibitors (ChEI) and memantine is limited to these three specialties. Insurance companies require Mini-Mental State Examinations (MMSE) every 3 months for the reimbursement of cognitive drug therapy. ChEI therapy is covered within the 13–25 range of MMSE score and memantine in the range of 6–17, allowing for dual therapy reimbursement in the range of 13–17, which is quite regularly prescribed [2]. In case of ChEI intolerance, memantine can be prescribed free of charge up to a MMSE score of 19.

With average catchment areas of 1500–1800 people per GP, it is estimated that one GP should have 15–20 patients with dementia (while only approximately 2–4 patients are actually referred to specialists who can prescribe ChEI) [4]. About half of dementia patients seek specialist help directly. There is still a relatively high use of nootropics, vasoactive substances and other non-evidence-based therapy. This might be partially due to insurance companies constraining the use of ChEIs to patients with MMSE scores below 25, yet are deemed clinically to have AD. It may also be the result of underdiagnosis by GPs, who aren't allowed to prescribe anti-dementia medication. Reimbursement of non-evidence-based medications is likely to be revoked during 2012 while insurance companies expect a gradual increase in usage – and therefore cost – of ChEIs. However, patents of ChEIs have expired, lowering the cost.

National recommendations for diagnosis and treatment are comparable to European guidelines [5], which were translated and adapted for the Czech Republic and its specific environment [6,7].

There are over 10 specialist sites dealing with AD, some involved in research and most attached to universities. There are four laboratories measuring cerebrospinal fluid tau, phosphorylated tau and beta-amyloid levels. The main obstacle for such tests to be freely available is the lack of reimbursement by health insurance providers and uncertainty about cut-off and normative values, yielding different results across laboratories. They are therefore used primarily for research rather than clinical diagnostic purposes [8].

The Czech Republic is participating in many European Union (EU) projects, such as the EU Joint Program on neurodegenerative diseases. One other key example of Euro-Atlantic cooperation is an EU-funded collaborative project in cardiology and neurology, that is, the International Clinical Research Centre Brno, which in part focuses on AD epidemiology and collaborates with the Mayo clinic, Rochester, USA. Czech researchers participate in the INTERDEM international research group on psychosocial interventions in dementia and are active in the field of palliative care, collaborating on recommendations for end-of-life care [9].

The Czech Alzheimer Society (CALS, established in 1997) is an active member of Alzheimer's Disease International and Alzheimer Europe (current vice-president of Alzheimer Europe is the delegate of CALS) and is involved in many national activities. Memory Days is a project focusing on early diagnosis and case finding of dementia, funded by different sponsors and supported by independent experts. Project GOS (Gerontological and Organisational Supervision) aims to improve care in residential facilities in Southern Moravia. Improvement of long-term care provision is one of the goals of CALS, and there is since 2011 an international collaboration: ELTECA (Exchange of Experiences in Long-term Care).

In 2011, leading experts established the Alzheimer Foundation with the objective of supporting young scientists and research in the field of AD and related disorders.

Although the Czech Republic is internationally very active in AD research, there is still no national Alzheimer or Dementia plan. In early 2011, a task force was approved by the Czech government to design concept solutions for AD and similar diseases ('Alzheimer Plan'), the aim being to analyse the current situation of people with dementia and their carers and to create health care, social, educational and research measures to improving their care. The various government departments involved pledged to finalise this plan by June 2011, but further steps were not taken until early 2012.

Acknowledgement

Supported by Grant Agency of the Czech Republic Grants 309/09/1053; European Regional Development Fund – Project FNUSA-ICRC (No. CZ.1.05/1.1.00/02.0123)

References

1. Goedert M (2008) Oskar Fischer and the study of dementia. *Brain* 132(4):1102–1111.
2. Sheardova K, Hort J, Rektorova I, Rusina R, Linek V, Bartos A (2012) Dementia diagnosis and treatment in Czech neurological and psychiatric practices. *Cesk Slov Neurol N* 75/108(2):208–211. in print.
3. Bartos A, Kalvach P, Trošt M, Ertsey C, Rejdak K, Popov L, et al. (2001) Postgraduate education in neurology in Central and Eastern Europe. *Eur J Neurol* 8:551–558.
4. Hort J (2011) Nová guidelines pro diagnostiku a léčbu Alzheimerlovy choroby. *Neurol Prax* 12(4):277–281.
5. Hort J, O'Brien JT, Gainotti G, Pirttila T, Popescu BO, Rektorova I, et al. (2010) EFNS Scientist Panel on Dementia. EFNS guidelines for the diagnosis and management of Alzheimer's disease. *Eur J Neurol* 17(10):1236–1248.
6. Sheardova K, Hort J, Rusina R, Bartos A, Linek V, Ressner P, et al., za Sekci kognitivní neurologie České neurologické společnosti ČLS JEP (2007) Doporučené postupy pro léčbu Alzheimerovy nemoci a dalších onemocnění spojených s demencí. *Cesk Slov Neurol N* 70/103(5):253–258.
7. Ressner P, Hort J, Rektorová I, Bartos A, Rusina R, Linek V, et al., za Sekci kognitivní neurologie České neurologické společnosti J. E. P. (2008) Doporučené postupy pro diagnostiku Alzheimerovy nemoci a dalších onemocnění spojených s demencí. *Cesk Slov Neurol N* 71/104(4):494–501.
8. Hort J, Bartos A, Pirttilä T, Scheltens P (2010) Use of cerebrospinal fluid biomarkers in diagnosis of dementia across Europe. *Eur J Neurol* 17(1):90–96.
9. Gove D, Sparr S, Dos Santos Bernardo AM, Cosgrave MP, Jansen S, Martensson B, et al. (2008) *End-of-Life Care for People with Dementia*. Luxembourg: Alzheimer Europe.

Hungary

Gábor Gazdag[a,b], Brigitta Baran[c] and Zoltán Hidasi[c]

[a]*Department of Psychiatry and Psychotherapy, Faculty of Medicine, Semmelweis University, Hungary*
[b]*Szent István and Szent László Hospitals, Hungary*
[c]*Department of Psychiatry and Psychotherapy, Faculty of Medicine, Semmelweis University, Hungary*

Epidemiology

To date no systematic survey has explored the prevalence of dementia in Hungary, but estimates can be extrapolated from two surveys conducted in general practice:

1. Linka et al. found dementia prevalence rates to be 7.4% (<65 years), 17.7% (65–75) and 38.7% (>75) [1].
2. Rates in the second survey were 7.3% (<60), 29.1% (60–69), 39.2 (70–79) and 54.6% (>80) [2].

Rates in both surveys are higher than internationally published data, probably because they were conducted in general practice rather than in general population cohorts [3]. Besides this selection bias, significant alcohol consumption in the Hungarian population may be contributing to the higher prevalence of dementia [4]. Based on the above, it was estimated that between 150,000 and 300,000 Hungarians suffer from dementia [5].

An important finding is the high prevalence of vascular dementia as a result of high overall vascular morbidity [6,7]. In a recent study, neurodegenerative pathology was found in 81% of the brains of patients with clinical dementia, with 43% showing vascular pathology and the rate of mixed cases being 25% [8].

In spite of the somewhat lower life expectancy in Hungary (70 for men, 78 for women [9]) the proportion of elders (≥65) has grown from 15.1% in 2001 to 16.3% by 2009, as a result of decreasing number of childbirths. Hungary is fast becoming one of the oldest countries in Europe, a significant burden on the economy [10].

Empirical evidence shows that health or social issues related to milder dementia are less important in Hungary compared to more developed countries. For instance, elderly Hungarians can manage their daily life without driving while their American counterparts cannot. Many old people live close to relatives in Hungary, which is less typical in, for example, the USA. A diagnosis of dementia is highly stigmatising and as such it discourages patients and their families to seek help early.

In 2002, there were 78,000 outpatient visits for dementia [11]. Based on these data, the estimated number of newly diagnosed cases was <5000. Of these, only about one-fifth were seen in specialist psychogeriatric services. Similarly low was the number of guardianship orders because of inability to manage affairs [12].

The development and present state of dementia care

Up to the late 1990s, patients with dementia were treated in the context of general psychiatry or neurology. The first professional recommendation for the examination and management of dementia was published in 1999. The first unit established for dementia opened in the National Institute of Psychiatry and Neurology (NIPN) in 1992, under the rather euphemistic name of 'Memory Clinic'.

By 2003, a network of specialised services called 'Dementia Centres' was set up with participation of 243 neurologists and psychiatrists in 84 countrywide centres. These new services were superimposed on existing general psychiatry or neurology outpatient services. Doctors affiliated with Dementia Centres were authorised to prescribe anti-dementia drugs with a national health insurance reimbursement of 50%. Certain criteria (e.g. abnormal CT scan and MMSE) for a diagnosis of dementia and administrative requirements for follow-up were also established. However, as the main aim of creating these centres was to control drug prescription and not to improve quality of care, limited capacity was provided by the centres and most patients could not access higher level dementia care [13]. Furthermore, increasing emigration of professionals after Hungary's entry into the EU seriously affected the workforce of both neurology [13] and psychiatry [14] resulting in further declines in levels of care. At present, usually only moderate or severe forms of dementia are detected and anti-dementia treatment is available only to a very small number. However, a positive development saw recently the authorisation for prescribing anti-dementia drugs extended to all psychiatrists and neurologists.

Social welfare for dementia patients in Hungary

Until the end of 2005, dementia patients in need of continuous care were admitted to nursing homes, or if severe symptoms made that impossible to long-term residential homes for psychiatric patients. The modification of the Social Welfare Act (1 January 2006) shifted placement of dementia patients to specialised wards of nursing homes tailored to their needs. As this Act did not specify where these wards are required, they were not established in several institutions, thus violating the legal rights of the residents with and without dementia [15].

In 2011, there were about 32,000 nursing home beds with some 10,000 patients waiting for beds. Most nursing homes are run by local government, churches, civil and for-profit organisations, and 543 institutions accept patients with dementia [16]. However, there are no data about the number of dementia patients living in nursing homes: a recent survey detected a rate as high as 60% in one home [2].

Non-governmental organisations (NGOs)

Of the numerous NGOs active in this field, two deserve special attention. The Society for Relatives of People with Memory Disturbances was founded in 1999 with the aim of helping relatives of patients with any type of dementia. The Society runs an information phone line and a website. Day-care services were provided for 5 years, but lack of financial support forced their suspension in 2006. Staff members and patients of the Memory Clinic of NIPN established in the mid-1990s the Memory Foundation [17]. Initially, the Foundation published information leaflets and organised meetings for patients and relatives. A day-care service for 10–12 patients started in Budapest in 1997.

Suggestions for future developments

In order to improve dementia care in the face of the worsening economic situation in Hungary, the authors regard the following as both necessary and achievable in the near future:

1. Separate centres for diagnosis and management of particular forms of dementia (e.g. Alzheimer's, Pick's etc.) should be set up.

2. To reduce the burden on families and increase the likelihood of patients remaining longer at home, it is vital to establish day-care services in all larger Hungarian cities.
3. It is important to establish specialised wards for patients with dementia in every nursing home that accepts such patients.

References

1. Linka E, Kispál GY, Szabó T, Bartkó GY (2001) A dementia szűrése és a betegek egyéves követése egy háziorvosi praxisban. *Ideggyogy Sz* 54:156–160.
2. Leel-Őssy L, Józsa I, Szűcs I, Kindler M (2005) Szűrővizsgálatok a dementia korai felderítésére. *Medicus Universalis* 38:149–160.
3. Lobo A, Launer LJ, Fratiglioni L, Andersen K, Di Carlo A, Breteler MM, et al. (2000) Prevalence of dementia and major subtypes in Europe: a collaborative study of population-based cohorts. Neurologic Diseases in the Elderly Research Group. *Neurology* 54(11 Suppl 5):S4–S9.
4. World Health Organization Deperment of Mental Health and Substance Abuse (2004) WHO Global Status Report on Alcohol 2004. Geneva.
5. Érsek K, Kárpáti K, Kovács T, Csillik G, Gulácsi AL, Gulácsi L (2010) A dementia epidemiológiája Magyarországon. *Ideggyogy Sz* 63:175–182.
6. Dementia – Etiology and Epidemiology (June 2008) *A Systematic Review*, Vol. 1. Stockholm: SBU, The Swedish Council on Technology Assessment in Health Care.
7. Józan P (2009) Halálozási viszonyok és életkilátások a XXI. század kezdetén a világ, Európa és Magyarország népességében. *Magy Tud* 170:1231–1244.
8. Kovács GG, Kővári V, Nagy Z (2008) Dementiával járó kórképek gyakorisága az Országos Pszichiátriai és Neurológiai Intézet hároméves neuropatológiai anyagában. *Ideggyogy Sz* 61:24–32.
9. WHO Countries: Hungary Available at: http://www.who.int/countries/hun/en/ (last accessed on 20 February 2013).
10. Bodrogi J (2009) Az idősödés néhány demográfiai, közgazdasági és társadalombiztosítási összefüggése. *LAM* 19:527–530.
11. Available at: http://www.gyogyinfok.hu (last accessed on 20 February 2013).
12. Hungarian College of Psychiatrists (2005) A demencia kórismézése, kezelése és gondozása. (Professional recommendations) Egészségügyi Közlöny 12th issue.
13. Bereczki D, Ajtay A (2011) Neurológia 2009: helyzetfelmérés a magyarországi neurológiai kapacitásokról, azok kihasználtságáról és a szakorvosokról a 2009-es intézményi jelentések alapján. *Ideggyogy Sz* 64:173–185.
14. Gazdag G (2008) Fenyegető humánerőforrás-krízis a pszichiátriai ellátásban. *IME* 7:23–29.
15. Betegjogi, Ellátottjogi és Gyermekjogi Közalapítvány: Demens betegek jogsérelmei és jogvédelme (2009) Jogvédelmi füzetek sorozat 6. szám második kiadás. szeptember hó.
16. Idősgondozási kézikönyv (2011) Magyarországi idősotthonok, otthoni ápolók és hospice-ok adatbázisa. Geriáter Service Kiadó.
17. Available at: http://www.memoriaalapitvany.hu/ (last accessed on 20 February 2013).

Poland

Jerzy Leszek[a,b] and Marta Sochocka[c]

[a]*Department of Psychiatry, Wroclaw Medical University, Poland*
[b]*Lower Silesian Association of Alzheimer's Patients' Families, Poland*
[c]*Laboratory of Biomedical Chemistry, Institute of Immunology and Experimental Therapy Polish Academy of Sciences, Poland*

Poland has a population of about 40 million, 16.5% of whom are aged over 65. This is expected to rise dramatically to 23.8% by 2035. The consequence is an increasing number of patients with age-related diseases, especially various types of dementia [1].

The Polish healthcare system

The political transformation in Poland at the end of the 1980s, together with socio-economic changes, led to alterations in the way care for people with mental illnesses is provided. On the one hand, access to psychiatric advice is limited, on the other – because of the low status of mental illness in public awareness – accepting such advice when accessible and willingness to take advantage of it is poor. Due to an increasing number of patients who needed support and professional care in mental health, it was essential to transform the mental healthcare system and move it from the previous institutional model towards a model of health care based on the person's environment. These changes are progressing slowly but efficiently. The number of beds in psychiatric hospitals is decreasing steadily, while in general hospitals, long-term medical care homes and nursing homes it is growing. Large centres are transformed into smaller ones, which improves the quality of patient care. At present, there are 29 teams operating in the community, mainly in large cities. These teams, however, often consist only of a psychiatrist, which means that they are not multidisciplinary. Moreover, access to this form of health service across the country is not equal. There are only about 3000 psychiatrists in university psychiatric clinics, psychiatric departments and in community practice, catering for all those with mental illness. This situation strongly endorses the need for further changes in psychiatric services [2].

Dementia care in Poland: Services and development

There are numerous care services designed for older people, while there is a lack of specific services for people with dementia. The only exception is the Alzheimer's Centre in Ścinawa, which has a neurological and psycho-geriatric department, is dedicated to research into dementia and is partially financed by the EU.

Care of patients with dementia takes place mainly in family homes and in long-stay medical care homes, nursing homes and welfare homes, psychogeriatric day hospitals, 24-hour psycho geriatric wards, municipal welfare centres and private welfare homes. These care settings are controlled by the Ministry of Health and Welfare. Support for people with dementia is also provided by clinics and Alzheimer's Associations as well as associations and support groups promoting understanding of mental health. There are a large number of private welfare homes, but costs are very high, making them accessible only to a small group of patients. There is a lack of effective scrutiny of these centres, resulting in reporting of many serious abuses.

Patient care at home

The largest 'long-term care institution' in Poland is the family. Almost 92% of patients with dementia remain at home in the care of their loved ones from the beginning of the disease to the end. Carers, mostly spouses, often have to give up work to provide such care which may be required for many years. Often carers themselves are aged and frail [3,4], and additionally, a heavy burden may be placed upon the children of the person with dementia. Unfortunately, family carers do not receive financial support nor any form of care insurance, and they are not entitled to benefits or allowances [5]. If the illness prevents the patient from living independently and making decisions autonomously, a carer can apply for 'incapacitation'. Those who are entitled to submit such an application are the spouse, relatives in a direct line and siblings or legal representative. They may apply for the incapacitated person to be placed in a welfare home or other such care setting [6].

Welfare homes provide housing, care and educational services that support the individual needs of patients. Residents are provided with various health benefits such as nursing care, medical assessment, advice and treatment, rehabilitation, psychological assessment and therapy, prevention and health promotion.

Chronic medical care homes and nursing homes offer 24-hour health services, such as care and rehabilitation of people who do not require hospitalisation, medical input appropriate for their condition, and cultural activities and recreational courses. Payment for residence in these institutions is determined individually according to income.

Temporary care

Usually short term and day care is provided by nurses or carers. Welfare agencies cooperate with the welfare centres which employ paid carers. Day care is offered by community organisations, local government and private organisations.

Associations and foundations

The Polish Alzheimer Foundation and other such organisations not only promote public understanding and awareness of dementia, but also provide various forms of assistance to patients and their families, including educating carers, working with national and international centres, setting up support groups and participating in efforts further to develop interventions, including diagnosis and treatment [7].

Binding acts

Poland has always used international classifications to define mental health disorders and applies international standards to mental health treatments. Currently, the 10th revision of the International Classification of Diseases (ICD-10), introduced in Poland in 1997, is used [8]. The program of Polish reforms of mental health services is outlined in two official documents: the 'National Health Care Program (NHCP) for the years 2007–2015' and the 'Regulation of the Ministry' pertaining to the NHCP and the National Alzheimer's Program (NAP-2011), which dates from 28 January 2010.

References

1. Central Statistical Office (CSO) (2010) Demographic Yearbook of Poland.

2. Meder J, Jarema M, Araszkiewicz A (2008) Psychiatryczna opieka środowiskowa w Polsce. Raport Instytut Praw Pacjenta i Edukacji Zdrowotnej.
3. Leszek J (2011) *Choroby otępienne. Teoria i praktyka*. Wroclaw: Continuo.
4. Ciałkowska-Kuźmińska M, Kiejna A (2010) Caregiving consequences in mental disorders – definitions and instruments of assessment. *Psychiatr Pol* 4:519–527.
5. Błędowski P, Pędich W, Bień B, Wojszel ZB, Czekanowski P (2006) *Supporting Family Carers of Older People in Europe – The National Background Report for Poland*. Hamburg: LIT Verlag, p. 1.
6. Jędrejek G (2008) *Kodeks postępowania cywilnego (Code of Civil Procedure)*. Warszawa: C.H. Beck.
7. Durda M (2010) Care arrangements for people with dementia in Poland and developed and developing countries. *Gerontol Pol* 2:76–85.
8. World Health Organization (2002) *Word Health Report 2002 – Reducing Risks, Promoting Healthy Life*. Geneva: WHO.

Turkey

Ahmet Turan Isik[a] and Engin Eker[b]

[a]*National Alzheimer Foundation, Turkey*
[b]*Faculty of Medicine, Department of Geriatric Medicine and National Alzheimer Foundation, Bezmialem Vakif University, Turkey*

With ageing populations around the world, the incidence and prevalence of dementia is increasing, and this is likely to continue in the forthcoming years. The same is true for Turkey: 7.2% of the population is over 65, and numbers of people with dementia are increasing [1]. Therefore, dementia will be one of the most important issues in the near future. However, it remains a somewhat hidden problem due to low levels of public awareness. There are no specialised services for older people except those run by departments of geriatric medicine in university hospitals. General practitioners are not trained to identify and manage dementia as the undergraduate medical curriculum pays little attention to geriatric medicine and dementia [2].

In the beginning of the new millennium the prevalence of dementia was reported to be 7.3% in a cross-sectional study of 265 community-dwelling persons over 65, living in Elazıg (a county in East Anatolia) [3]. However, with increasing life expectancy, the prevalence and incidence of dementia has been increasing in recent years: a cross-sectional population-based two-stage prevalence study of 1019 community-dwelling persons over 70 living in Istanbul reported a prevalence of AD of 20.0% and the prevalence of probable AD was reported as 11.0% [4]. In other words, it was estimated that there will be more than 300,000 people with dementia in Turkey [5].

Most are being cared for at home, thanks to high levels of traditional family support and a culture in which relatives afford due respect to their aged loved ones; unfortunately, there are few specialist dementia centres, with those few having poor facilities and poor services [6]. Although awareness is increasing, all those with suspected dementia are typically evaluated by specialist services (neurology, geriatric medicine and psychiatry) based in university hospitals.

To increase awareness of dementia and to improve the care, support and treatment of persons with dementia and their caregivers, the Turkish Alzheimer Foundation was founded in 2000 by Engin Eker and colleagues. Since 2003, it operates a care centre for people with dementia in Istanbul, this being the first specialist care centre for people with dementia in Turkey [7].

Virtually all people with dementia are being cared for in general care settings, mainly in the public and charitable sector. The above-mentioned specialist care centre expanded its operations in May 2011 to include day care, which further expanded later that year [8]. The expanded centre provides extensive home-based care and actively supports caregivers.

Outpatient dementia care services in developing countries will have to take the added responsibility of supporting home-based care for people with dementia. This is crucial, as institutional care is neither available nor affordable for most families. The need for such a service was evident from the eagerness with which caregivers make use of it [2].

Dementia care is in its infancy in Turkey, as probably is the case in most developing countries. Development of specialised dementia services, including dementia clinics, dementia specific nursing home care and care centres is essential. Such services should aim to establish case registers, capable of guiding further service development. Dementia clinics can provide a setting in which clinicians and researchers, who are interested in dementia, can undergo further training. There is obviously a need for many more such centres, so that clinicians can be trained, services developed and impetus can be given to establish overarching national dementia strategies.

References

1. Turkish Statistical Institute (2011) Available at: http://www.tuik.gov.tr (last accessed on 20 February 2013).
2. Shaji KS, Iype T, Praveenlal K (2009) Dementia clinic in general hospital settings. *Indian J Psychiatry* 51(1):42–44.
3. Bulut S, Ekici İ, Polat A, Berilgen S, Gönen M, Daş E, et al. (2002) Elazığ İ li Abdullah paşa Bölgesinde Demans Prevalansıve Demans Alt Grupları. *Demans Dergisi* 2:105–110.
4. Gurvit H, Emre M, Tinaz S, Bilgic B, Hanagasi H, Sahin H, et al. (2008) The prevalence of dementia in in urban Turkish population. *Am J Alzheimers Dis Other Demen* 23(1):67–76.
5. Eker E, Ertan T (2005) The practice of dementia care: Turkey. In: Burns A (ed.), *Standards in Dementia Care*. London: Taylor and Francis, pp. 105–111.
6. Cankurtaran ES, Eker E (2007) Being elderly in a young country. *Int J Ment Health* 36(3):66–72.
7. Turkish Alzheimer Foundation (2012) Available at: http://www.alz.org.tr (last accessed on 20 February 2013).
8. Turkish Alzheimer Society (2012) Available at: http://www.alzheimerdernegi.org.tr (last accessed on 20 February 2013).

Chapter 14

Western Europe

In Germany, first contact is usually with a primary care physician, who rarely refers patients with dementia to psychiatrists or neurologists, and only 15% of dementia patients receive anti-dementia medication. Geriatric day care is an important part of services, but not many patients access them. Specialist dementia care in nursing homes is either a segregated or a partially segregated model. Results are presented comparing various types of services.

Spain has a complex political structure with 17 Autonomous Regions, but it also has a National Health Service (SNS). However, the political structure hampers generalised implementation of dementia care strategies, although the Autonomous Regions of Catalonia and Galicia are pioneers in this respect. Despite many examples of excellent services, the development of a National Strategy for the Care of Dementia is deemed of high importance.

Sweden has a national quality register, SveDem (Swedish Dementia Register), which is the world's largest dementia case register with more than 15,000 people registered. It links to national evidence-based guidance for diagnosis, treatment and care. However, service provision is at times disconnected, being provided by county councils and municipalities, with increasing involvement of the private sector complicating matters. A common form of accommodation is group homes with 6–10 people per unit, but there are concerns about staffing levels.

In the UK, memory services have gradually moved towards community-based services and are often nurse-led, in part because of increasing numbers of referrals. The publication of the National Dementia Strategy has emphasised the importance of dementia and with the national accreditation programme of the Royal College of Psychiatrists is helping to develop and improve existing memory services.

Designing and Delivering Dementia Services, First Edition. Edited by Hugo de Waal, Constantine Lyketsos, David Ames, and John O'Brien.
© 2013 John Wiley & Sons, Ltd. Published 2013 by John Wiley & Sons, Ltd.

Germany

Siegfried Weyerer

Zentralinstitut für Seelische Gesundheit, Deutschland

Long-term care insurance and medical care of dementia patients

At present more than 1 million people in Germany have moderate to severe dementia. Most live in private households, while about 40% are institutionalised. Statutory health insurance covers the cost of medical services. To alleviate the enormous costs involved in long-term care for elderly patients with chronic disorders such as dementia, the long-term care insurance law was established in 1994. While health insurance is a fully comprehensive system, long-term care insurance only provides limited cover. All members of the health insurance system are automatically covered by long-term care insurance. Employees who are not covered by the social insurance system (i.e. civil-servants, the self-employed, etc.) are usually members of a private insurance scheme. Long-term care insurance follows three principles:

1. all measures that prevent, treat or rehabilitate diseases and thus reduce the need for care have priority
2. home care is given preference so that people can stay at home as long as possible
3. outpatient care and geriatric day care have precedence over long-term institutional care [1].

Evaluation of after care needs leads to a person being assigned to one of three care levels: considerable (I), intensive (II) or highly intensive (III) care. The long-term care insurance law went through several revisions and in 2008 a major reform was introduced. It included an increase in benefit payments and provision of more thorough care for severely impaired persons, including those with dementia. At present, the total number of beneficiaries is about 2.36 million, 69.2% of whom receive home care and 30.8% institutional care, almost exclusively in nursing homes [2].

Almost all patients with dementia first contact a primary care physician, many of whom are not well enough trained to deal with psychogeriatric disorders. They rarely refer patients with dementia to psychiatrists or neurologists. Only 15% of dementia patients receive anti-dementia drugs [3].

Outpatient services

Community nursing services were established in Germany in the early 1970s. They provide primarily medical care (dressing of wounds, administration of injections, etc.) and basic nursing care (personal hygiene, etc.). Staff – mainly nurses – frequently encounter elderly patients with psychiatric disorders, and many of those have dementia. Based on a national survey, 25.8% of dementia patients living at home use such outpatient services. A further 20% use other professional services providing delivered meals and performing basic housework. Apart from very few exceptions, dementia patients using professional outpatient services were mainly cared for by an informal caregiver. More than half of the dementia patients were only cared for by informal caregivers [3].

Specialised outpatient services have been established at many state and university psychiatric hospitals, focusing on early recognition of cognitive disorders, pharmacological treatment, provision of cognitive training programs, training of primary care physicians and psychiatrists, as well as counselling for care-providing relatives.

Geriatric day care

Institutions offering geriatric day care are an important constituent in the system of care provision. In general, trained nurses at these units offer everyday-life activities, games, individual training and outings, aiming to enhance patients' well-being and skills and to reduce caregiver burden. A study carried out in 17 geriatric day-care facilities revealed that 58.6% of clients suffered from moderate to severe dementia. In addition, symptoms of depression and behaviour problems were observed among a substantial number of attendees [4]. A longitudinal study reported significant positive effects of day care on well-being and dementia symptoms [1]. However, compared to outpatient services and nursing homes, geriatric day-care units play only a minor role. A national study revealed that only about 2% of dementia patients living in private households use geriatric day care [3].

Nursing home care

Care provided by old-age homes has changed greatly over the last 30 years: the original focus on residential care has since given way to a focus on nursing care. Most recent statistics indicate that this trend persists: the number of nursing homes increased from 9165 (2001) to 9700 (2009). Parallel to this development, the number of nursing home residents rose from 604,000 (2001) to 711,000 (2009) [2]. Nursing homes are key providers of dementia care: a national study revealed that 68.6% of all nursing home residents have moderate to severe dementia [5]. More than half of all nursing homes in Germany provide traditional care (dementia patients and non-dementia patients live in the same residential unit). Special dementia care in nursing homes can be realised on the basis of either a segregated or a partially segregated model:

- the segregated model involves specialised, segregated round-the-clock care for dementia patients living in a special care unit
- the partially segregated arrangement means patients with dementia share a residential unit with non-demented residents but spend part of the day in a special group for dementia patients.

Political efforts have been made to improve the institutional care of dementia patients. At present, 28% offer segregated care, and 15% partially segregated dementia care [5]. The forerunner of special dementia care was the city of Hamburg. To fulfil the special needs of dementia patients with behaviour problems, a segregative and a partially segregative programme was established for 750 residents. Each is characterised by much higher staffing ratios, specialised staff training, regular psychogeriatric care and enhanced milieu-therapeutic concepts, including architectural changes. The extra costs that such specialised dementia care entails are, in general, passed on to the resident [6].

Comparison of segregated and partially segregated dementia management in Hamburg

The activity rates of dementia patients, the number of visits from relatives and their involvement in nursing and social care were much higher in the partially segregative care arrangement as opposed to segregative care. Among the residents in segregative care, however, significantly more biographical information was collected and the proportion of patients receiving psychogeriatric care was also higher. Dementia patients in these homes received more psychotropic medication with significantly more prescription of anti-dementia drugs and antidepressants and less frequent prescription of antipsychotic drugs.

Comparison of special dementia care in Hamburg to traditional dementia care in Mannheim

Compared to traditional integrative care, the special dementia programme in the city of Hamburg revealed a better quality of life and quality of care: a higher level of volunteer caregiver involvement, more social contact with staff, fewer physical restraints and more involvement in home activities. In both settings, about three-fourths of the dementia patients received psychotropic drugs. However, residents in special dementia care were treated significantly less often with antipsychotics and more often with antidepressants [6].

Summary and conclusions

The number of dementia patients is expected to double within the next 40 years: in 2050 between 2.2 and 2.7 million cases are expected [7]. At the same time, the number of family caregivers will decrease, giving rise to an enormous demand for professional dementia care, particularly nursing homes. Significant differences in some indicators of quality of life point in favour of the model pioneered in Hamburg. However, there are still quality indicators (e.g. activities offered within nursing homes, appropriate medication and use of anti-dementia drugs) where special care was not significantly better than traditional care. Since these areas can be modified by intervention, improvements to the special care programme should be made. It could be shown that only about 10% of the dementia patients in traditional nursing homes fulfil the criteria for special dementia care as applied in the Hamburg approach. It is also important to provide adequate care for the vast majority of patients in traditional nursing homes who do not benefit from special care programmes because they are immobile or do not exhibit severe behavioural problems [6].

Acknowledgements

This work was supported by the INTERREG IVB project 'Health and Demographic Changes'.

References

1. Zank S, Schacke C (2002) Evaluation of geriatric day care units: effects on patients and caregivers. *Journal of Gerontology: Psychological Sciences* 57B(4):348–357.
2. Statistisches Bundesamt (2011) *Pflegestatistik 2009. Pflege im Rahmen der Pflegeversicherung. Deutschlandergebnisse*. Wiesbaden: Statistisches Bundesamt.
3. Schäufele M, Köhler L, Teufel S, Weyerer S (2006) Betreuung von demenziell erkrankten Menschen in Privathaushalten: Potenziale und Grenzen. In: Schneekloth U, Wahl H-W (eds), *Selbständigkeit und Hilfebedarf bei älteren Menschen in Privathaushalten*. Stuttgart: Kohlhammer, pp. 103–145.
4. Weyerer S, Schäufele M, Schrag A, Zimber A (2004) Demenzielle Störungen, Verhaltensauffälligkeiten und Versorgung von Klienten in Einrichtungen der Altentagespflege im Vergleich mit Heimbewohnern: Eine Querschnittsstudie in acht badischen Städten. *Psychiatrische Praxis* 31:339–345.

5. Schäufele M, Köhler L, Lode S, Weyerer S (2009) Menschen mit Demenz in stationären Pflegeeinrichtungen: aktuelle Lebens- und Versorgungssituation. In: Schneekloth U, Wahl H-W (eds), *Pflegebedarf und Versorgungssituation bei älteren Menschen in Heimen. Demenz, Angehörige und Freiwillige, Beispiele für Good Practice*. Stuttgart: Kohlhammer, pp. 159–221.

6. Weyerer S, Schäufele M, Hendlmeier I (2010) Evaluation of special and traditional dementia care in nursing homes: results from a cross-sectional study in Germany. *International Journal of Geriatric Psychiatry* 25:1159–1167.

7. Doblhammer G, Ziegler U (2011) Perspective for dementia trends: predictions derived from demographic research. In: Dibelius O, Maier W (eds), *Versorgungsforschung für dementiell erkrankte Menschen. Health services research for people with dementia*. Stuttgart: Kohlhammer, pp. 11–18.

Spain

Raimundo Mateos[a], Manuel Sánchez-Pérez[b] and Manuel Franco[c,d,e]

[a]*Department of Psychiatry, University of Santiago de Compostela, USC, Spain*
[b]*Psychogeriatric Unit, CHUS University Hospital, School of Medicine, Spain*
[c]*University of Salamanca, Spain*
[d]*Psychiatric Department, Zamora Hospital, Spain*
[e]*Iberian Research Institute, Intras Foundation, Spain*

Demographic and epidemiological aspects

Just over 17% of the Spanish population is over 65, approaching 25% in several regions. Those over 80 comprise 5.3% with a third living in rural areas. Prevalence ranges between 5% and 10% [1], which means that 3.5 million people are affected. The resulting expenditure is estimated to be approximately €30,000 per year per patient.

The Spanish national health service (SNS)

Spain has a complex political structure consisting of 17 Autonomous Regions. The SNS guarantees free and universal health care, and patients are only required to pay part of the cost of prescribed medications [2].

Recently, an act was passed recognising the universal right to social benefits for all senior citizens and persons with disabilities who need assistance for their basic daily activities, thus providing a legal foundation for long-term care [3]. However, the Autonomous Regions are responsible for the organisation and funding of social and health care, resulting in significant differences in the care provided to people with dementia, leading to sharp criticism. Over the last two decades there has been a remarkable growth in social awareness of the challenges posed by dementia. This has led to the development of a variety of educational programs (ranging from university degrees to the training of informal carers), handbooks and monographs describing the basic principles of dementia care and a number of consensus documents [4]. Recently, the Spanish Ministry of Health included these in its Clinical Guidelines [5].

Health and social care models

In the 1990s, Catalonia pioneered the development of a bio-psycho-social model of dementia care, called 'Socio-Sanitario'. In 2000, a report published by the Ombudsman analysed the challenges faced by older people, specifically addressing the needs of and care resources required by people with dementia and calling for the government to take a number of specific measures.

The Catalan model inspired other regions, but in most cases, nothing came to fruition because of funding problems: it established a network for the diagnosis and treatment of dementias, but it has not been replicated elsewhere.

Catalonia implemented a Socio-Health Master Plan, co-financed by the Department of Health and the Department of Welfare and Family, which is being further developed under the Program for the Prevention and Care of Chronicity (PPAC) [6]. This model consists of outpatient and inpatient services, the inpatient services being of two types: psychogeriatric long-stay and medium-stay units. The latter are for patients with dementia and behavioural problems who cannot be managed at home or in nursing homes. Outpatient services include psychogeriatric day hospitals for mild to moderate cases, home-care teams (PADES) and Outpatient Teams for Cognitive Disorder Assessment (EAIA-TC), consisting of neurologists, geriatricians, psychiatrists, neuropsychologists, social workers and, in some cases, nurses. There are 30 such teams across Catalonia [7].

Galicia has also pioneered a model of psychogeriatric care and formulated a Dementia Plan [8]: it has put in place an important public network of Day Centres catering mainly for people with dementia [9].

A recent study by the Spanish Society of Psychogeriatrics (SEPG) shows that the situation in most other regions is more precarious. With family carers as the main source of support for patients with dementia, the Spanish Confederation of Relatives of Alzheimer Patients (CEAFA) not only asks for more action, but also provides guidance and care. Funded by the respective regional governments, it runs day centres or 'Relief Units', but this is not coordinated with the wider care sector.

Dementia in primary care

Professional associations have long recognised the key role of primary care in early detection, follow-up and the provision of support to patients and relatives [10]. In spite of this, it is recognised that primary care is not sufficiently involved in dementia care. This has been attributed to pressure on healthcare services, difficulties in coordinating with specialist services, scientific and technical shortcomings and educational deficits.

How dementia patients are referred to specialist services

A GP may refer a patient to a relevant consultant (psychiatrist/neurologist/geriatrician). Generally, neurology focuses on diagnosis and initial treatment while psychiatry and gerontology aim to provide continuing care.

Two shortcomings should be mentioned: (1) patchy establishment of geriatric services in several regions (an issue the Spanish Society of Geriatrics and Gerontology [SEGG] has frequently complained about) and (2) the limited number of psychiatrists devoted to the treatment of dementias, an issue the SEPG is trying to address.

The SNS funds anti-dementia medication, but this can only be prescribed by consultants in Psychiatry, Neurology or Geriatrics.

There is no shortage of examples of best practice in dementia care, whether in primary care, specialist care or day centres and nursing homes. However, various associations are highlighting the need for such services to be more generally available and the development of a National Strategy for the Care of Dementia is deemed of high importance [11].

References

1. Del Barrio JL, De Pedro-Cuesta J, Boix R, Acosta J, Bergareche A, Bermejo-Pareja F, et al. (2005) Dementia, stroke and Parkinson's disease in Spanish populations: a review of door-to-door prevalence surveys. *Neuroepidemiology* 24(4):179–188.
2. Wikipedia contributors (2012) Spanish National Health System. Available at: http://en.wikipedia. org//wiki/Spanish_National_Health_System (last accessed on 28 March 2013).

3. Gutiérrez MF, Jimenez-Martin S, Sánchez RV, Vilaplana C (2010 June) The Long-Term Care System for the Elderly in Spain. ENEPRI Research Report No. 88, CEPS, Brussels. Available at: http://www.ceps.eu/book/long-term-care-system-elderly-spain (last accessed on 28 March 2013).

4. Martin M, Agüera L, Sánchez I, Mateos R, Franco M, Castellano M, et al. (2005) Consenso Español sobre Demencias. Sociedad Española de Psiquiatría y Sociedad Española de Psicogeriatría. Barcelona: Exter Comunicación & Marketing Muntaner. Available at: http://www.sepg.es/actividades/LibroConsenso.pdf (last accessed on 28 March 2013).

5. Grupo de trabajo de la Guía de Práctica Clínica (2009/2007) Guía de Práctica Clínica sobre la atención integral a las personas con enfermedad de Alzheimer y otras demencias 2010; Guías de Práctica Clínica en el SNS: AIAQS Núm. pp. 1–508. Available at: http://www.gencat.cat/salut/depsan/units/aatrm/pdf/gpc_alzheimer_demencias_pcsns_aiaqs_2011vc.pdf (last accessed on 21 February 2013).

6. Generalitat de Catalunya, Departament de Salut (2006) *Pla Director Sociosanitari*. Barcelona: Departament de Salut.

7. Sánchez Pérez M (2002) Asistencia sociosanitaria en salud mental: evaluación de una experiencia. *Informaciones Psiquiátricas* 167(1):95–103.

8. Comisión Asesora en materia de Psicoxeriatria (1999) *Plan Galego de atención ó enfermo de Alzheimer e outras demencias*. Santiago de Compostela: Xunta de Galicia.

9. Vázquez Piñeiro A, Campos Pérez X, Alvarez Gallego E, Consorcio Galego de Servizos de Igualdade e Benestar (2008) *Os centros de día en Galicia, un apoio as persoas maiores con dependencia: documento técnico*. Santiago de Compostela: Consorcio Galego de Servizos de Igualdade e Benestar.

10. Sociedad Española de Medicina Familiar y Comunitaria (2005) *Demencias desde la Atención Primaria*. Barcelona: semFYC.

11. Mateos R, Franco M, Sánchez M (2010) Care for dementia in Spain: the need for a nationwide strategy. *International Journal of Geriatric Psychiatry* 25(9):881–884.

Sweden

Lars-Olof Wahlund

Department of Neurobiology, Care Sciences and Society, Section of Clinical Geriatrics and Section of Nursing, Karolinska Institutet, Sweden

Background and demography

Sweden, while large in geographical area, has a population of only about 9 million and is therefore sparsely populated. As elsewhere, the population is ageing and predictably, the prevalence and incidence of dementia are high: approximately 180,000 and 25,000, respectively [1].

There are about 90,000 places in various forms of institutional living for the elderly, around 70% of which cater for people with dementia. Approximately 25,000 people have access to housing specifically built for the care of people with dementia, so-called 'group homes'. Over the past 25 years, the number of places in care homes has declined rather sharply, with increasing numbers being cared for in their own homes with the support of their family and home-care services. Some municipalities have specialist home-care teams for people with dementia.

National guidelines

The National Board of Health and Welfare recently published National Guidelines on services for people with dementia, providing evidence-based guidance for diagnosis, treatment and (nursing) care. The guidelines are explicit about the fact that dementia care needs to be person-centred. There is a national quality register (SveDem: Swedish Dementia Register) linked to these guidelines. All patients with a diagnosis of dementia are registered at the point of diagnosis, as well as at annual follow-up. This register can freely be used for research and epidemiological enquiries and includes information from primary care, specialist care and sheltered housing. It is currently the world's largest dementia case register with more than 15,000 people registered.

County councils

Responsibility for diagnosis and pharmacological treatment of people with dementia resides with county councils. All people with suspected cognitive impairment receive further investigation, which is usually carried out within primary care. If no diagnosis can be established or the case is complex, the patient will be referred to a specialist memory clinic with geriatric expertise. However, more and more primary and specialist care is being transferred to private companies.

Municipalities

All care and accommodation is provided by municipalities, and particularly in the larger ones, continuity of care with health services can be problematic, an issue given high priority in the above-mentioned guidelines. A key principle is that people with dementia can live at home as long as possible, for which purpose the municipality provides home-help, food, travel to and from day care and provision of respite care. District nurses provide medication and people are monitored annually within primary care. There is therefore a possible disconnect between services provided under the supervision of county councils on the one hand and municipalities on the other.

Great emphasis is placed on supporting relatives, and many areas provide specialist consultants and educational programmes for relatives [1]. As mentioned earlier, carers are supported further through provision of respite care. A trend in primary care is to work more in teams. Specialist nurses are at times involved in data collection throughout the care pathway, facilitating research.

Special accommodation

A common form of accommodation consists of group homes with 6–10 people per unit, usually staffed by auxiliary nurses or care assistants with access to nurses, occupational therapists and physiotherapists. About 80% of staff have studied the care and nursing programme at upper secondary school [1]. There is an ongoing debate concerning optimal staffing levels at group homes, but the basic requirement is good education and leadership. However, a recent inspection by the National Board of Health and Welfare found that more than half of group homes had inadequate staffing at night and many residents were left alone for long periods at night.

Medical responsibility for group homes generally lies within primary care, but there is a strong desire that physicians with geriatric competence should assume this. A thorough national review of medications, aimed at reducing cognitively harmful drugs and optimising others, is currently underway: many people with dementia have co-morbidities, and this often results in polypharmacy, necessitating regular monitoring. More than two-thirds of people with dementia are prescribed psychotropics: about 25% neuroleptics and over 50% antidepressants. Physically frail people with dementia receive highly specialised nursing care, either in nursing homes or specialist geriatric homes.

Continuity of the care pathway

The need for a cohesive well-functioning care pathway cannot be overstated. This can be found in many places, but not all. Where it works best, there will be dementia nurses responsible for early identification of people with cognitive impairment, but subsequently able to provide guidance through the continuum of care from investigation and pharmacological treatment via home care to specialist nursing care: this dementia coordinator plays an important role in guiding and helping people with dementia and their families through the long duration of the illness.

As mentioned above, the National Guidelines advise on the implementation of evidence-based medical and nursing care and specifically attempts to ensure continuity of care, avoiding someone being passed back and forth in the system. An extensive effort is now under way to implement these guidelines across the country, but it will take several years to do so. In urban areas, the situation is particularly complex, with many municipalities and private providers involved in care provision.

While dementia care is mainly publicly financed, care can be provided by both public and private providers. Recently, a series of scandals have highlighted reduced staffing levels in the for-profit sector, leading to neglect [1]. Another important issue is coercion and deprivation of liberty in dementia care. There is currently a government investigation ongoing with a view to formulating guidelines for the way in which coercion may be used.

Dementia centre (www.demenscentrum.se)

About 5 years ago, a Swedish Dementia Centre was established to gather and disseminate evidence-based best practice in dementia care. An important step was to provide online education for nursing staff, based on the National Guidelines: in January 2012 nearly 30,000 people had completed the education.

Future challenges

One of the most challenging issues in dementia care in Sweden is the implementation of the National Guidelines. Work to introduce and adjust these national guidelines into local guidelines for each county council and municipality has been ongoing for the past 2 years. The problem is to reach all units, memory clinics, GPs and group homes with information. This challenge is enhanced by the fast privatisation of both memory clinics and GP units.

References

1. Swedish National Guidelines (2010) *Nationella riktlinjer för vård och omsorg vid demenssjukdom.* Available at: http://www.socialstyrelsen.se/publikationer2010/2010-5-1 (last accessed 28 March 2013).

The United Kingdom

Stephen Curran[a,b] and John Wattis[b]

[a]*South West Yorkshire Partnership NHS Foundation Trust, UK*
[b]*Centre for Health and Social Care Research, School of Human and Health Sciences, University of Huddersfield, UK*

Introduction

Until the 1960s, interest in old age psychiatry was largely confined to research. In 1973, a Special Interest Group was formed by the Royal College of Psychiatrists and in 1978, the Psychiatry of Old Age became a Specialist Section. Although the first survey of old age psychiatry services was published in 1981 [1], it only became an official specialty in the National Health Service (NHS) in 1989 [2,3]. Today, mental health services for older people are well established and mental illness in older people is recognised as a major health issue. The numbers of old age psychiatrists have increased in parallel with increasing referral rates to old age psychiatry services and memory clinics in particular. Memory services in the UK have gradually developed. Initially, community-based services were supported by a large hospital bed base which has gradually reduced over the past 20 years. There is now a greater emphasis on supporting patients in the community with a focus around the memory clinic.

Memory clinics in the UK: Background

Memory clinics in the UK are a relatively recent innovation. In the mid-1970s, a large number of potential drugs were being developed for the treatment of patients with Alzheimer's disease, and the early clinics had predominantly a research focus and were largely funded by the pharmaceutical industry. In the UK, one of the first memory clinics was set up at St Pancras' Hospital in London in 1983 [4]. By 1995, the number of clinics had risen to 20 [5] and to nearly 60 by 2002 [6]. To some extent, the development of memory clinics seemed to be at odds with the philosophy and clinical practice of the 'psychogeriatric movement' which emphasised, from the late 1960s, taking specialist care and expertise out of the hospital and into the community [7]. However, the introduction of the cholinesterase inhibitors and ever-increasing numbers of referrals ensured that memory clinics continued to develop despite the lack of sound research evidence. The emphasis was on hospital clinics with a strong medical focus. Over time, clinics have become more community and nurse-led and have evolved into multi-professional services. The precise number of services is not known. In a recent survey, the number of clinics was estimated to be around 330 in England. In Scotland, a similar survey only identified 18 clinics [8].

There has been little research evidence to support the development of memory clinics, and the very existence of memory clinics has been questioned [8,9]. One study undertaken by the authors compared a traditional hospital clinic with a community service. Both services were equally compliant with National Institute for Health and Clinical Excellence (NICE) guidance [10], but the community service was cheaper and was preferred by patients, carers and general practitioners [11].

Memory services: The current position

Memory Clinics in the UK offer a wide range of assessments, diagnosis and treatments for people with memory impairment, especially in patients with dementia or suspected dementia [12]. In recent years, there have been a large number of policy documents in the UK culminating in the National Dementia Strategy (NDS) [13] which helpfully also summarises the policy framework (Annex 2 of the NDS). The NDS outlined 17 objectives for improving the quality of services including

- improving professional awareness and understanding
- improving diagnosis and interventions
- improving the provision of good quality information and support for patients and carers
- the development of a specific carers' strategy
- improving the experience of patients with dementia in general hospitals, care homes and at the end of life.

A considerable amount of work has increased awareness of the behavioural and psychological symptoms in patients with dementia and has raised concerns about the use of antipsychotics because of severe unwanted effects. This campaign has been championed by the Dementia Action Alliance [14] and has widespread national support.

A typical memory service has a lead clinician (usually an old age psychiatrist but occasionally this might be a neurologist, a geriatrician or a psychologist) and a team including mental health nurses, dieticians, psychologists and other healthcare professionals. The composition varies depending on historical and local needs, and there is currently no agreed national standard for staffing. Most services are NHS-funded and focus on assessment, diagnosis and treatment, especially with the cholinesterase inhibitors and memantine in accordance with NICE guidance [10]. The first assessment is often done by a nurse followed by diagnostic and treatment appointments. Referrals are rising steadily and this trend seems likely to continue: it is currently estimated that there are approximately 700,000 people with dementia in the UK, and this is expected to rise to 1.4 million over the next 30 years. Costs will rise from approximately £17 billion per year now to £50 billion over the next 30 years [13]. In a recent survey, the average number of patients using individual services in 2008–2009 was 605, and this had increased to 951 in 2010–2011 [15].

Other services typically provided by a memory service include support for patients in general hospitals (Hospital Liaison Team) and in care homes (Care Homes Liaison Team). Most services also provide day and respite care, but these are increasingly being provided through social services.

Most memory services have close links with social services and the voluntary sector such as the Alzheimer's Society [16]. This allows for a detailed assessment of patient and carer needs and in particular helps to target practical support tailored to the needs of individual families.

Accreditation

No two memory services are the same and in the UK these have evolved often in isolation to meet the needs of local people and have been heavily influenced by local geography, funding and history. The Centre for Quality Improvement (CCQI) of the Royal College [17] aims to improve standards in mental health through a variety of mechanisms including national audits and Accreditation of Services. The Memory Services National Accreditation Programme (MSNAP) works with memory services in the UK to assure and improve their quality. It engages staff in a comprehensive review process and services are supported to identify areas for improvement by a comparison of their service with a comprehensive set of national standards covering all aspects of service design and delivery. Accreditation assures staff, patients, carers, commissioners and regulators of the quality of the service provided.

Looking forward

With increasing numbers of people likely to develop dementia, new drugs becoming available and new diagnostic technology improving diagnosis, costs will increase. Patient and carer expectations and influence will rise and scrutiny and performance monitoring from commissioners and regulators are likely to increase. Referrals will increase but resources are likely to fall or fail to keep pace with increasing demand. These factors will put memory services under enormous pressure, and services will need to evolve and adapt to meet the challenge. It is likely that more work will be done by nurses and other healthcare professionals and nurse prescribing will increase. It is also likely and expected that all services will eventually be accredited by the Royal College of Psychiatrists ensuring that while individual services may vary in the way they are organised and deliver the service, they will all meet the same set of agreed national standards. GPs will probably be asked to do more monitoring. It is likely that in most services the trend towards 'ageless' services will continue with a tendency to develop separate dementia services – a so-called dementia or memory pathway, and this will be linked to payment by results – PbR [18]: services will be paid for what they do rather than relying on the traditional block contract. This might help to meet increased demand, provided the tariff is set at a realistic level. Assistive Technology will also increasingly play a part: telephone monitoring is already an important part of many services, and reminders via text messages and telephone calls to reduce the number of missed appointments are already established. There is more detail on this topic in Chapter 17 in this book. One thing is certain: we will all be expected to do more for less!

References

1. Wattis J, Wattis L, Arie T (1981) Psychogeriatrics: a national survey of a new branch of psychiatry. *British Medical Journal* 282:1529–1533.
2. Arie T (1994) The development in Britain. In: Copeland JRM, Abou-Saleh MT, Blazer DG (eds), *Principles and Practice of Geriatric Psychiatry*. Chichester: John Wiley and Sons, pp. 7–10. Chapter 2.
3. Hilton C, Arie T, Nicolson M (2010) A witness seminar; the development of old age psychiatry in Britain, 1960–1989. Themes, lessons and highlights. *International Journal of Geriatric Psychiatry* 25:596–603.
4. Philpot MP, Levy R (1987) A memory clinic for the early diagnosis of dementia. *International Journal of Geriatric Psychiatry* 2:195–200.
5. Wright N, Lindesay J (1995) A survey of memory clinics in the British Isles. *International Journal of Geriatric Psychiatry* 10:379–385.
6. Lindesay J, Marudkar M, Van Diepen E, Wilcock G (2002) The second Leicester survey of memory clinics in the British Isles. *International Journal of Geriatric Psychiatry* 17:41–47.
7. Jolley D, Moniz-Cook E (2009) Memory clinics in context. *Indian Journal of Psychiatry* 51:70–76.
8. Foy J (2008) A survey of memory clinic practice in Scotland. *Psychiatric Bulletin* 32:467–469.
9. Simpson S, Beavis D, Dyer J, Ball S (2004) Should old age psychiatry develop memory clinics? A comparison with domiciliary work. *Psychiatric Bulletin* 28:78–82.
10. National Institute for Health and Clinical Excellence (NICE) (2011) Donepezil, galantamine, rivastigmine and memantine for the treatment of Alzheimer's disease. NICE technology appraisal guidance 217, March 2011. Available at: http://www.nice.org.uk (last accessed on 20 February 2013).
11. Timlin A, Gibson G, Curran S, Wattis JP (2005) Memory Matters; A Report Exploring the Issues Around the Delivery of Anti-Dementia Medication. University of Huddersfield. Available at: http://www.hud.ac.uk/research/staff (last accessed on 20 February 2013).
12. Ellis AM (2004) The role of the memory clinic. In: Curran S, Wattis JP (eds), *Practical Management of Dementia; A Multiprofessional Approach*. Oxford: Radcliffe Medical Press, pp. 161–177.
13. Department of Health (2009) Living Well with Dementia; A National Dementia Strategy. Available at: http://www.dh.gov.uk (last accessed on 20 February 2013).

14. Dementia Action Alliance (2012) The Right Prescription; a call to action on the use of antipsychotic drugs for people with dementia. Institute for Innovation and improvement. Available at: http://www.institute.nhs.uk/dementiac2a (last accessed on 20 February 2013).
15. Information Centre for Health and Social Care (2011) Establishment of Memory Services; Results of a Survey of Primary Care Trusts. Available at: http://www.ic.nhs.uk (last accessed on 20 February 2013).
16. Alzheimer's Society (2012) Home Page. Available at: http://www.alzheimers.org.uk (last accessed on 20 February 2013).
17. Royal College of Psychiatrists (2012) Memory Services National Accreditation Programme. Available at: http://www.rcpsych.ac.uk/quality/qualityandaccreditation.aspx (last accessed on 20 February 2013).
18. Payment by Results – PbR (2012) Arrangements for 2011–2012. Department of Health. Available at: http://www.dh.gov.uk/en/Publicationsandstatis (last accessed on 20 February 2013).

Section 5
Designing and developing services

Chapter 15

Developing a business case, negotiating, securing funding

Hugo de Waal[a,b], John Beaumont[c,d] and Claire Mitchell[e]

[a]Norfolk Dementia Care Academy, The Julian Hospital, UK
[b]Postgraduate School of Psychiatry, East of England Deanery, UK
[c]School of Management, University of Bath, UK
[d]Applied Management Systems, University of Stirling, UK
[e]Durham University Business School, UK

Why is drafting a business case important?

In a book with health service design and development as its main topic it is pertinent to give some attention to the process of persuading any potential funding authorities on the desirability of any proposed development, whether funding might have to come from governmental departments, public health providers, health insurance industries, healthcare providers or simply budget-holding managerial colleagues. Ideas about services and service development will range from practical changes or innovations with limited scope, which may simply address shortcomings in a particular clinical setting or care team, to configurations of care involving any number of provider systems delivering comprehensive services to large numbers of people, who present with a wide range of service needs and preferences.

The first step in trying to transform an idea into practical reality is to gather evidence and explore what has been tried before: many initiatives, including how they fared, are featured in the chapters in Sections I and II of this book; there is an ever-expanding literature highlighting all sorts of developments and an (almost) random selection shows how such efforts can range from quite specific issues, such as reports on attempts to improve the management of time and tasks on a ward [1], via the organisational context which supports the delivery of high-quality nursing care in acute stroke units [2], to highly sophisticated analyses involving a number of partner organisations, such as the evaluation of a collaboration between clinical practice and research, which leads to the formulation of guiding principles and strategies for initiating, designing and implementing programme evaluation research [3].

Ideas on all sorts of service improvements often originate in the minds of those who deliver care or are otherwise interested and involved (such as patients and carers – often through patient organisations – or colleagues in charitable sectors). There will be enthusiasm and passion and a lot of clinically relevant knowledge, but often there is a lack of the necessary managerial expertise or

Designing and Delivering Dementia Services, First Edition. Edited by Hugo de Waal, Constantine Lyketsos, David Ames, and John O'Brien.

decision-making power to translate the idea into reality, and all too often, such a practitioner or interested party winds up abandoning a proposal, simply because it is difficult to navigate the relevant system of resource allocation or to put the proposal in such clear terms that it is difficult for the 'budget holder' to ignore the case being put. Those who hold the purse-strings may well be genuinely interested in service development, but they are likely also to occupy a position from which any allocation of scarce resources has to be defended in a world where there is constant competition for them. They therefore may require the enthusiastic service developer to present an evidence-base supporting the proposed change and/or to formulate a business case, which details whatever is being proposed and why it should be supported.

Regarding the former, the chapters in Sections I and II of this book contain comprehensive accounts of evidence for various types of dementia services and particularly Chapter 10 in Section III on health economic aspects, healthcare funding and service evaluation provides more insight into how evidence-bases can be supported by evaluations of the outcomes of certain projects and the difficulties pertaining to such matters.

This chapter deals in more detail with the issue of how to translate an idea into a business case, which can underpin efforts to persuade certain authorities to part with the necessary funding. It should be noted that any business case which does not present at least some evidence why something should be done is likely to fail to persuade, while on the other hand, the uncovering of evidence ideally should inform further service design and development, quite probably at some point in the process taking the form of a business case: these two aspects are therefore closely intertwined.

In principle the development, submission and implementation of a business case should be straightforward. In practice the process is usually time-consuming, frustrating and often seemingly unnecessarily repetitive (and for health carers the message 'Please submit a business case' can be positively daunting, as such activity is not usually part of a clinician's competencies and skills). Frustration generally arises because the business case is not clearly presented and the formal process is not comprehended fully. In some organisations it can be actually unclear where requests or cases for investment have to be taken for support, and this is very likely the case in complex healthcare systems, such as exist in most countries. It must also be appreciated that in the health sector funding is always in short supply, and usually any specific investment has to compete with other deserving projects.

For any investment decision a sound business case is needed to provide the organisation (or a potential external funding authority) with the clear evidence to support management's decision-making about a specific project. In so doing, it should offer assurance that the decisions are aligned with their fiduciary responsibilities. Thus, the underlying premise of the business case is that, whenever resources (not only money, but also people's time and effort) are invested, these should be in support of an explicit business or health service need. For instance, while an IT investment is expected to improve the scheduling of patient appointments and associated follow-ups by enhancing system performance and functionality, the business case should actually revolve around identifying the better performance which would improve patient satisfaction. For the purposes of this book we therefore regard healthcare outcomes and health service impacts as legitimate and identifiable 'business needs'.

Size is not necessarily important. Business cases are not solely required for large-scale investments, but are equally relevant to small projects. Moreover, it should be viewed as a management process to aid decision-making, rather than simply the creation of a document and presentation. The process must involve detailed examination of all pertinent financial and non-financial dimensions of a proposed project to ensure that the most appropriate solution is chosen against a range of potential circumstances and options, including of course the option of 'doing nothing': a choice which many international contributions to this book report as the main hurdle encountered when attempting to improve dementia care (see Section IV).

The usual shortcomings of a business case, especially in the health sector (even if they are actually funded), are a recurrent failure to achieve their stated objectives and deliver their expected benefits. The underlying causes are all too frequently an inadequate scoping of the project, specifying, planning and scheduling of the necessary tasks, too singularly a focus on delivery of the work, insufficient attention on the benefits to be realised and a failure to understand associated risks of delays and non-full completion.

In this chapter the straightforward, albeit common, checklist or template approach is disregarded, not only because of its naïve misguided simplicity, but also because practice is about both objectivity and subjectivity. Indeed, if there is not personal passion by the lead proposers, why should any 'investment committee' say 'yes'? Notwithstanding this basic observation, a systematic and objective approach is essential, which actually can be independently audited if required [4].

It is impossible to exaggerate the importance of a business case. It is the management planning process which enables all stakeholders to support and justify a particular case along a number of different dimensions, including

- strategic – alignment with the organisation's or wider strategy
- clinical – relevant in terms of healthcare outcomes
- economic – justifiable on cost-benefit grounds
- financial – affordable with available resources
- managerial – achievable with available resources

Thus, the business case is not simply a vehicle for gaining approval for an investment or some health service development: it continues by supporting the development, implementation and subsequent monitoring of the project. A single project should not be viewed in isolation: any interdependencies between projects (and in dementia services such interdependencies are often present in abundance) should be identified explicitly at the outset.

In the next section, we present an overview of the business case management process, including some suggested 'dos' and 'don'ts'. There follows then a description of a business case as a document, followed by a brief discussion on presentation and negotiation. As an illustration, there are two examples of actual business cases (the first quite limited in scope, the second considerably more complex), which set out the environmental factors leading to the need, the process which then has to be followed and the potential pitfalls, including gaining the appropriate advice, ensuring budget holders' 'buy-in', keeping to the original scope and following the organisation's guidelines, whatever they may be. Some concluding comments are made in the final section.

Development of a business case

The objective of any business case is to generate the information to support defensible decisions about investment, transformation, service development and service improvement. The business case process must ensure all stakeholders understand what is proposed to be undertaken and why. Importantly, the business case process should not stop when the investment is made: there should be formal monitoring of outcomes against the original plan and also any lessons learnt during the whole process.

In most organisations there is not one single business case document for investment or service proposals. Instead, a formal iterative process comprises gates or hurdles as the outline original case is supported and more detail is required, not only to justify the investment, but also to demonstrate the management resources to implement successfully. As listed below, it is possible to differentiate the various stages through which a business case may evolve and any enthusiastic proposer should feel reassured that initially all is needed is stage 1: subsequent fine tuning of the proposal will ensue, while the proposer collects requests for more information and the necessary responses gradually along the way:

1. Outline Business Case
   - identifies the opportunity and/or the problem
   - links explicitly to corporate strategies or national initiatives or guidelines
   - indicates preferred solution
2. Full Business Case
   - develops the Outline Business Case arguments, with more supporting information
   - incorporates a detailed financial plan, with a number of sensitivities including a detailed project plan
3. Final Business Case
   - finalises the Full Business Case (includes tendering details, if required)
   - includes necessary sign-offs.

In each of these stages the logic for an investment should continue to be stated explicitly, highlighting value as well as risks. This can of course be quite difficult, particularly in dementia care services, where certain benefits may be intangible and difficult to quantify, as was outlined in Chapter 10: the quoted Dutch study highlighted in its discussion the difficulty as follows [5]:

> The intangible aspects of benefits were difficult to capture, since quality of life metrics tend to provide a single measure of well-being and may not pick up important changes caused by the intervention, such as the benefit of having your own choice in where you receive care.

In such a situation the difficulty should not be avoided, but highlighted and explained, so that those reviewing the merits of the business case can assist in finding ways around such unquantifiable outcomes.

In trying to develop a cogent and consistent business case, there will likely occur a self-culling of what had been thought initially to be a sensible and justifiable project, and quite often the iterative process in itself will identify aspects or components which are not useful or do not stand the test of further scrutiny: this can again cause frustration (as the original 'dream' has to be taken down a peg or two on the ladder of imagination), but the business case is likely to gain in coherence and rationale as a result.

It goes without saying that any business case should be a well-structured and self-contained written document. While needing to be comprehensive, it does not necessarily need to be long. One can reassure oneself that a draft proposal is on the right track if it is remembered that it should be the single place where all relevant facts are documented and integrated to enable decision-makers to make the correct decision. Simply stated, it should cover the 'why', 'what', 'how', 'when' and 'where'. As mentioned before, there should always be an explicit examination of the option of doing nothing, including the associated costs and risks of inactivity, if such figures are available; if need be it might be prudent to carry out a literature search of similar projects or initiatives to see what others have identified as the costs and risks of not doing something.

In viewing a business case as a management process (as well as an outcome), it is therefore essentially about supporting decision-making, and it comprises a range of ongoing and parallel activities for initiating, developing, refining, approving and implementing investments and service developments. A range of different individuals and groups obviously play important roles in the life cycle of a project, with responsibilities often varying depending on the stage of the project: an important part of the process is identifying the key authorities and individuals, who are in a position to take the process from one stage to the next.

The business case process

As with a management process, the business case process should have generic features, including

- general purpose – suits different-sized investments: the proposal can be adjusted to some degree if the original plan overestimated available funds or resources, while at least some of the original idea remains achievable
- business focus – emphasises business, rather than technical impacts[1]
- all inclusive – incorporates all relevant factors
- comprehensible – allows sound and logical evaluation and decision-making
- objective – permits direct measurement of milestones and outputs
- clear – provides transparency, enables independent audit (if required)
- accountability – specifies responsibilities and authorities.

The business case process should ideally be managed by a dedicated project manager (although this may not always be possible). However, the actual production of the business case document should not be regarded as an output of the project manager's role: their task is to focus on the progress of the project and managing the various components and relationships in such a way that stipulated timelines are as much as possible being adhered to and important milestones are achieved as planned. Suitable governance structures must be in place to ensure processes, procedures and decisions are properly followed, involving interrelated issues of approvals and responsibilities. Ultimately the type and quality of business case management is also affected by the skills and competencies of the people involved, as well as the tools and techniques that are deployed. For example, while the Initial Business Case has to be developed before any process-based method for effective project management can be used, a management tool such as 'PRINCE2' (PRojects IN Controlled Environments) may be relevant later: originating in the British public sector it has become a de facto standard, which is applied extensively by the UK Government and the private sector, both in the UK and internationally. This method is in the public domain [6] and offers a non-proprietorial best practice project management guidance, which is characterised by

- a focus on business justification
- product-based planning approach
- manageable and controllable stages for project division
- flexible multi-level application
- organisational structure of the project management team

Even though it contains business case components, the management of the business case process is much more than just an implementation of the PRINCE2 method and by itself it must be appreciated that it will not generate robust and defensible business cases: it simply offers a framework enabling and facilitating sound project management.

The ownership of the business case process (for which the associated documents represent the key repository for information) must ideally remain within the organisation and for significant investments, the project's direction should have a Board-level sponsor, assuming that a structure such as a Board of Directors is present. In many areas an alternative 'owner' will have to be identified. Moreover, while it does too frequently occur, the responsibility for the development of a

---

[1] As mentioned before: healthcare outcomes and health service impacts are legitimate and identifiable 'business needs'.

business case must never be 'outsourced' to external consultants. Abdication of management responsibility can never be defended. Obviously, external consultants can provide invaluable assistance and experience to a project team, primarily when the required skills are unavailable internally, but such involvement should be strictly in an advisory and supportive capacity.

The timescales for the process will vary by organisation, healthcare environment and investment size. It should be noted that in some situations during the process, internal and external factors change. Consequently, at regular intervals, the business case should be reviewed to ensure that:

• the justification remains valid
• the project can deliver the desired solution.

The result of any review may be amendment of the project (and therefore amendment of the business case) or even termination of the project.

The business case document

A major (and the most obvious) reason for writing a business case is to justify the resources and capital investment required. This should not be interpreted to imply that the business case is simply a financial document: it should include the financial justification, but it should not be the sole purpose.

Regarding business case document(s), a variety of different templates exist, but – as stated earlier – we will desist from simply recommending a particular template and rather describe in more fluent terms the essential components that need to be covered. However, we do note that there are many books, articles and online modules, such as Harvard's *ManageMentor* [7], which provide easy-to-follow steps to creating a soundly reasoned and compelling case for a desired investment. While it is not necessarily essential to follow one structure religiously, a template can help as an aide-memoire to check that all aspects have been included. Moreover, in the private sector (and increasingly in the public sector), it is common that an organisation will have its own specific requirements for the structure and contents of a business case (as is implicit in Figure 15.1). It helps decision-makers to make more consistent decisions, especially when deciding between competing projects, and it aids the subsequent evaluations of any implementations. To summarise, the following topics will usually feature in a business case document:

1. Background
   a. definition of the opportunity/problem
   b. description of expected benefits
   c. alignment with strategic considerations
2. Project Scope
   a. objectives
   b. alternative options (including 'do nothing')
   c. recommended solution
3. Benefits and Costs
   a. financial
   b. non-financial (services/products/organisation/societal)
4. Project Management
   a. human resources (internal and external)
   b. tools
   c. plan (milestones)

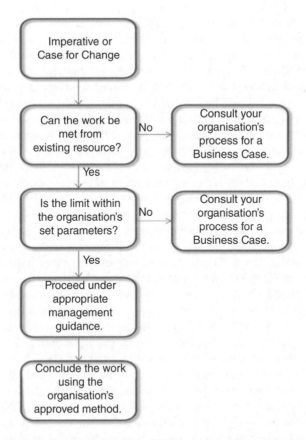

Figure 15.1 An example of a typical management decision process leading to a business case being prepared

   d. procurement approach, if relevant
   e. reporting
5. Critical Success Factors
   a. identification of specific outcomes
   b. identification of risks and methods of mitigating against risks
6. Approvals
   a. sign-off timings
   b. lines of accountability

It was noted above that the business case process is usually iterative and therefore the associated documentation is 'live': there must be a stipulated structure which facilitates formal change control and acceptance, meaning that the 'owners' of the project should be able to amend and change the document whenever necessary, but there should be a process whereby such changes are endorsed and accepted by a supervising managerial level above the level of project management. This ensures proper governance of the process and clear accountability when things get difficult or certain aims or milestones are not being met.

In the **Background** section an overview of why the project is required should be presented, along with the expected benefits and how it is aligned with the agreed business or service strategy of the organisation and therefore its priorities or simply how it is aligned with national strategies and frameworks with respect of health service development and delivery.

In the **Project Scope** section, which can be thought of as a self-contained summary of the proposed project with an explicit description of its size and complexity, different options should be covered and a clear justification stated for the recommended solution. Assumptions as well as any constraints and dependencies should be highlighted. For the 'recommended solution' the delivered outcomes should be specified explicitly, along with their associated planned benefits.

In the **Benefits and Costs** section it should be presented clearly how much money, people and time will be needed to deliver the proposed project and where and when the benefits will be realised. Inevitably, assumptions will have to be made, and these should be stated explicitly. For any project the benefits and costs have both financial and non-financial dimensions. Business cases in health care crucially include financial calculations, but the investment decision is not only about money. The nature of public sector organisations in general, and in our case, health services in particular (whether in the public sector or not), necessitate that other factors, such as social inclusion, quality of life, independence and public and societal values, will be examined to assess the most appropriate use of scarce resources. The traditional 'cost-benefit analysis' is a comparative evaluation tool that can include the relative assessment of different potential projects. Non-quantifiable characteristics of a proposed project should also be included. It is an appraisal method attempting to put monetary values on all benefits arising from a project, which are then compared with the project's total cost. The technique is widely used, especially for large-scale infrastructure projects in the public sector, but there are problems, particularly with putting quantitative values on essentially qualitative outcomes: these difficulties are discussed in detail in Chapter 10.

The objective of the **Project Management** section of the business case document is to demonstrate that it is achievable with the proposed resources. What are the required resources and how will the project team be managed? If there are any non-project dependencies, such as IT implementations, then these must be highlighted and discussed and interdependencies with wider service environments, such as social services or insurance frameworks, which may impact on the proposal, should be clarified or at least identified. There has to be a detailed project plan and work schedules, with workload estimates and critical paths broken down into manageable steps. Project controls and reporting must be clear.

In the **Critical Success Factors** section a discussion of the factors critical for a successful outcome should be presented. These ought to include any risks that can be identified as potentially jeopardising a successful completion of the project, and in listing these risks, it is essential to indicate how each one will be managed and what possible ways there are to mitigate against them.

In the **Approvals** section the formal sign-offs for different aspects of the project, including dependencies, should be presented formally: this ensures that at any stage it is clear who is responsible and accountable for ascertaining that a particular milestone has or has not been achieved.

Thus, as a document, the business case should demonstrate that all issues have been considered thoroughly and in a balanced manner. There will sometimes be an accompanying short formal presentation, which should leave sufficient time for questions and answers. Cases do not succeed on presentation skills per se, but a good presentation can help to focus minds and steer the decision-makers' thinking in the right direction. If a presentation is planned, one should try and anticipate any reasonable critique or likely questions and prepare answers and rebuttals as much as possible.

We present two case studies to illustrate the above characteristics in more practical detail.

The first case study highlights the need for the practitioner to understand the decision-making processes necessary to achieve his objectives, that is, to ensure his patients' safety and to improve the patient care environment. He needed to seek out those individuals who could assist him with completing the documentation as quickly and smoothly as possible, but he encountered 'scope

Case study 1 Re-fitting a dementia care unit

Adam, a qualified dementia nurse, was a newly promoted manager of a Dementia Care Unit. This unit was specially built in 2001 for people with severe dementia, accommodating 36 patients at any one time. It had not had any improvements or significant repair work carried out since it was opened.

One Monday morning Adam was informed of a serious incident that had taken place over the weekend: a patient had fractured her hip when a chair had collapsed under her and she was now in the general hospital. His first meeting that morning was with the hospital safety inspector who would advise on the action he needed to take.

The safety inspector told him that all furniture had to be checked, and it was possible that much would have to be replaced as a matter of urgency. To avoid the risk of a repeat of the weekend's incident, Adam was tasked with ensuring this work would be carried out as a priority with a deadline of 2 weeks.

He first called the Works Department to ask for someone to check all the furniture and the outcome of this 'risk assessment' was that by and large all furniture in the day area had to be replaced. The Works Department informed him he needed to have authorisation from the Finance Department before they could go ahead with ordering replacements so he rang them and explained what was needed. He was advised that the work likely involved an amount of money over the spending threshold of £2000, which meant they needed him to submit a Business Case. He was provided with a form and was told to submit the completed form to his manager for budgetary approval, before returning the form to Finance.

The form was daunting: Adam was a nurse and some of the terms used on the form, such as 'financials' and 'benefits realisation' were completely new to him. He decided to go onto the ward to have another look and to collect his thoughts and realised that the unit itself was looking generally 'tired' (to put it politely): not only was the furniture worn out, the place itself had not been touched in 11 years. Curtains were looking faded and walls could do with freshening up. He made some notes, decided that he might as well try and draft a business case for a more comprehensive revamp of the unit and attacked the form with renewed enthusiasm. Needing some assistance with this, he arranged to meet up with someone from 'Finance', and during this meeting he explained why there suddenly appeared to be more to the business case than just replacement of potentially dangerous furniture. 'Finance' explained to him that any project is driven by three key elements and these needed to be 'in balance' if the project was to succeed:

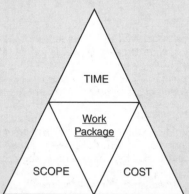

Adam's enthusiasm for re-decorating the unit along with replacing all the furniture was changing the SCOPE of the original work package. This would have a direct effect on the other two: TIME and COST. He was conscious of the fact that he faced a non-negotiable deadline of 2 weeks, and he realised that it was of course unlikely he could achieve the aim of a full revamp within that timeline. A bit disheartened he decided to focus on replacing the dangerous furniture, limiting his business case to the original scope of the work package. After obtaining some costings he completed the business case: 'scope', 'cost' and 'time' were in balance. He submitted the form for budgetary approval, and the furniture was replaced within the time limit.

(Continued)

> *However, he was still disappointed about the missed opportunity of having the unit refurbished. He realised the importance of achieving the TIME element of his original work package in order to comply with the safety inspector's requirement and as such he fully understood he had had to reduce the SCOPE of the work, but he still had a vision for the newly decorated unit.*
>
> *He decided to submit a second business case, this time for the full refurbishment, so in effect he was phasing the work in a way he had not foreseen. Given that the earlier pressure of the TIME element was now not an issue, he expanded the SCOPE according to his earlier plan, again obtained quotes for the COST and then re-estimated the TIME it would take to complete the work. He now felt reasonably at ease with drafting a business plan, more so than he would have expected prior to the unfortunate incident. At this point the success of 'phase 2' was likely to be dictated by the COST element, but here is where this story ends ...*

creep': his enthusiasm led him to expand on the work to the point where the 'time' factor became an obstacle. Having adjusted the management of his business case and in effect inserting a 'second stage' allowed him to continue work on his second aim, and he therefore learned to navigate the management process successfully.

A far more complex scenario follows in case study 2, where a whole-systems approach is reflected in a business case to invest funds in a scheme, designed to decrease avoidable emergency admissions to a general hospital of vulnerable older adults with complex co-morbidities. The 'executive summary' clearly shows that negotiations with a number of stakeholders have been ongoing for some time at probably a high level, and it bears the hallmarks of a proposal that has undergone quite a bit of iteration and fine tuning.[2]

Case study 2 Decreasing emergency admissions

EXECUTIVE SUMMARY

1. Introduction

  i) Three main healthcare providers (a district general hospital, a mental health service and a primary care community service) agreed proposals for utilisation of the CQUIN[3] 1% monies to target avoidable emergency admissions.

  ii) The proposal will focus on the list of patients frequently accessing acute services and a specific allocation of funds from each of the three provider services to fund the proposal were agreed.

2. Historical context

  i) Demographic pressures may account for some or all of the increase in emergency admissions, but at best it would appear that previous schemes designed to reduce emergency admissions have not been able to date completely to prevent demographic and other pressures leading to a year-on-year increase in total numbers

  ii) The challenge for all the organisations in the local health and social care system therefore is to find an effective way of reducing emergency admissions as an absolute number over time so that the whole system can provide effective services within the resources available. This has been expressed as an aspiration over time to return to 2008/2009 levels of admissions which would mean a reduction of approximately 10%

---

[2]The case study is based on a real-life proposal and was therefore 'anonymised'.

[3]'Commissioning for Quality and Innovation' (CQUIN) is a UK-wide payment framework which enables commissioners to reward excellence by linking a proportion of providers' income to the achievement of local quality improvement goals [8].

3. Current work

i) There are a number of small initiatives already in place at the district general hospital, designed to prevent emergency admissions, such as GPs working in the Casualty Department and a range of liaison services. The picture is fragmented though, and while all successful in their own right, none of these initiatives have really achieved the outcomes desired around preventing admissions. In addition, these schemes are focused on the hospital's 'front door', which clinicians and managers alike have identified as too late to make interventions maximally efficient.

ii) There is a strong view, therefore, that for the greatest impact to be achieved, prevention and avoidance has to begin in the community, within the patients' own home.

4. Principles and rationale

i) The commissioners outlined the imperative for all providers to work together across the system to reduce emergency admissions to the district general hospital and highlighted the fact that genuine pooling of resources between providers and shared, integrated approaches was lacking.

ii) Clinicians and commissioners all support this approach and are keen to adopt the same principles by genuinely pooling resources and having one joint business case.

iii) Subsequently it was agreed that the system-wide business case likely to have the greatest impact on admission rates is a multidisciplinary FAP (Frequently Admitted Patients) scheme, able to reduce the numbers of admissions for frail and elderly patients. The preferred approach from community providers is to work to the principles of integration and a focus on admission prevention at the patient's front door, rather than the hospital's front door.

iv) The district general hospital itself initially submitted a number of separate business cases to the commissioners, with a total value of £2.426m, focusing on improved access and assessment within the hospital, discharge planning and service reconfiguration.

v) Subsequently the hospital has agreed for £400k of their proportion of the initial incentive/investment proportion of the 1% CQUIN allocation to be used for FAP schemes, in partnership with the mental health provider.

5. System wide CQUIN Funding

i) A total of £2.31m is available through CQUIN to the three organisations. These funds are only available to the provider organisations if the single target of achieving the same (or fewer) emergency admissions in 2012/2013 as in 2011/2012 is met. All the 'reward' funding is dependent on the achievement of this target.

ii) The schemes all have part year costs. Full year costs (for 2013/2014) have also been shown for illustrative purposes at this stage. There will need to be funds for project management and expertise around informatics and performance as part of the FAP scheme, to coordinate the approach and to ensure that there is robust data analysis to evidence outcomes.

6. Governance

i) Robust project governance will be required to ensure the schemes are meeting the required outcomes. It is suggested that a Programme Board with the relevant senior representation (or equivalent) is required, with an appropriate project team/implementation group as the delivery agent.

ii) Clear reporting mechanisms and governance will be essential.

7. Service principles

i) The FAP project will focus on decreasing the number of A&E admissions for this specific target group. The team will be based in the community, but will work closely with hospital staff to focus on preventative planning in order to reduce the prevalence of admissions.

ii) There will be three main elements to the service:

(a) Clinical Evaluation of the Client Group: fact finding, identifying need, outlining the reasons, behaviours and triggers for frequent presentation and admission, making recommendations regarding multi-agency care plans, coordinating and utilising some of the existing resources and services within the three organisations.

(b) Integrated Case Management: an intensive multidisciplinary approach, providing support for 6–8 weeks to enable re/engagement with local services, develop shared crisis plans, minimise triggers to admission, and so on.

(Continued)

(c) *Practical Support: drawing on the work/principles from various previous initiatives, the FAP service will also offer practical, hands-on support for 6–8 weeks.*

8. *Outcomes*
   i)   *earlier patient discharge*
   ii) *reduced re-attendances*
   iii) *improved staff attitudes and knowledge*
   iv) *stabilise clinical challenging situations*
   v)   *improve quality of care and well-being*
   vi) *avoid unnecessary admissions to secondary care or independent sector*
   vii) *avoid breakdown of placements in independent sector*

9. *Cost*

Full establishment	Total		Mental Health Service		Primary Care Community Service	
	£	WTE	£	WTE	£	WTE
Team leader	(59)	1.00	(59)	1.00	–	–
Qualified nurses	(234)	4.00	(117)	2.00	(117)	2.00
Support workers	(121)	3.00	(81)	2.00	(40)	1.00
Social workers	(46)	1.00	(46)	1.00	–	–
Admin support	(30)	1.00	(30)	1.00	–	–
Total	(606)	12.00	(450)	9.00	(176)	3.xx

(We truncate the original business case at this point.)

Some interesting features can be gleaned from this more complex example of a business case. The following is presented to illustrate how a critical decision-maker might be interpreting a business case, which in and of itself appears perfectly laudable.

1. There is evidence that previous efforts have undergone some analysis regarding efficacy and efficiency, and it appears that in the wider scheme of things, although successful to some degree, these efforts did not yield the desired effect (2i). Therefore, this business case is founding itself on actual evidence and is designed to address the shortcomings identified in other work.

2. There is implicit recognition in point 2ii that a whole systems approach is needed. However, there appears no clear partnership for social services: while it is abundantly clear that high-quality provision of home care from social services plays an important role in keeping people at home, these appear not to be mentioned as a fourth partner in the project. This may be implicitly recognised in point 7iic where 'practical support' is mentioned as a component of the services to be provided. One assumes that 'practical support' may refer to the type of assistance provided by social workers and home carers, rather than medical or nursing staff. Decision-makers are likely to query why social services are not party to the project. A possible 'rebuttal' may lie in the fact that it may prove very difficult to merge funds from the relevant budgets: social services in the UK (where this case study originates) are funded through local authority or municipal streams; the three partners mentioned here all derive their funding from the UK NHS funding streams, and it is known to prove difficult to combine the two.

3. The outcome mentioned in point 2ii of a desired decrease in admissions by approximately 10%, based as it is on a comparison of numbers of admissions of the year 2008/2009 with the projected numbers for 2012/2013 appears arbitrarily chosen. There may be a good reason for that choice (for instance, a 10% decrease in anticipated numbers may lead to a workload for which there is sufficient capacity), but it is not stated. Decision-makers may well enquire what the rationale for that number was, and they may even challenge the definition of a successful outcome in this respect. They may even require a higher number for the funds invested.

4. In point 3i it is explained that fragmentation of previous and ongoing but 'smaller' initiatives has led to a failure in decreasing emergency admissions. Decision-makers might want to know why there appears to be no provision in this business case to try and deal with that fragmentation, particularly if it is thought that a higher cohesion between those initiatives could have led to a successful decrease.

5. The target set in point 5i appears different from the earlier stated target in point 2ii. There may be good reasoning behind this, but it is not clear in the business case and may therefore well lead decision-makers to challenge.

6. Under point 8 it appears that there is 'outcome creep': while previously decrease in emergency admissions was mentioned as the main, even the only, driver for the business case, we now suddenly see as outcomes 'earlier patient discharge' and 'improved staff attitudes and knowledge'. The latter could be construed as a workforce development issue, which might even warrant its own business case, rather than being tacked onto this proposal. It runs the risk of appearing to decision-makers as an 'afterthought' and if that occurs, it may decrease the impression of cohesive thinking. On the other hand, it might be that the staff subject to this outcome are those that provide home care and that it is realised that more intensive home support can be more efficacious if staff are specifically trained for this purpose. If that is the case, then one wonders why it is not mentioned earlier as a target in its own right.

7. All these points arise in the 'Executive Summary'. Of course, some or all of them may well be addressed to some degree in subsequent documentation. However, decision-makers and other interested parties are likely to turn to this summary in the first instance, particularly if a business case is large. It would be advisable to avoid questions arising in inquisitive minds at an early stage, because it is tiresome to have to read documents that make the impression of a fact-finding puzzle. If these questions can be addressed elsewhere, they should be addressed here or amended.

Concluding comments

In conclusion, a business case presents the rationale to start a particular project. Any investment proposals should be justified by a well-structured business case, and the length and detail of a business case must be proportionate to the scale and complexity of the estimated expenditure involved. Simply stated, the logic is that a specific business need drives and justifies the proposed consumption of scarce resources (money, time, etc.). The implications of 'doing nothing' must be understood explicitly, and in practice there are always quantifiable and non-quantifiable dimensions which have to be evaluated.

Proposers need to realise that this sort of 'process is usually time-consuming, frustrating and often seemingly unnecessarily repetitive'. One would do well to understand the need for such irritating iteration as an integral part of the process of thinking through clearly why scarce resources should be put to use in this particular way and why competing projects may have to be abandoned as a result.

Having taken into account these more technical aspects of a potentially complicated process, one must not lose sight of the most important requirement: a good business case is dependent on people and their passion. Identifying an opportunity or need, recognising an implementable solution, following internal management (business case) processes, securing a positive decision, implementing well and reviewing the implementation and operation: none of these steps have any chance of being carried out successfully if there is no passion and passion translates best in carefully crafted narratives, which then receive logical and rational underpinning as a result of a detailed process of thinking through what should be done, why, by whom, when and where. As important as these rational aspects are, the narrative which communicates the passionately held convictions is as much deserving of attention. In Chapter 9 in this book a cogent explanation is being offered regarding 'building the narrative', even if the background to that expose is slightly different from the topic of this chapter.

References

1. Morrow E, Robert G, Maben J, Griffiths P (2012) Implementing large-scale quality improvement: lessons from The Productive Ward: releasing time to care. *J Health Care Qual Assur* 25(4):237–253.
2. Burton CR, Fisher A, Green TL (2009) The organisational context of nursing care in stroke units: a case study approach. *J Nurs Stud* 46(1):85–94.
3. Secret M, Abell ML, Bertlin T (2011) The promise and challenge of practice-research collaborations: guiding principles and strategies for initiating, designing, and implementing programme evaluation research. *Soc Work* 56(1):9–20.
4. Gifford WA, Davies B, Graham ID, Lefebre N, Tourangeau A, Woodend K (2008) A mixed methods pilot study with a cluster randomized control trial to evaluate the impact of a leadership intervention on guideline implementation in home care nursing. *Implement Sci* 3:51.
5. Wolfs C, Dirksen C, Kessels A, et al. (2009) Economic evaluation of an integrated diagnostic approach for psychogeriatric patients. *Arch Gen Psychiatry* 66:313–323.
6. Available via: http://www.prince-officialsite.com/ (last accessed on 21 February 2013).
7. Available via: http://harvardbusiness.org/harvard-managementor (last accessed on 21 February 2013).
8. More information via: http://www.dgoh.nhs.uk/quality/cquins/ (last accessed on 21 February 2013).

Chapter 16

Workforce planning and development

Dorothy Kennerley[a] and Hugo de Waal[b]

[a]Norfolk & Suffolk Dementia Alliance, UK
[b]Norfolk Dementia Care Academy, The Julian Hospital, UK

The best way to predict your future is to create it (Abraham Lincoln)

Introduction

Many contributors to this book highlight the need for dementia care services to be provided and delivered by highly skilled, motivated and compassionate carers, who are able to understand and meet the needs of their patients or clients. The actual needs of a person with dementia are only in part predicted by the diagnostic category itself. People with the same type of dementia and a similar level of severity often have different problems, may have found different solutions to some of their problems and respond to the challenges they face in very different ways. Furthermore, needs change over time and care has to be adapted accordingly.

It can immediately be seen that this unpredictability and changeability means that any carer, professional or informal, has to be flexible and able continuously to reassess and review what is going on and what needs to be done. On top of that comes the realisation that people with dementia often experience a threat to their personhood and even if they themselves have lost insight, that threat is still a constant concern to their loved ones. People want to enjoy their lives in their own way and want to make their own decisions about lifestyles as far as possible. These are complex matters, and it is beyond the purview of this book to discuss them in detail (for a careful analysis and review of them we refer to a recent publication by Julian Hughes [1]). But we are clear that any care must have as an overarching aim the preservation and protection of that personhood, as well as the provision of pragmatic solutions and coping strategies for more practical problems.

Inevitably this means that professional dementia carers must have a wide range of competencies, that is, skills, knowledge, emotional intelligence and judgement, in order to carry out their work properly. This is all the more important because they will invariably need to support others, particularly family carers: integral to their work must be the ability to assess and appraise the needs of those who live with and care for the person with dementia, and this task is all too often not sufficiently understood or acknowledged.

In most countries and healthcare systems a sizeable part of the workforce delivering dementia care undergoes constant change: many lower-paid carers spend a limited part of their working career in dementia care, moving on to other opportunities as time goes by. Staff replacing them may often

Designing and Delivering Dementia Services, First Edition. Edited by Hugo de Waal, Constantine Lyketsos, David Ames, and John O'Brien.
© 2013 John Wiley & Sons, Ltd. Published 2013 by John Wiley & Sons, Ltd.

be relatively inexperienced and young. This phenomenon is even more prevalent in non-specialist services, where the skills base may be relatively low and many people with dementia receive their support mostly from such services. This means that, even if procured from elsewhere, education, training and wider workforce development should be a constant, if ever-changing, core component of dementia care services.

Good care and poor care can be equally expensive but with overwhelmingly different results, and the difference is not only the result of poor training and education: the culture of societies and organisations appears to be a significant determinant to the quality of care. The culture in a particular organisation can have a detrimental effect on the workforce: someone may be quite competent but feel that they are not empowered to exercise their competence, often if the organisational culture is overly defensive, too focused on avoiding risks, overly bureaucratic or managed by people who have difficulty in interpreting guidelines and governance structures other than in a literal and regimented fashion. Regulators of health and social care often comment on culture and compassion, and there are early studies [2,3] which tried to identify the components which constitute a compassionate and caring culture: creating a culture rich in compassion is a key part of the development of the workforce [4], and there are a number of instruments that claim to measure the organisational culture in health care using quantitative measurements [5].

These are just a few of the compelling reasons for those who design, deliver or commission services to pay particular attention to workforce development, and no service can hope to be efficacious, compassionate or indeed efficient without it.

Workforce planning and workforce development

Workforce planning, that is, the process by which an understanding of future needs is used to prepare for that future by building on existing provision, implies an appraisal of the ability of the existing workforce to deliver the necessary quality care. In that sense workforce planning and 'future proofing' can only be successful if deficiencies as well as successes in the present delivery are understood and, where necessary, addressed: it has a longitudinal component, rooted in the present, and this directly links workforce planning to workforce development.

A traditional view of workforce development focuses on providing a sufficient number of suitably qualified staff to deliver sustainable services. We propose that this definition is not nearly ambitious enough when applied to dementia care, as it fails to include several important factors, which we deem fundamental to high-quality care for people with dementia:

1. the 'army' of informal carers, family members, friends and volunteers who deliver increasingly significant and important care to people with dementia
2. the contribution of the general public to improving the lives of people with dementia
3. the need to increase productivity, engagement and a compassionate culture, which makes fuller use of existing competencies
4. the need for leadership to motivate the workforce to achieve ever better outcomes
5. the embedded use of 'talent management' to ensure consistency of workforce development over time.

This chapter focuses by and large on the development of a professional workforce, but with reference to the first two points we would like to make a few specific comments:

1. Given the central role of informal carers and the importance of at least some level of understanding of dementia in the general public, one could argue that comprehensive workforce develop-

ment minimally ought to try and raise the profile and awareness of dementia at a larger scale than just within dementia services: the wider community (or at least segments thereof) can contribute to help people with dementia to live well and in that sense can be thought of as part of the 'workforce'.

2. Family carers, volunteers, support workers and other 'non-professional' carers have often closer and more sustained contact with a particular individual with dementia than qualified health and social care professionals. Therefore, these carers need to be supported and developed at least as much as professionals. Furthermore, in order to ensure their health and well-being, attention should be given to their ability to look after themselves (self-care) and avoid carer burnout (Norfolk & Suffolk Dementia Alliance[1] Competency Framework [6]: 42, 43, 44; see Appendix). This area of development and support are invaluable to both the carer and the person with dementia.

3. Recently the UK government launched an initiative, which recognises the important role non-professionals can play. The Dementia Friends Scheme, led by the Alzheimer's Society, is the UK's biggest ever project to change the way people think about dementia: volunteers will be given free awareness sessions to help them understand dementia better, changing the way they think, talk and act, and become Dementia Friends with the know-how to make people with dementia feel understood and included in their community. The Scheme aims to recruit 1 million people as Dementia Friends by 2015. It forms part of the 'Dementia Challenge', which was launched by the UK's Prime Minister in 2012 and supplemented by another ambitious initiative: the creation of Dementia Friendly Communities through which society can make the change to enable people with dementia to go about their daily lives confidently, safely and free from stigma [7].

It is quite clear that within these wider initiatives there is a compelling opportunity for the professional workforce to become engaged and to cascade understanding and awareness throughout the wider community, and this will be discussed in more detail in the later section on the Norfolk Dementia Care Academy.

In essence, an effective workforce enables people with dementia to stay as independent as possible, living life to the full, for as long as possible and to maximise their quality of life in all care settings and communities. It cannot be static or based on historical data or patterns of need: earlier we made the point that things constantly change, at the level of individual need as well as at the level of communities, not in the least as a result of the demographic trends described in many contributions to this book. The aim therefore must be to produce a flexible workforce with contemporary understanding of the evidence base, able to detect changes and respond to them, with competency and compassion evident in every act of care. It must include the skill of allowing someone with dementia as much freedom, fun and decision-making opportunities as is possible within their overall level of functioning and their mental capacity.

All of this implies that planning and development needs to be strategic and it is to this we now turn: we emphasise that the workforce element of a dementia strategy should underpin all training and education.

The need for a strategic approach: Vision, planning and ownership

Ideally, strategic workforce planning and development should flow from an overall strategy for dementia care and the latter – where present – should function as a continuous driver for the former.

---

[1]The Norfolk & Suffolk Dementia Alliance consists of more than 20 local partner organisations (including patient and carer organisations). It coordinates a cohesive campaign to improve caring for people with dementia.

Some countries have such overall strategies in place, if at varying levels of sophistication (see particularly Chapters 8 and 9 and the various contributions in Section IV of this book). Where such a strategy has been formulated, there will clearly be a futurist vision of what good dementia care must look like and that will greatly aid efforts to plan and develop the workforce. But particularly when this is not the case, the issues of *vision and ownership* become more pertinent.

First and foremost a workforce development strategy should describe what best practice and competence looks like and – where possible – what the evidence base is. It should result in a Dementia Care Competency Framework (such as the one developed by the Norfolk & Suffolk Dementia Alliance – NSDA), which describes the reasonable expectation of competencies for all involved in dementia care. It will take time and effort to formulate a comprehensive description, and it can really only be complete if it is the result of a full engagement between people with dementia, their carers, providers of health and social care, providers of education and training, the voluntary and/or charitable sector, commissioners, and so on. These stakeholders need to describe good practice and define an agreed dementia competency framework in accessible language: without a clear vision of what good practice looks like, the whole workforce development strategy will be disjointed and ineffective. It means that such a framework is the result of an active, genuine and open discussion, led by local experts (including patients and carers, who are of course the experts of what it is like to live with dementia).

As said, this process takes time and is labour intensive, but it ensures 'buy-in' by all those involved and a high level of ownership, without which any strategy will become just another document or a vague set of good intentions without an agreed view of how to realise its objectives. The NSDA went through this process painstakingly, insisting that all stakeholders literally signed up to the end product: the ensuing Competency Framework is available online and can be downloaded for free: it may give some helpful ideas for those who want to embark upon the process of establishing their own version [6]. Most importantly, it contains performance indicators, which break competencies down into accessible, bite-sized steps, and this is important to underpin and support a learning process (see appendix). Once a Competency Framework has been formulated, it will form the basis for virtually all other workforce development activities.

However, establishing competency frameworks, which enable charting and monitoring someone's progress through an educational pathway, is not sufficient to ensure a strategic approach to educational workforce planning: that requires educational providers to make sure that dementia is an integral part of their curricula where relevant. In those healthcare systems where there is a defined role to commission services (such as in the UK), the relevant commissioning bodies should be equally engaged in demanding their educational providers reserve a place for dementia within their programmes. Obviously those authorities (commissioners as well as providers of education and training) should determine what they think are desirable, necessary or essential competencies for particular workforce segments and that will depend on the nature of the interaction staff are expected to have with people with dementia and their carers, as well as the frequency and intensity of that interaction. Again, a competency framework can aid in this task. It is recommended that specific 'occupational standards' are developed, the attainment of which then may lead to accreditation and credentialing. Institutions such as the Norfolk Dementia Care Academy or indeed any educational provider, can offer assessment and appraisals of those being educated and trained, leading to some form of certification, and that certification must be recognisable in the wider care system.

Within existing professional education (nursing, medical training, allied health professionals, social workers, etc.), occupation-linked standards should therefore be built in to ensure learners of all levels (pre-professional, professional, pre-graduate, graduate or postgraduate) have the opportunity to gain relevant exposure to dementia: the demographic expansion in demand, reported in many contributions in this book, predicts that all such professionals will need to be familiar with dementia at some level or other. It should not be too difficult to link particular dementia competencies to existing modules or themed educational programmes, perhaps under existing headings, such as 'dignity and respect', 'palliative care', 'long-term conditions' and so on.

There is a need for a catch-up for the generation of professionals who missed out on such opportunities in the past, and this poses a challenge in itself for educational providers and planners. A starting point would be to ensure that at least a basic level of dementia awareness is being incorporated in development of the general workforce, be it in health care, social care or even in other sectors of the community where one can expect to come across people with dementia. With regard to the latter, the UK Dementia Friends Scheme, as mentioned above, is an example of an imaginative way in which basic awareness can be cascaded throughout the community.

Lastly, those in leadership positions in education, training and service development must have the ability to lead such efforts and influence policy. They should be able to appraise the competency of their workforce and motivate and inspire practitioners not to neglect any educational and professional development needs they may have, making dementia and dementia care part and parcel of educational workforce development strategies.

Competencies and training needs analysis

It may be useful to clarify what exactly is meant by the term 'competency'. Being competent in a particular area means that the practitioner or carer is able to deliver a defined and measurable level of effective care by the habitual and judicious use of

- communication
- knowledge
- skills
- reasoning
- emotions
- values
- reflections on practice.

It is important to note that many competencies are gained throughout life and through personal and professional experience: every person entering dementia care has a variety of life and/or professional competencies, which are likely to be transferable to the new caring role and should indeed be identified, welcomed and fostered as such: these are possibly most powerfully deployed along the dimension of 'common sense' and there is no doubt that these competencies play an important role in the armamentarium of carers [8]. It is therefore possible to distinguish many different competencies in dementia care, and the need for these will vary from one person to the next: a receptionist in a family doctor's practice will need a different set of competencies from a nurse or a family carer, and so on. In specialist dementia care those 'extra' competencies are often indicated by the term 'dementia differentials'.

There are two interesting difficulties one can distinguish with respect to identifying competencies:

1. not knowing what is known, that is, underestimating one's competence (unconsciously competent)
2. not knowing what is not known, possibly overestimating one's competence (unconsciously incompetent).

In the professional workforce the latter can present a significant safeguarding, management and regulatory challenge. The former is encountered even in the most specialist care environment and some professionals seem to underestimate their specialist skills, often identifying them as 'common sense'.

Even if carers suspect there is more they ought to learn to provide the best possible care, they may not have the conceptual framework to recognise or express their own needs, and this then hampers any efforts to carry out a training needs analysis: it is difficult to delineate one's competency profile if there is no background against which to 'measure' it. A competency framework can assist with this (the NSDA website features a 'Learning Location', specifically to aid people to 'diagnose' their learning needs (free and completely confidential) and it further assists in pointing to a range of suitable educational resources [9]). The recognition of existing competencies is important as building upon them will increase confidence as a person moves from the known to the unknown. Obviously it also avoids unnecessary repetition, making development opportunities more productive and more interesting.

This brings us in more detail to the role of training needs analysis, which can be carried out with respect of an individual practitioner or carer or at a service level: the NSDA for instance completed a comprehensive training needs analysis of the wider health economy, which established a shared understanding of the 'dementia differentials' in competencies, as needing to be present in a number of different staff groups in varying roles and working in different organisations (available upon request from the corresponding author). Such a wider and more systemic training needs analysis leads to a clearer background against which an individual learner can chart their current position and desired development. But even if a training needs analysis only pertains to an individual practitioner, it is clear that the process of identifying competencies and any gaps or deficits needs to be structured and guided by the cohesion of the same competency framework. It can be done simply by going through the competencies and decide where the gaps are. However, this presumes a readiness and ability to engage in practice reflection and an understanding of the subtleties prevalent in dementia care, so it is often advisable to carry out training needs analysis in a wider context of clinical supervision or overall professional appraisal: one might call that a 'holistic' approach to learner-centred education and continuous professional development. Central to the latter are the formulation of personal learning or development plans, underpinned by facilitated reflective practice.

Personal learning plans and reflective practice

Once training needs have been identified the practitioner can move on to construct a personal learning plan: it should be realised that developing 'bite-sized' skills should support developing someone's overall competence. The actual overall performance will be the result of the carer or practitioner being able to integrate these 'bites' and use them together, delivering complex care and support. A more advanced, but crucially important, competency lies in the ability *not* to use a skill or approach if the situation is appropriately judged to be better dealt with in a way different from what one perhaps otherwise would do. This is recognising the idiosyncrasies a practitioner may come across and directly reflects the ability to identify when person-centred care may legitimately lead to deviate from usual practice. This skill is not easily learned through traditional teaching approaches, such as lectures or courses: there is ample evidence that such 'meta-level' skills are best achieved through a structured and facilitated programme of practice reflection [10]. It involves the ability to make an unconventional decision while being mindful of the need to avoid untoward risk, and although such decision-making has historically received more attention in the business world [11], it can be found directly as a topic of reflection within, for example, nursing:

'As I stated before (. . .), whenever I had to make a decision, I was a searcher. I first would look inward to see what was there. When I found that what I saw was distorted or unclear, I would look outward. Where could I go to find the answers that would clear up the distortion? Once I found what I thought I needed, I would take that knowledge and return to my inner self to see if the distortion was still present or if the picture was clear. What I learned is that for any decision, the comfort of coming to a decision was always short lived. It only lasts for a moment in time because every moment brings newness (. . .)' [12].

We could not express better the role of reflection as a basis for decision-making in ambiguous circumstances and consider this to be a competency all 'leaders' should possess in abundance. As an example of incorporating reflective practice within an educational and training strategy, which underpins the process of learners formulating their personal learning plans and ensures the holistic approach to learner-centred education we mentioned earlier, we now turn to a description of the Norfolk Dementia Care Academy.[2]

The Norfolk dementia care academy

The Norfolk Dementia Care Academy (NDCA) was established in 2011 in recognition of the fact that increased demand on dementia services is inevitable, while resources are likely to stagnate, which of course means resources relative to demand will decrease. Although previously in this chapter the importance of family and other informal carers were highlighted, it is equally assumed that a specialist dementia care provider is likely to have many highly skilled staff members, who should be able to disseminate their skills to the wider health economy and support others in providing dementia care, thereby increasing the capacity in the wider healthcare system. At the same time, specialist practitioners can learn immensely from others. Figure 16.1 captures the two-way process through which the NDCA attempts to increase the quality of care in the whole healthcare system.

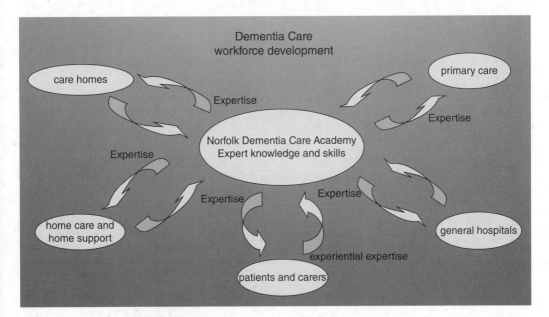

Figure 16.1 The Norfolk Dementia Care Academy

[2]NDCA is an initiative of the Norfolk & Suffolk NHS Foundation Trust, a secondary care specialist psychiatric provider in the UK.

While the NDCA is heavily engaged in dementia workforce development in the widest possible sense, it is crucial that the specialist staff it uses in education and training are constantly engaged in professional development themselves. To embed this into professional practice we formulated the following concepts.

Dynamic dementia care

This professional model combines the concepts of 'person-centred care', 'personalised care' and 'learner-centred education' with the high-quality clinical care the specialist services aim to provide for people with dementia: while 'person-centred care' focuses on the patient and the care received and 'learner-centred education' focuses on education and the learner, Dynamic Dementia Care combines the two and adds in practice reflection as an integral component. This creates an 'educational workforce', which continuously and consciously deploys a theory-to-practice-to-theory model, with a heavy emphasis on experiential learning methods. In short: clinical care is informed by delivering education and receiving it (from ourselves to ourselves and from learners to ourselves), and our learning is informed by our clinical practice, as is our teaching (see Figure 16.2).

The term 'dynamic' expresses the idea that through this continuous loop all components are constantly subject to reflective scrutiny, influence each other and therefore benefit from informed and reciprocal improvement, with learning and teaching being embedded in the whole practice model.

The NDCA has two core components: a dedicated Dementia Training Team (DTT) and a Practice Development Team (PDT).

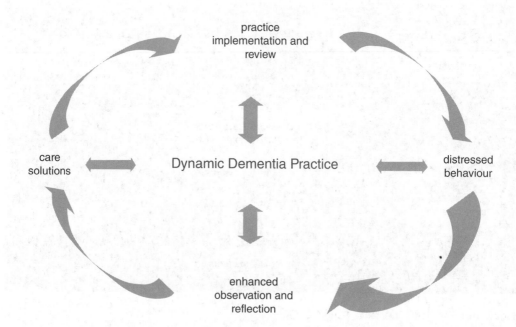

Figure 16.2 Dynamic Dementia Practice

The dementia training team

The DTT provides a range of educational opportunities developing skills and confidence in care workers and deploys a range of learning styles to ensure an effective learning experience, but it places an emphasis on experiential and reflective learning. Learning opportunities are designed to be accessible and relevant to new and novice members of care services and teams, right through to more experienced and advanced practitioners. To illustrate the DTT's usage of various methodologies, it offers among other educational opportunities a 'Searching for Connections' workshop in which participants aim to understand the need for meaningful occupation, exploring a range of approaches, such as memory boxes, short interventions, the use of objects to engage with, supporting mealtimes and specific cognitive stimulation therapy. Participants put the learning material into practice with a person with dementia they already are involved with and are taught to match activities to the abilities of the person with dementia. They are then required to reflect and record their application of the learned strategies in the clinical interaction and share this with fellow participants.

The team furthermore offers opportunities for learners to have experiences alongside more expert practitioners, such as shadowing colleagues, engaging in supported care giving, co-facilitating a Cognitive Stimulation Therapy group or participate in dementia care mapping (a few team members are accredited Dementia Care Mappers[3]).

It can be seen that the Academy's educational philosophy is heavily influenced by the need to judge progression in competency through measuring improved outcomes for the person with dementia and their carer, not just through easy-to-measure training inputs, and there exist a number of tools to measure outcomes, with one of the easier to use being the Quality of Interactions Schedule (QUIS). This observational tool codes the quality and number of social interactions between individuals and care staff [14]. An example of measuring training inputs is the so-called sheep dip approach to learning: many organisations assume that sending their staff on short courses will result in increase in competencies and better performance. As educators we strongly doubt the efficacy of that approach, and for a more detailed critique we refer to a thoughtful analysis from the world of 'human resources' [15].

The NDCA emphasises the importance of experiential learning as a process of making meaning from direct experience and reflecting-while-doing. Such a depth of learning offers confidence that learners will rationalise and apply their learning, again having a positive effect on the outcome of improved care provision [16]. The NDCA adopts the three learning strategies, which Stern et al. described as being essential to effective practice and skills development [17]:

1. Opportunities to gain perspective in the lives of patients through the use of, for instance, Dementia Care Mapping and other tools, ensuring people with dementia are included in the learning events. Such learning experiences seem to have the greatest impact on care workers [18].
2. Structured reflection on these experiences by self-reflection, guided reflection within workshops, facilitated group reflection and formalised practice reflection within other learning opportunities.
3. Focused mentoring: each learner is given the opportunity to access support from an allocated 'practice supervisor'. This helps in replicating structures of support in their working environment, such as supervision and mentoring, and these are important to sustain and develop learning.

[3]Dementia Care Mapping (DCM) is a method designed to evaluate quality of care from the perspective of the person with dementia [13].

In developing these unique opportunities for learners to engage with experiential learning situations we heavily lean on expert practitioners to engage as educators: by supporting our own practitioners continually to engage with their learning and reflect upon both learning and practice, their expertise is readily incorporated into their care work and can be meaningfully transferred to others. But it is of course not always easy to extract staff from the busy world of clinical care, so the Academy has initiated the PDT through which it aims to build capacity.

The practice development team

The PDT consists of practitioners from various parts of the specialist dementia service, who are 'seconded' part-time to the Academy: it meets regularly with facilitation from a clinical psychologist. The agenda is set by the participants themselves and sessions are confidential. Any topic can be brought to the table by any member of the team, but the essence of the exercise is to discuss and debate matters of clinical interest. It can be seen that the activity of this team is closely intertwined with the educational ethos of the Academy, and it aims to inform in a two-way interaction its overall activity.

One important and recurring theme is the distress many people with dementia and their carers experience. It is recognised that carers who need to respond to this are themselves often 'irradiated by distress' [19], a phenomenon which some experts explain through the use of the psychoanalytic defense mechanism of 'projection': the person in distress, who may well have problems in communicating their feelings and because of their illness are less able to think their emotions through or deal with them by talking about them as they might have done otherwise, projects the unwanted unpleasant feeling out into others. In care settings this will usually mean care staff, while at home the person's family members and friends may find themselves feeling distressed and helpless. Often staff (or family members and other informal carers) do not quite understand the reasons why and in professional care settings this contributes to staff not functioning well and suffering burnout. Understanding of all of this can help prevent stress and sickness, and it is through practice development exercises that these phenomena can be brought into focus, discussed and understood. It is clear that here lies a wider task for the PDT: to construct a method in which it can assist and support informal and formal carers alike. With respect to the former, attempts are being made to establish peer support networks, hosted by the NDCA: groups of carers who have been previously involved in Cognitive Stimulation Therapy (which is routinely provided by NDCA throughout its catchment area) are invited to continue to meet up, and it is hoped this will grow into a larger network of 'alumni' and 'peer supporters'.

Staff and informal carers are called upon to 'contain' the distress and agitation people with dementia experience, and Bion's concept of 'containment' can be helpful in dementia care: people with dementia who are agitated and distressed need containment of those emotions by the care staff, who in turn need containing by their colleagues, their management and their employing organisations. These concepts, and others, can greatly enrich care of patients with dementia, and they therefore feature in the regular proceedings of the PDT.

Compassion

Exploration of the more intense emotions occurring in dementia care leads us to the topic which in many reports on the quality of care provided in certain dementia services features all too prominently as an issue: compassion or the lack thereof. It has close links to the discussion on the culture in organisations (see above) but is difficult to use in a competency framework, a personal learning plan or a workforce development strategy: it is intangible, but everyone knows when it is absent and it has recently been identified as a major area of concern in the Care and Compassion Report by the UK's Health Services Ombudsman [20]. It can be recognised in many competencies in the NSDA Competency Framework (see Appendix) but is not defined as a competency in its own right: it is a value and a human trait which weaves itself through everything else. Compassion has been viewed by some people as a passive feeling, but Archbishop Desmond Tutu stated [21]:

'Compassion is not just feeling with someone, but seeking to change the situation. Frequently people think compassion and love are merely sentimental. No! They are very demanding. If you are going to be compassionate, be prepared for action!'

There are views that compassion has somehow been washed out of health care. One Maori website in New Zealand expressed the following opinion:

'The Maori name "Waiatawhai" can roughly be translated as "healing waters of compassion". It's our belief that all health practitioners enter their profession with a genuine desire to provide caring and compassionate service to patients and families. Unfortunately, the evolution of our health professions and institutions has seriously limited the expression of that humanity and compassion. Clinical detachment and objectivity are emphasised over and above compassionate caring. Our hospitals are overcrowded and under stress. Resources are limited. There doesn't seem to be time to care'.

We can do no better than to quote further from the relevant website:

'The Maori people have a very holistic concept of health and wellbeing including the four dimensions of physical, mental, emotional/relationship, and spiritual health. The incorporation of Maori traditional spiritual ceremonies and practices within our healthcare institutions is found to strengthen meaning and commitment of our healthcare practitioners and this is a wonderful alignment with our goals to strengthen compassion in healthcare' [22].

There is a lot to be learned from the Maori people, and it is even more humbling to find the website reporting that

'leaders in the National Health Service in the UK have recently revised the core values that underpin the service. 'Compassion' is now identified as a core value, having been invisible for many years.'

People with dementia and their carers want compassionate care, and they need compassion desperately from every person with whom they interact. Therefore, workforce development without compassion will not meet any of the desired outcomes for people with dementia and particularly not 'I am treated with dignity and respect', which is at the core of 'outcomes' mentioned in another recent report from the UK's Department of Health [23].

It is perhaps noteworthy that this chapter ends with a concept, which refuses to let itself be captured under the category of 'competencies'. No matter how useful and important in our analysis the various aspects of workforce development may be, high-quality care is not just the result of well thought-through competency frameworks and educational strategies: at the core of good quality care we find the human trait which transcends such structures, but which is of vital importance to our fellow humans who happen to have dementia.

References

1. Hughes JC (2011) *Thinking through Dementia*. Oxford, UK: Oxford University Press.
2. Davies HTO, Nutley SM (2000) Organisational culture and quality of health care. *Qual Health Care* 9:111–119.
3. Scott T, Mannion R, Davies HTO, Marshall MN (2003) Implementing culture change in health care: theory and practice. *Int J Qual Health Care* 15(2):111–118.
4. Griffin R (2012) *Changing the Culture for Dementia Care*. Eau Claire, WI: PESI Healthcare: PHC Publishing Group.
5. Scott T, Mannion R, Davies H, Marshall M (2003) The quantitative measurement of organisational culture in health care: a review of the available instruments. *Health Serv Res* 38(3):923–945.
6. Available at: http://www.dementia-alliance.com/Media/framework.pdf (last accessed on 28 March 2013).
7. Available at: http://dementiachallenge.dh.gov.uk/ (last accessed on 28 March 2013).
8. Lipton AM, Marshall CD (2013) *The Common Sense Guide to Dementia for Clinicians and Caregivers*. New York: Springer.
9. Available at: http://www.dementia-alliance.com/learning_location.html (last accessed on 28 March 2013).
10. Mamede S, Schmidt HG (2004) The structure of reflective practice in medicine. *Med Educ* 38: 1302–1308.
11. Buchanan L, O'Connell A (2006) A brief history of decision making. *Harv Bus Rev* 84(1):32–41, 132.
12. Truglio-Londrigan M, Lewenson SB (2006) *Decision-Making in Nursing. Thoughtful Approaches for Practice*, 1st edn. Sudbury (MA): Jones & Bartlett Publishers.
13. Available at: http://www.brad.ac.uk/health/dementia/dcm/ (last accessed on 21 February 2013).
14. Dean R, Proudfoot R, Lindesay J (1993) The quality of interactions schedule (QUIS): development, reliability and use in the evaluation of two domus units. *Int J Geriatr Psychiatry* 8:819–826.
15. Available at: http://www.hr.com/en/communities/training_and_development/avoiding-the-sheep-dip_ead0rt08 .html (last accessed on 21 February 2013).
16. Moon JA (2004) The framing of learning: approaches to learning. In: *A Handbook of Reflective and Experiential Learning: Theory and Practice*. London: Routledge Falmer, pp. 58–69.
17. Stern DT, Cohen JJ, Bruder A, Packer B, Sole A (2008) Teaching humanism. *Perspect Biol Med* 51(4):495–507.
18. Brandes D, Ginnis P (1986) *A Guide to Student Centred Learning*. Cheltenham: Stanley Thorne Ltd.
19. Hinshelwood RD, Skogstad W (2002) Irradiated by distress: observing psychic pain in health-care organizations. *Psychoanal Psychother* 16(2):110–124.
20. UK Health Services Ombudsman Moon JA (2004) Care and compassion. Available at: http:// www.ombudsman.org.uk/__data/assets/pdf_file/0016/7216/Care-and-Compassion-PHSO-0114web.pdf (last accessed on 21 February 2013).
21. Tutu D, Armstrong K (2009) *Guardian*, 25 September 2009. Available at: http://www.guardian.co.uk/ commentisfree/belief/2009/sep/25/charter-compassion-tutu-armstrong (last accessed on 21 February 2013).
22. New Zealand Centre of Compassion in Healthcare (2008, May) Available at: http://health.groups.yahoo.com/ group/iatrogenic/message/4111 (last accessed on 21 February 2013).
23. Quality outcomes for people with dementia: building on the work of the national dementia strategy. Available at: http://www.dh.gov.uk/en/Publicationsandstatistics/Publications/PublicationsPolicyAndGuidance/ DH_119827 (last accessed on 21 February 2013).

Appendix

Some important competencies (from the Norfolk & Suffolk dementia alliance competency framework)

A. Memory matters – know the characteristics of dementia and understand the experience of a person with dementia

Explain what is meant by the term dementia and identify the primary causes of dementia. 1

Recognise the key characteristics of dementia, including the early signs of dementia, and appreciate that these signs can be associated with other medical conditions and/or changes to the person's general circumstances. 2

Understand the definition and significance of delirium and depression and how this differs from dementia. 3

Recognise the differences between irreversible and reversible dementia. 4

Describe how brain changes affect the way a person functions and behaves. 5

Know the current research findings into cause, prevention and recommended diagnostic procedures. 6

Discuss why it is important to personalise the care you provide to someone with dementia. 7

Demonstrate that you understand the use, effects, side effects and undesirable effects of medication used to manage symptoms of dementia. 8

Demonstrate a knowledge and understanding when caring for people with dementia. 9

Recognise that there are different ways of thinking about dementia. 10

Demonstrate an understanding of the legal and ethical issues involved in caring for people with dementia and designed to protect people with dementia. 11

Understand why a person with dementia may be more vulnerable to abuse and neglect. 12

B. Remember the person – person-centred care

Discuss the characteristics of person-centred care. 13

Describe how you can give care to help the person with dementia be comfortable and secure, as well as live a full and meaningful life. 14

Describe how knowing a person's background, culture, and experiences can help you give the best possible care. 15

Describe how your background, culture, experiences, and attitudes may affect how you give care. 16

C. Care interactions

Provide help with physical care tasks in ways that match the needs and abilities of the person and support disability. 17

Recognise and report on changes to physical and cognitive function. 18

Support a variety of care options, which may be available to the person with dementia. 19

Understand the importance of positive interactions with people with dementia. 20

Support advance care planning. 21

D. Communicate sensitively to support meaningful interaction

Identify and support the feelings – whether spoken or otherwise expressed – of the person with dementia. 22

Show effective ways of listening to and communicating with someone who has dementia. 23

Understand the factors, which can affect interactions and communication of individuals with dementia. 24

Understand that individuals with dementia may communicate in different ways, verbally and non-verbally. 25

E. Understand distressed behaviours

Understand that how a person behaves is a form of communication. Behaviours may   26
reflect emotions or unmet needs or may be triggered by physical illness.

Recognise that what a person thinks is acceptable behaviour is his or her own reality. Many   27
things, including their cultural background and family dynamics, may influence this. These
influences can affect behaviour related to gender roles, eye contact, and personal space.

Recognise distressed behaviours and describe helpful responses to distressed behaviours   28
that you find 'challenging' or 'difficult'.

F. Enrich the lives of people with dementia

Consider the person's abilities, needs, desires and interests while providing comfort, a   29
sense of living well and independence.

Support and encourage the person to continue their usual activities, social life and   30
community involvement.

Recognise how important it is for people to do activities that give meaning and purpose.   31
The activities are often a part of their culture and background.

Recognise how important pleasurable activities are in a person's life. These may include   32
sexual activities, intimacy and feeling close to others.

Support the person with dementia to retain safe independence and a good quality of life through   33
adapting their home or the area in which they are living and/or using assistive technologies.

G. Support and look after family members and other carers

Respond respectfully to the family's unique relationships, experiences, cultural identity   34
and losses.

Use a positive and accepting approach with family members or when talking about the   35
family with other staff.

Get and use information about the individual's personal history; personal, religious and   36
spiritual preferences, and cultural and ethnic backgrounds.

Ensure carers have access to assessments of their own needs.   37

H. Work as part of a multi-agency team including the carers

Learn about the services available to the person with dementia.   38

Plan care based specifically on the needs of the individual.   39

Recognise the family as part of the caregiving team.   40

Explain positive ways to talk with supervisors and co-workers to address differences and   41
ideas about caregiving and what you believe is best for the person with dementia.

I. Caregiver self-care

Identify your own feelings, beliefs or attitudes that may affect your caring relationships.   42

Identify helpful ways to prevent and cope with your own stress and burnout.   43

Identify the ways you cope with grief and loss.   44

J. Managers ensure members of their team are trained and well supported

Promote an environment that encourages people to grow, develop and use their full   45
potential by balancing support and accountability.

Provide opportunities and encourage caregivers to develop a quality relationship with   46
each individual, which gives work meaning and purpose.

Give caregivers the information and tools they need to effectively work with people with   47
dementia at all stages.

Chapter 17

The role of assistive technology in the care of people with dementia

June Andrews[a] and Louise Robinson[b]

[a]*School of Applied Social Science, University of Stirling, UK*
[b]*Institute of Health and Society, Newcastle University, UK*

Introduction

Our rapidly ageing population has led to considerable concern as to whether existing health and social care provision will cope with such an increased future demand and established an urgent need to explore alternative, innovative solutions to this challenge [1]. This chapter will use examples of research and innovation in the provision of assistive technology in dementia care from the UK, but we hope that these will be helpful to our international readers. In the UK, national policy has over the last two decades continued to emphasise the need for the care of older people, including those living with dementia, to be based in the community and for them to remain in their own homes for as long as possible [2–6]. Assistive (or enabling) technologies provide one possible solution to promote autonomy and independence for older people [7], but in the UK they are still underutilised in routine care [8,9]. A series of current UK research studies is exploring the effectiveness of assistive technologies in the care of older people and those with long-term illness and how they can become better integrated into usual care. In England, the Department of Health Whole System Demonstrator (WSD) programme was set up in 2009 as a randomised controlled trial of telecare and telehealth in chronic illness management on three sites [10]. In Scotland the Joint Improvement Team ran a National Telecare Development Programme from 2006 to 2011. The aim was to consider the range of devices and services that harness developing technology to enable people to live with greater independence and safety in their own homes, and to support the implementation of the use of those devices [11].

The words that are used to describe the use of assistive technology include

- Telecare: to facilitate independence and enhance personal safety. Devices include community alarms, sensors and movement detectors, and the use of video conferencing or 'Skype' to allow visual and auditory communication with carers. This has been described by the WSD programme as a 'service aimed at vulnerable people who need the support of Social Care or Health Services to keep living on their own. For example, those with physical disabilities, the frail and elderly or those suffering from dementia or epilepsy' [10].

Designing and Delivering Dementia Services, First Edition. Edited by Hugo de Waal, Constantine Lyketsos, David Ames, and John O'Brien.

- Telehealth, which facilitates the monitoring of long-term health conditions and bodily functions for clinicians at a distance to offer support and is described by the WSD as a 'service aimed at helping people manage their long term conditions in their own home' [10]. Dementia is not listed as an example of a long-term condition at this point.
- Environmental controls, which are often used to give a disabled person the capacity to control many aspects of the home environment from a single unit. For a person with dementia the environmental controls may eventually be operated by someone else or automated.
- Leisure equipment such as touch screen monitors which can be an easy way to access reminiscence materials or entertainment such as music, films or photographs, or games specifically designed considering the impairments that are associated with dementia. They are also used for communication.
- Dementia-friendly design, where the whole environment is considered as a way of helping the person with dementia to live independently or to reduce the burden of care on the family, or others who provide care and support. Environmental design equipment can also include innovations such as the controlled emission of odours to signal the time of day and to encourage appetite [12].

The term 'assistive technology' is often assumed to refer only to sophisticated equipment that uses electronic information and communication technology. In reality the term can refer to quite simple devices such as a modified sink plug, which can prevent flooding when someone is forgetful in the kitchen and bathroom and leaves an unattended bath or sink. The plug is activated by the pressure of the water or the sink and will open and release the excess water down the plughole to avoid flooding (http://www.magiplug.com). It is a small, inexpensive, easily available, mechanical device requiring no maintenance and no new skills to use. It presents no ethical dilemmas. By the definition assumed in this chapter, that plug is both 'assistive' and 'technology'.

Another assumption in this chapter is that the 'kit' or equipment that is brought into use should never be introduced in isolation, but only as part of a strategy of care that includes the provision of information and support, health advice and advice on design of the environment:

'We've put in a movement sensor in my mother's bed room which means that when she gets out of bed during the night, the toilet light switches on automatically. We know her really well and that is usually where she is planning to go when she gets up at those times. In an attempt to reduce the number of times she gets up at night, I have started to take her for a walk in the daylight every morning, which helps to set her body clock. We've also changed the light bulbs. They are still energy saving, but her old ones had lost their luminosity over time, and were a bit dull, so these new ones light up faster and provide stronger light to help her orientate herself. And we've put a sign on the toilet door. We're not sure how significant any of these things are individually, but the situation is better now at night.'

In this example, the sensor that switches on the light is the only electronic part of the assistive technology solution, but works with the advice on exercise, design and lighting to alleviate a nocturnal problem which is very common for people with dementia and their carers (although telecare can of course help all older people).

The quality of life of people with dementia and those who care for them can be enhanced significantly by the thoughtful use of assistive technology. It is an important part of normal dementia care to provide access to aids, particularly when the technology is low cost and accessible. It is important for people with dementia, their families and professionals who support them to be aware of the sort of technological equipment that is available and to develop the skills needed to use the equipment well, including the capacity to undertake simple maintenance tasks. As well as knowing what is already on the market, health and social care professionals and other workers including service managers should be aware of emerging useful devices and have a strategic approach to keeping up to date with what is being developed in this dynamic field. It is also their responsibility to communicate with designers, inventors and entrepreneurs to make sure that increasing energy is put into the creation of new technologies [13] which, because it is useful and taken up by care organisations and individual people, will be of commercial value to the industry, which in turn will stimulate greater inventiveness and ultimately benefits for patients and clients.

Why is assistive technology in use in dementia care?

There is considerable variation in how assistive technology is used in dementia care. In some countries a wide range of technology is readily available, with assessment of individual need and implementation integrated into a routine social care assessment. For example, in 2009, a programme of provision of telecare was implemented in Scotland for anyone living at home over the age of 60 who wanted it, thus 'mainstreaming' a strategy of capacity building and encouraging people to grow old where they are. The evaluation noted positive effects on

- staff working in a new culture of care, emphasising support and capacity building
- client satisfaction
- quality of life for both older people and unpaid family caregivers
- the ability of a local (municipal) authority to deliver on performance indicators and the supply of good-quality services at low cost [14].

There was clear learning from the programme. Early intervention appears to be important in housing solutions for people with dementia. People with dementia can build capacity in this way. The role of committed and skilled staff is crucial because of the need to focus on what people with dementia can do, rather than focusing on their disabilities. The researchers were keen to point out that 'mainstreaming' (a term which indicates that everyone is being given some basic assistance) carries the danger that those with particular needs such as those with dementia wind up being marginalised. Their greatest emphasis was on the fact that it was not the assistive technology in isolation that enabled the success of the programme, but the whole system. However, it is clear that using assistive technology improved cost and quality of care.

The role of assistive technology in supporting family carers

In the UK (as in many countries) most people with dementia live independently in the community, with one-third residing in care homes; around half a million family carers provide the mainstay of community support to the former [15]. Carers of people with dementia are more likely to experience worse physical and mental health and to report a higher care burden compared with carers of people with other long-term conditions [16]. A systematic review of the effectiveness of networked technology in supporting family carers of people with dementia revealed that the technologies had moderate effects on carer stress and depression [17].

Assistive technologies have the potential to help reduce the burden of care for family carers. Describing care as a 'burden' shapes our frame of reference in a negative way. In order to get improved services and to raise money for third-sector organisations, the negative aspects of caring are often emphasised in public. The perception of many health and social care workers is further shaped by the fact that they are more often involved when the situation is in crisis. Looking after your family is actually still an important part of our society across many cultures (see the chapters in Section IV) and people do it willingly in general. Many families are glad to care for a person with dementia for as long as possible. Having a carer living with you at home has been said to reduce the likelihood of institutionalisation by up to seven times [18]. Carers mostly do not undertake this work under duress, but out of loyalty and long-standing commitment, and a sense that this is what life is about – caring for each other. But for many of them care is more burdensome than it needs to be. Without some basic information and advice the carer spends more time, has more adverse incidents and opportunity costs and may spend more money than is absolutely necessary. Carers need access to assistive technology so that the energy they are devoting to the person with dementia can be focused on other aspects of their own, and their family's needs, such as getting a decent night's sleep.

For staff working in hospitals and care homes or other residential settings, a concern is often expressed that technology 'replaces caring'. Of course this is theoretically possible. The invention of a robot nurse might give rise to concern that dependent people might one day never see a human again [19]. As it happens, the robot nurse, if the face was not painted on it, and it did not have a voice generator in it, is really a rather splendid hoist, for moving and handling physically dependent people in a way that is superior to the mechanical cranes that have been commonly used in hospital and other settings. When in production this may turn out to be safer for staff as well as being comfortable for patients.

Other concerns are expressed about movement sensors and methods of electronic observation, which are seen to replace the watchful eye of the friendly nurse. Again, the framing of the dichotomy is misleading. The question is not whether we would prefer a person to be watching over us or a machine. The real question is whether we would like to be protected at all, and in what way? In reality a nurse or carer cannot be watching all the time, unless the patient or resident is in an open plan area like an old Nightingale hospital ward and the staff have nothing else that they have to do. If you want privacy in an individual room, but you are vulnerable, the compromise may be that you agree to unobtrusive electronic monitoring. Any staff time and energy can then be focused on those things for which there is no satisfactory assistive technology application, like dancing with or sharing a meal with the person with dementia.

The ethics of the use of assistive technology

In practice, there are mental capacity issues and decision-making responsibilities that arise at some point along the journey of the person with dementia. However, not all are raised with everyone and in some cases some issues arise quite late on, or not at all, if sufficient preparation has been made and advanced directives and proxy forms of decision-making have been put in place in good time. Giving maximum control to the person for as long as possible is crucial. The person with dementia may be reluctant or refuse to accept assistive technology and even if staff or families wish to overrule them because the decision being made seems unwise, the person may want to retain their right to control their environment. If the decision is taken to overrule the person with dementia, this should be done cautiously and with a proper understanding of how serious this is. In particular, a difficulty in communicating with a person with dementia must never be interpreted as making them incompetent to make a decision. There are mechanisms that can be used to find out what people with dementia think and want which are easily available and simple to use, for example, talking mats (http://www.talkingmats.com). In addition, some skilled communicators have a highly developed capacity to hear the voices of people with dementia who others think are beyond contact.

A recent literature search on the use of assistive technology in the care for community-dwelling elderly people suggested that the necessary ethical debate appears not to be a priority [20], with the exception of care homes [21]. Issues in the public domain which give greatest rise to debate are often centred on tracking devices, seen as problematic because of the association of their use in the criminal justice system for tagging offenders on parole. The families showed higher support for tracking devices both for the independence and safety of the relative in their care and for their own peace of mind, particularly if the device is user-friendly, whereas professional staff are particularly concerned about the autonomy of the person with dementia and minimising their risk of harm [22]. This balance between a person with dementia's right to independence and a professional carers' duty to minimise harm is a core issue in decision-making about the use of assistive technology [23]. This short chapter is too brief to cover ethical issues in depth, but it is important to highlight that for many people with dementia the views of family or professional carers are taken as a proxy for their own views, even when they are still competent to express a view [24]. This is clearly not acceptable unless the person with dementia has delegated this responsibility and is no substitute for consulting that person.

Because it is important to remember that the person's individual choices and beliefs are an important consideration, health and social care staff need to be conscious and aware of their own beliefs and prejudices. Because these situations are complex, it is difficult to produce a checklist or guide that will make clear what is right or wrong in every situation. Cox et al. describe a set of core values when making decisions concerning people with dementia: people should make sure that

- the person using the service should have the maximum control
- real and informed choice should be a key part of any service
- people who use the service should be valued and respected as unique individuals
- continuity of care is built into service delivery in a way that keeps the person in touch with their past and present
- the person is not discriminated against because they have dementia or because of any other differences and they receive their fair share of good quality and appropriate services [25].

Assessment of the person with dementia for use of assistive technology

The concept of risk assessment and risk management would appear to be a key component when considering the use of assistive technology as part of the care planning process in dementia [23]. In England recent multidisciplinary guidance on how to best assess and manage risk in dementia care has been released to supplement existing practice on the care planning and safeguarding of potentially vulnerable adults. The Department of Health guidance *'Nothing Ventured, Nothing Gained: risk guidance for people with dementia'* combines a summary of research evidence and current best practice to provide guidance for people with dementia, their families and practitioners on a more positive approach to risk management via the process of risk enablement [26]. Risk enablement combines a more individualised person-centred approach to risk assessment and acknowledges that

1. Dementia and the potential risks of living with a condition where mental capacity is impaired can fluctuate and affect different people in different ways.
2. The concept of risk goes beyond physical components, such as falling or getting lost, and should include psychosocial aspects such as diminished well-being or loss of self-identity.

Shared agreement about the degree of risk may not always be possible, but it is important to ascertain everyone's views about the potential risks and reach at least a shared understanding. Individualised assessments should be carried out with a balanced consideration of both the benefits and the risks of the situation to the person with dementia.

People with dementia are often subject to a wide range of assessments over time from a range of health and social care professionals. The possibility of the use of assistive technology should be introduced at the earliest possible time. The decision to include assistive technology as part of a package of care must involve the person with dementia, so it is important to use language that the person and their carer can understand. Consider the situation described in a particular area in Scotland where in sheltered housing some equipment is installed routinely regardless of the state of the person's health, to promote a more proactive approach to the care of older people. This might include a community alarm, smoke and flood detectors and a security device for the front door. Opinion is divided about whether this global community approach is cost-effective: it depends on the individual assessment [27].

People need to be clear about the question of whether installation is feasible in the place where the person lives and who will respond to any calls. This is relevant because factors such as the design of the property and the availability of networks and signals will vary [27]. The person as an individual will vary in how much new equipment they want or can cope with. As part of the assessment of the personal need, portable activity monitoring equipment can be used. Movement sensors in the home generate a 24-hour activity chart, which can be accessed via the Internet. The system is reusable and so can be moved from the home of one person with dementia to another, after the assessment has been undertaken. Sensors are installed in each of the main rooms: bedroom, bathroom, kitchen and living room, for example. Door catches are fitted to record when external doors are opened and closed. Sometimes people with early dementia who are a source of worry to their relatives can be discovered to be managing better than anyone expected in their own homes. Keeping them in their familiar environment is a good way of maximising function.

Observing the person using their own home over 24 hours provides extremely useful information: it can help with the timing of home visits and interventions or simply reassure concerned carers. An accurate picture can be created of the extent to which the person is leaving the home (which is sometimes over-reported) or leaving the door open, by using the 'just checking' system (http://www.justchecking.co.uk). Supportive protection and care arrangements can then be made. Informal or family carers can be involved in this process, bringing them together with professionals and the person with dementia to communicate about what is happening, and what could help. When undertaking a risk assessment, the dangers of the cooker, flooding and scalding are key, along with the risk of unwelcome visitors, getting lost and vulnerability to crime or abuse.

Information about assistive technology: How to find out what is currently available

People with dementia and their families require information on a wide range of topics, including information about their illness and its prognosis, the range of therapies and support services available, legal and financial support, and where to seek help in a crisis [28]. In terms of disseminating information about assistive technology, a great deal has been done in the UK to help professionals and families discover the range of devices currently available. The Social SCIE website (http://www.scie.org.uk/publications) provides updated lists of resources available. For example, it gives links to the Assistive Technology Dementia website (http://www.atdementia.org.uk), which brings together information about assistive technology with a searchable database of products. SCIE also provides links to guides such as *Telecare and Dementia*, a book which explores how telecare can contribute to quality of life. This book is also available as a free download from http://www.dementiashop.co.uk.

The devices that are currently commercially available can be viewed at the many conference exhibitions that take place around the world, which are often free and offer an opportunity to examine and discuss the equipment. The following list is not exhaustive but gives a sense of what is available. It has been constructed using the categorisation from the AT dementia website, which divides technology into Prompts and Reminders, Communication, Leisure and Safety (http:// www.atdementia.org.uk).

Prompts and reminders

- Devices that can remind you of the date and time if you have problems keeping track. These include large easy-to-see items, produced for people with visual impairment and talking clocks. In addition there are clocks that include the day and date and an indicator of whether it is night or day.
- Devices that can help you to find things that are commonly mislaid. These include simple ideas like a pocket that hangs on the doorknob into which crucial items can be placed or a battery-powered electronic locator.
- Dispensers for medication that can remind you when to take medication and which can stimulate a reminder call from someone else if you fail to take it when the alarm tells you to.
- Voice recorders that will give you a message, in your own voice or the voice of someone you know, which plays to you when you activate it through a passive infrared beam, for example, 'don't forget your keys!', when you go near the door.
- Signs and notices. These are not very high tech, but they can be made to light up when the person passes them or can be as simple as a note held on the fridge with a magnet.

Communication devices

- An intercom for use between rooms, or between houses or for the front door could be useful.
- Phones are now available in big, easy-to-use formats and can incorporate help for hard of hearing or visual signals if the person is deaf. Retro-design phones are available for people who may have forgotten the push button technology and prefer a round dial. Simple phones with fast dial can help. The telephone company can sometimes help if the person with dementia is making unhelpful calls, and incoming calls can be blocked if the person is vulnerable to callers from a known number.
- Communication aids such as Talking Mats are very low tech (they are made of carpet and card), but they are a superb tool for finding out what people with dementia want and need.
- Internet-based communication systems such as Skype or touch screen programmes allow families to communicate directly with each other.

Leisure

- Computer aids are of increasing interest as the people who are entering into their dementia journey increasingly includes people who have already worked computers or have used them at home. In addition, designers are producing touch screen technology which is very intuitive and easy to use.
- TV, radio and music and computer games: the AT Dementia website describes easy-to-use remote controls and other devices. The importance of music and appropriate diversion cannot be over emphasised, particularly if one has observed residents stuck in front of television broadcasts that are not entertainment or pleasurable distraction for them.
- Reminiscence materials are extremely popular when presented through assistive technology because of the ease with which they can be shared across wide distances with family members who can contribute to their compilation. A particularly good example can be found at http:// www.caringmemories.net.

Safety

- Activity monitors including the 'Just checking' system described earlier and passive infrared movement monitors that can be connected to a call centre or the pager of an attendant or the phone of a relative. Pressure mats are a relatively simple form of this and the more sophisticated models may be body worn.
- Alarm and pager units are available which will inform a call centre or a carer if the person with dementia who is being monitored requires assistance. This can be as specific as a pager message. This sort of technology, combined with passive infrared sensing, could replace the noisy and visually disturbing nurse call systems in our hospitals and care homes.
- Fall detectors are increasingly sophisticated, ranging from bed or chair occupancy sensors that will tell you if the person does not go back to where you expect them to be, through to body worn sensors with sophisticated technology that will register a fall and can include GPS tracking so that the person can be quickly found, even outside of the home.
- Flood detectors and water temperature monitors are crucial elements of care at home. The technology ranges from simple pressure plugs that avoid floods to sophisticated flood detectors that can set off an alarm or alert a carer.
- Gas and extreme temperature monitors can be procured on the market, including, for example, a wireless gas detector with a shut off system, in addition to the smoke detectors and carbon monoxide detectors with which we are all familiar, and they can be enhanced with a facility to text message alerts to carers.
- Safe lighting has to be brighter for older people and in addition low-energy bulbs have to be changed more often than others because they lose their luminosity. Motion detectors need to be correctly positioned to allow the low-energy bulb to light up completely.
- Other safety and security devices, including key safes into which an emergency key can be placed or door locks that are operated by a thumb print to reduce the number of house keys that are circulating among paid and family carers.
- Wandering and safer walking technologies which include Global Positioning Technology.

Assistive technology in dementia care: Implications for future research and service provision

Potential areas for future research in this aspect of dementia care include how we can more routinely integrate assistive technologies into peoples' usual housing and care environments [29] and also how we can better involve people with dementia in the design and evaluation of new assistive technologies to improve compliance. A systematic review found that people with dementia were very rarely involved in studies evaluating the acceptability and effectiveness of technology interventions, while the views of family carers were sought more often [30]. People with dementia appear to be very positive about the use of technologies, if such devices allow them to lead a normal life for as long as they are able to and they are also able and interested in being involved in the design and development of new technologies that promote independence while minimising the stigma of living with dementia [13].

With the costs of dementia care in the UK currently estimated at £20 billion, assistive technology has been suggested as a possible means of providing more cost-effective care [31]. However, recent reviews still stress the need for stronger evidence from randomised controlled trials to confirm clinical and cost-effectiveness before more widespread implementation [32,33]. Within the UK, the strongest evidence to date comes from an uncontrolled study: the 'Safe at Home' project [34]. This study found that 58% of a sample of 233 people with dementia was still living in the community after 21 months compared to 24% in a comparison group, with savings equivalent to £3690 per person per year. In addition, it also found that the vast majority of carers in the intervention group were less concerned and felt the use of technology had led to improvements in their quality of life. Although promising, such findings need to be further tested and confirmed via large-scale, multi-site, randomised trials before routine practice can better align with national policy recommendations.

At an international level, such emerging evidence on the effectiveness and cost-effectiveness of assistive technologies within dementia care could provide a possible solution for more efficient care, especially for countries with less well-developed social care systems and those with high numbers of rural inhabitants. The cost of individual devices is relatively low, and currently these can be purchased directly from the manufacturers. However, there is a danger that the time and resources required to set up the infrastructure and support systems for monitoring people using such technologies, and also the professional expertise to assess which devices are most appropriate to meet individual needs, is neglected. In the UK key policy documents on dementia care continue to emphasise the potential of assistive technology to support people with dementia to live independently [3–6]. Notwithstanding this, it is interesting to note that although an increasing number of national governments are developing strategies to create the infrastructure and accountability to sustain the care of people living with dementia, very few of these policy documents mention telecare as a specific intervention [35].

Additional resources: Useful websites

- http://www.dhcarenetworks.org.uk/independentlivingchoices/telecare/ which is the website of the Telecare Learning and Improvement Network supported by the Health Tech and Medicines Knowledge Transfer Network. It is the national network supporting local service redesign in England through the application of telecare and telehealth to aid the delivery of housing, health, social care and support services to older and vulnerable people.
- http://www.jitscotland.org.uk/action-areas/telecare-in-scotland which is a website offering practical support to partnerships across Scotland to deliver better health, housing and social care services.
- http://www.atdementia.org.uk which is a website bringing together information about assistive technology that has the potential to support the independence and leisure opportunities of people with dementia. It includes a questionnaire that people can fill in to get advice online about practical problems that can be helped with assistive technology.
- http://www.dementia.stir.ac.uk which is a website for the Dementia Services Development Centre. It includes a library and information service and a bookshop with free downloadable materials.

References

1. Wanless D (2006) *Securing Good Care for Older People: Taking a Long Term View*. London: King's Fund.
2. Department of Health (2006) *Our Health, Our Care, Our Say: A New Direction for Community Services. Health and Social Care Working Together in Partnership*. London: Department of Health. Available from: http://www.dh.gov.uk/policyandguidance/organisationalpolicy/modernisation (last accessed on 20 February 2013).
3. Department of Health (2009) Living well with dementia: a national strategy. Available from: http://www.dh.gov.uk/en/SocialCare/Deliveringadultsocialcare/Olderpeople/NationalDementiaStrategy/index.htm (last accessed on 20 February 2013).

4. Alzheimer's Society/Welsh Assembly Government (2011) National dementia vision for Wales: dementia supportive communities. Available from: http://wales.gov.uk/docs/dhss/publication/110302dementia.pdf (last accessed on 20 February 2013).
5. The Scottish Government (2010) *Scotland's National Dementia Strategy*. Edinburgh: The Scottish Government. Available from:: http://www.scotland.gov.uk/topics/health/health/mental-health/servicespolicy/dementia (last accessed on 20 February 2013).
6. Department of Health Social Services and Public Safety (2011) *Improving Dementia Services in Northern Ireland: A Regional Strategy*. Deparment of Health, Social Services and Public Safety, Northern Ireland. Available from: 4http://www.dhsspsni.gov.uk/improving-dementia-services-in-northern-ireland-a-regional-strategy-november-2011.pdf (last accessed on 21 February 2013).
7. Department of Health (2006) *A New Ambition for Old Age: Next Steps in Implementing the National Service Framework*. A resource document from Prof Ian Philp, National Director for Older People. London: Department of Health.
8. Audit Commission (2004) *Assistive Technology Independence and Well Being*. London: Audit Commission.
9. House of Lords Select Committee on Science and Technology (2005) *Science and Technology: First Report*. London: House of Lords.
10. Department of Health (2011) Whole system demonstrator. Available from: http://dh.gov.uk/health/tag/whole-system-demonstrator-programme/ (last accessed on 20 February 2013).
11. Joint Improvement Team (2011) National development programme. Available from: http://jitscotland.org.uk/action-areas/telecare-in-scotland/ (last accessed on 20 February 2013).
12. The Design Council (2011) *The Scents Clock, Rodd Design and the Crossmodal Research Lab*. Oxford: University of Oxford. Available from: http://www.designcouncil.org.uk/dementia (last accessed on 20 February 2013).
13. Robinson L, Brittain K, Lindsay S, Jackson D, Olivier P. (2009) Keeping in Touch Everyday (KITE project): developing assistive technologies for people with dementia and their carers to promote independence. *International Psychogeriatrics* 21:494–502.
14. Bowes A, McColgan G (2009) Implementing telecare for people with dementia: supporting ageing in place in West Lothian, Scotland. *Journal of Care Services Management* 3:227–243.
15. Alzheimer's Society (2007) *Dementia UK: The Full Report*. London: Alzheimer's Society.
16. Brodaty H, Green A (2002) Who cares for the carer? The often forgotten patient. *Australian Family Physician* 31:833–836.
17. Powell J, Chiu T (2008) A systematic review of networked technologies supporting carers of people with dementia. *Journal of Telemedicine and Telecare* 14:154–156.
18. Banerjee S, Murray J, Foley B, et al. (2003) Predictors of institutionalisation in people with dementia. *Journal of Neurology, Neurosurgery and Psychiatry* 74:1315–1316.
19. Kuo T, Broadbent E, MacDonald B, (eds) (2008) Designing a robotic assistant for healthcare applications. Health Informatics New Zealand Conference; Rotorua, New Zealand.
20. Zwijsen SA, Niemeijer AR, Hertogh CM (2011) Ethics of using assistive technology in the care for community-dwelling elderly people: an overview of the literature. *Aging and Mental Health* 15: 419–427.
21. Niemeijer AR, Frederiks BJ, Riphagen LJ II, et al. (2010) Ethical and practical concerns of surveillance technologies in residential care for people with dementia or intellectual disabilities: an overview of the literature. *International Psychogeriatrics* 22:1129–1142.
22. Landau R, Werner S, Auslander GK, et al. (2008) Attitudes of family and professional care-givers towards the use of GPS for tracking patients with dementia: an exploratory study. *The British Journal of Social Work* 39:670–692.
23. Robinson L, Hutchings D, Corner L, et al. (2007) Balancing rights and risks – conflicting perspectives in the management of wandering in dementia. *Health, Risk and Society* 9:389–486.
24. Nuffield Council on Bioethics (2009) Dementia: ethical issues. Available from: http://www.nuffieldbioethics.org (last accessed on 20 February 2013).
25. Cox S, Anderson I, Dick S (1998) *The Person, the Community and Dementia; Developing a Value Framework*. Stirling: Dementia Services Development Centre.

26. Department of Health (2010) Nothing ventured, nothing gained: risk guidance for people with dementia. Available from: http://www.dh.gov.uk/publicationsandstatistics/publication/publicationspolicyandguidance/DH_121492 (last accessed on 20 February 2013).
27. Kerr B, Cunningham C, Martin S (2010) *Telecare and Dementia: Using Telecare Effectively in the Support of People with Dementia.* Stirling: Dementia Services Development Centre.
28. Wald C, Fahy M, Walker Z, et al. (2003) What to tell dementia caregivers – the rule of threes. *International Journal of Geriatric Psychiatry* 18:313–317.
29. Torrington J (2009) Extra care housing: environmental design to support activity and meaningful engagement for people with dementia. *Journal of Care Services Management* 3:250–257.
30. Topo P (2009) Technology studies to meet the needs of people with dementia and their caregivers: a literature review. *Journal of Applied Gerontology* 28:5–37.
31. House of Commons All Party Parliamentary Group on Dementia (2011) The £20 billion question; enquiry into cost effective dementia services.
32. Lauriks S, Reinersmann A, Van der Roest HG, et al. (2007) Review of ICT-based services for identified unmet needs in people with dementia. *Ageing Research Reviews* 6:223–246.
33. Bharucha AJ, Anand V, Forlizzi J, et al. (2009) Intelligent assistive technology applications to dementia care: current capabilities, limitations and future challenges. *American Journal of Geriatric Psychiatry* 17:88–104.
34. Woolham J (2005) *The Effectiveness of Assistive Technology in Supporting Independence of People with Dementia: The Safe at Home Project.* London: Hawker.
35. Norwegian Ministry of Health and Social Care Services (2011) Dementia Plan 2015. Available from: http://www.alzheimer-europe.org/Policy-in-Practice2/National-Dementia-Plans (last accessed on 20 February 2013).

Index

Page numbers in *italic* refer to figures. Page numbers in **bold** refer to tables.